BC
Van
Libr
600 West 10th Ave.
Vancouver, B.C. Canada
V5Z 4E6

D0803180

OXFORD MEDICAL PUBLICATIONS

GASTRIC CANCER

Dose schedules are being continually revised and new side effects recognized. Oxford University Press makes no representation, express or implied, that the drug dosages in this book are correct. For these reasons the reader is strongly urged to consult the pharmaceutical company's printed instructions before administering any of the drugs recommended in this book.

GASTRIC CANCER

Edited by

TAKASHI SUGIMURA
President Emeritus, National Cancer Center, Tokyo, Japan

and

MITSURU SASAKO
Professor, National Cancer Center, Tokyo, Japan

This publication was supported by a generous donation
from the Daido Life Foundation.

OXFORD NEW YORK TOKYO
OXFORD UNIVERSITY PRESS
1997

Oxford University Press, Great Clarendon Street, Oxford OX2 6DP

Oxford   New York

Athens   Auckland   Bangkok   Bogota   Bombay   Buenos Aires
Calcutta   Cape Town   Dar es Salaam   Delhi   Florence   Hong Kong
Istanbul   Karachi   Kuala Lumpur   Madras   Madrid   Melbourne
Mexico City   Nairobi   Paris   Singapore   Taipei   Tokyo   Toronto
and associated companies in
Berlin   Ibadan

Oxford is a trade mark of Oxford University Press

Published in the United States
by Oxford University Press Inc., New York

© T. Sugimura, M. Sasako & the contributors listed on p. ix, 1997

All rights reserved. No part of this publication may be
reproduced, stored in a retrieval system, or transmitted, in any
form or by any means, without the prior permission in writing of Oxford
University Press. Within the UK, exceptions are allowed in respect of any
fair dealing for the purpose of research or private study, or criticism or
review, as permitted under the Copyright, Designs and Patents Act, 1988, or
in the case of reprographic reproduction in accordance with the terms of
licences issued by the Copyright Licensing Agency. Enquiries concerning
reproduction outside those terms and in other countries should be sent to
the Rights Department, Oxford University Press, at the address above.

This book is sold subject to the condition that it shall not,
by way of trade or otherwise, be lent, re-sold, hired out, or otherwise
circulated without the publisher's prior consent in any form of binding
or cover other than that in which it is published and without a similar
condition including this condition being imposed
on the subsequent purchaser.

A catalogue record for this book is available from the British Library

Library of Congress Cataloguing in Publication Data

(Data available)

ISBN 0 19 2626205

Typeset by EXPO Holdings, Malaysia
Printed in Great Britain by
Bookcraft (Bath) Ltd
Midsomer Norton, Avon

Contents

Preface

Gastric cancer is still the most common neoplasia in many countries. This volume offers a comprehensive but concise coverage of the experimental approaches, epidemiology, biology, etiology, histopathology, diagnosis, and treatment of this disease.

Gastric cancers are strongly associated with environmental factors and are more frequently found in people of socioeconomically deprived classes. In most developed countries, gastric cancer morbidity has sharply declined over the past decades, providing a good example of how this particular cancer is largely preventable. The recent discovery that the *Helicobacter pylori* infection rate is positively related to high incidences of gastric cancer in various populations is very important in giving clues to causative factors. Thus, inflammation resulting from infection may facilitate the condition, yielding atrophic gastritis and intestinal metaplasia in which genetic alterations are frequently found.

Many changes at the DNA level have in fact been detected in cancers of the human stomach and the existence of a predisposing genetic background is indicated by the relatively frequent concomitant occurrence of gastric polyps and cancers, analogous to the colon.

Gastric cancers can be experimentally produced in rats and other animal species by administering directly-acting genotoxic substances such as N-methyl-N′-nitro-N-nitrosoguanidine and N-methyl-N-nitrosourea. These are known to cause genetic alterations in gastric mucosa cells which accumulate and then culminate in gastric neoplasia. This suggests that a similar situation is likely to also exist in man.

Different histopathological types of gastric cancers may reflect different genetic alterations as indicated by K-*SAM* gene amplification in diffuse type lesions and c-*erb* B-2 gene amplification in those with intestinal characteristics.

In diagnosis, great advances have been achieved using double contrast radiography. Endoscopic imaging and biopsy sampling are also powerful and precise weapons in this respect. Surgical removal of early lesions under endoscopic observation, without the necessity for laparotomy, means that the treatment load on the patient is minimal and a few days hospitalization is often sufficient before return to normal social activity. Many patients are cured by extended surgery, even if they have metastasis to regional lymph nodes (N2 disease). Further evaluation of extended surgery is one of the current topics in dispute.

Overall, gastric cancer provides us with a success story with victory of control over malignancy. However, the recurrence rate after surgery and advanced gastric cancer cases not suitable for operating on, as well as scirrhous type lesions, remains as a challenge to new treatment approaches like gene therapy, immunotherapy, and combined chemotherapy. The search for effective chemotherapeutica is still a high research priority.

The editors sincerely hope that this volume will provide readers, including students, fundamental scientists, physicians, and surgeons, with an up-to-date, solid, and well-balanced knowledge of gastric cancer in all of its aspects.

National Cancer Center   *T. Sugimura*
Tokyo, Japan
January 1997

Contributors

W. Achterrath
Klinik und Poliklinik fur Allgemeine
Chirurgie, Westfalische
Wilhelms-Universitat, Munster, Germany

S. Ahmedzai
Professor, Palliative Medicine Section,
Royal Hallamshire Hospital,
Sheffield, UK

Yasumasa Baba
Division of Internal Medicine, Cancer
Institute Hospital, Tokyo, Japan

David Cunningham
Consultant Medical Oncologist,
The Royal Marsden Hospital,
London and Sutton, UK

Jean Bernard Dubois
Professor, Department of Radiotherapy,
C.R.L.C., Val d'Aurelle, Montpellier,
France

P. Ellis
Department of Medicine, Royal Marsden
Hospital, London, UK

John W.L. Fielding
The Queen Elizabeth Hospital, Birmingham,
UK

Isaburo Fujimoto
Department of Cancer Control and Statistics,
Osaka Medical Center for Cancer and
Cardiovascular Diseases, Osaka, Japan

Aya Hanai
Japanese Association of Cancer Registries,
Osaka, Japan

J.C. Harvey
Scottish Cancer Intelligence Unit,
Edinburgh, Scotland

Setsuo Hirohashi
Deputy Director, National Cancer Center
Research Institute, Tokyo, Japan

Tomohiko Hiyama
Department of Cancer Control and Statistics,
Osaka Medical Center for Cancer and
Cardiovascular Diseases, Osaka, Japan

Yae Kanai
Pathology Division, National Cancer Center
Research Institute, Tokyo, Japan

Hitoshi Katai
Department of Surgical Oncology, National
Cancer Center Hospital, Tokyo, Japan

Keiichi Maruyama
Department of Surgical Oncology, National
Cancer Center Hospital, Tokyo, Japan

Masakazu Maruyama
Division of Internal Medicine, Cancer
Institute Hospital, Tokyo, Japan

C.S. Muir
Scottish Cancer Intelligence Unit,
Edinburgh, Scotland

C. Meystre
Consultant Physician, Leicestershire
Hospital, Leicester, UK

Atsushi Ochiai
Pathology Division, National Cancer Center
Research Institute, Tokyo, Japan

Hiroko Ohgaki
National Cancer Institute, Bethesda, USA

Hisanao Ohkura
Department of Medical Oncology, National
Cancer Center Hospital, Tokyo, Japan

Akira Oshima
Department of Cancer Control and Statistics,
Osaka Medical Center for Cancer and
Cardiovascular Diseases, Osaka, Japan

Peter Preusser
Klinik und Poliklinik fur Allgemeine
Chirurgie, Westfalische
Wilhems-Universitat, Munster, Germany

Takeshi Sano
Department of Surgical Oncology, National Cancer Center Hospital, Tokyo, Japan

Mitsuru Sasako
Department of Surgical Oncology, National Cancer Center Hospital, Tokyo, Japan

Takashi Sugimura
President Emeritus, National Cancer Center, Tokyo, Japan

Eiichi Tahara
The First Department of Pathology, Hiroshima University School of Medicine, Hiroshima, Japan

Norishige Takemoto
Division of Internal Medicine, Cancer Institute Hospital, Tokyo, Japan

Suketami Tominaga
Aichi Cancer Center Research Institute, Nagoya, Japan

Shoichiro Tsugane
Epidemiology Division, National Cancer Center Research Institute, Tokyo, Japan

Hideaki Tsukuma
Department of Cancer Control and Statistics, Osaka Medical Center for Cancer and Cardiovascular Diseases, Osaka, Japan

Asgaut Viste
Department of Surgery, Haukeland Sykehus University of Bergen, Norway

Shaw Watanabe
Department of Nutrition, Tokyo University of Agriculture, Tokyo, Japan

H. Wilke
Department of Oncology, Kliniken Essen-Mitte, West German Cancer Center, Essen, Germany

Naohito Yamaguchi
Epidemiology Division, National Cancer Center Research Institute, Tokyo, Japan

Shigeaki Yoshida
Deputy Director, National Cancer Center Hospital East, Kashiwa, Japan

Part I: Epidemiology

1

Cancer of the stomach: overview

C.S. Muir and J.C. Harvey

Globally, stomach cancer is currently the second most common cancer with approximately 755 000 incident cases each year. In developing countries, the cancer is in first rank in males and third rank in females. While incidence falls into three bands, there is no consistent geographical pattern. The highest levels are observed in Japan. World-wide, there is considerable intra-country variation. Relative frequencies are presented for those areas not covered by incidence or mortality data. Irrespective of incidence level, mortality rates have been declining in most countries, the onset of the fall differing from country to country. Socio-economic disparities are examined: there is an excess risk in incidence in the most deprived areas compared to the most affluent. Changes in risk on migration, notably in Japanese are demonstrated. The significance of differences in histological type is considered—as is survival.

1. INTRODUCTION

Although ancient civilizations were aware of cancer and its symptoms, the causes and geographical distribution were unknown. The first serious attempts to determine these were made in the 19th (Hirsch 1864) and early 20th centuries (Hoffman 1915). For over 100 years, gastric cancer has been recognized as an important form of malignant disease with significant geographical, ethnic, and socio-economic differences in distribution. Stomach cancer has repeatedly been shown to be more common in the lower socio-economic strata of society.

In this chapter, the past and present incidence and mortality rates in selected countries are presented. For populations covered neither by incidence nor mortality, relative frequency data are provided. When appropriate, information on various ethnic and migrant groups residing in the same country is presented. Causation is not considered in detail.

2. METHODS AND MATERIALS

There are two prime sources of information—incidence and mortality. The more useful measure of the cancer burden is incidence (i.e. the number of newly diagnosed cases of cancer occurring in a defined population). Mortality (i.e. the number of deaths from cancer occurring in a defined population) is influenced by the success of treatment. In many countries with survival rates of about 8–12%, mortality provides a reasonable approximation of incidence but in Japan, where survival is much greater, mortality no longer provides an accurate assessment of the burden of the disease.

In this chapter, emphasis is given to incidence statistics derived from population-based cancer registries extracted from the *Cancer incidence in five continents* monographs, the latest of which covers the years 1983–87 (Parkin *et al.* 1992). When appropriate, mortality statistics extracted from cause of death registrations are cited. The most convenient compendium of such data is that by Aoki *et al.* (1992). All rates given are age-standardized to the 'world' standard and are average annual rates per 100 000. For brevity the words 'average annual per 100 000' are omitted. Unless stated otherwise, rates are for males. In developing countries with restricted health service infrastructures, these sources are often not available and recourse must be made to relative frequency data, usually collected by pathologists, which present the proportion of a given cancer in relation to all cancers seen. Such data are subject to many biases; the most useful compilation of this type of information is that by Parkin (1986).

Changes over time in the incidence and mortality of gastric cancer have been exhaustively reviewed by Coleman *et al.* (1993) and by Correa and Chen (1994).

3. GLOBAL PERSPECTIVE

Until recently, stomach cancer was estimated to be the most frequently diagnosed malignancy in the world. The tumour was displaced in the mid 1980s from the first rank by lung cancer, with an estimated 896 000 incident cases; at this time there was held to be some 755 000 incident cases of gastric cancer (Parkin *et al.* 1993). Stomach cancer is still in first place in the developing countries in males (473 000 incident cases) being in third rank (148 000 incident cases) in females, lying behind cervix uteri (344 000 incident cases) and breast cancer (298 000 incident cases) in such countries. In Japan and China the tumour is in the first rank in both sexes.

Table 1.1 shows estimates of the number of incident cases around 1985 and of the age-standardized incidence rates for stomach cancer in 4 of the 24 demographic areas recognized by the United Nations Demographic Bureau. In brief, incidence in males seems to fall into three bands: less than 15 per 100 000, less than 40 per 100 000 and over 40 per 100 000. There is no consistent pattern. While higher rates are to be found in some developing countries, such as those of tropical South America; in India, Pakistan, and Iran (Southern Asia in Table 1.1) rates are low and of the same level as those in North America. Southern and Eastern Europe exhibit intermediate rates, whereas the former USSR and China have similar high rates. Japan has much higher rates than anywhere else in the world. These rates, applied to populations of vastly varying size, result in China having many more cases of gastric cancer than any other country: the numbers in the former USSR and Japan are about the same.

Table 1.1. Estimated numbers, in thousands, of incident gastric cancers (*c*.1985)

Region	Estimated numbers		Estimated ASR	
	Male	Female	Male	Female
East Africa	4	5	11	11
Southern Africa	1	1	13	6
Caribbean	2	1	15	7
Central America	4	4	17	12
Temperate South America	6	3	25	12
Tropical South America	27	14	41	19
North America	14	9	9	4
China	176	85	43	19
Japan	54	31	75	35
Southern Asia	27	14	8	4
Eastern Europe	17	11	26	12
Northern Europe	11	7	17	8
Southern Europe	23	15	25	12
Former USSR	54	44	44	19
World	473	282	25	13

Estimated rates are per 100 000 age-standardized (ASR) to the 'world' population, by sex, for selected UN demographic areas. (From the United Nations Demographic Bureau.)

4. INTER-COUNTRY VARIATION

The highest recorded incidence is in Japanese males with rates of around 85 (93.3 in Yamagata Prefecture and 73.6 in Osaka). Comparable levels have been reported from parts of the former USSR (Napalkov *et al.* 1983). Recent figures from St. Petersburg, Belaurs, Krygyzstan, Estonia, and Latvia give the incidence as 52.8, 46.7, 44.6, 37.0, and 34.1, respectively.

Elsewhere in Eastern Europe, rates are in the 20–30 range. There are considerable contrasts within Italy ranging from 40.2 in Florence to 16.1 in Ragusa, Sicily, a difference confirmed in studies of southern Italian migrants to the north of the country (Vigotti *et al.* 1988). In Villa Nueva de Gaia in Portugal, risk is high (47.8) in contrast to Spain with rates between 15 to 27.

During the period 1981–90, stomach cancer was ranked fifth for both sexes in Scotland, accounting for 6.6% and 4.8% of cancer registrations for males and females, respectively. Incidence rates were higher in Scotland (M = 19.2; F = 9.3) than in England and Wales (M = 16.8; F = 6.5). The twofold differences in rates observed within Scotland are thought to be linked to socio-economic circumstances (see below).

Fairly high rates have also been reported from parts of China (Shanghai, 51.7) and Latin America (Costa Rica, 46.9, Colombia, 36.3, Porto Alegre, 33.8). Conversely, incidence in Cuba (9.8) is close to US Whites' levels (SEER, 8.0),

(SEER is an acronym for the Surveillance, Epidemiology and End Results program of the US National Cancer Institute, which measures incidence for around 10% of the US population).

In Western Europe, age-standardized incidence rates are generally in the range of 15–25. Low levels are recorded in the Gambia (3.9) and parts of India (Ahmedabad 2.1).

5. MORTALITY

Irrespective of the level of risk, mortality rates have been declining in most countries. However, stomach cancer is still one of the major causes of death in many countries including Japan, China, South America, the Caribbean, and the non-White population of the United States.

Table 1.2 presents the top, fourth, and bottom sextiles of age-standardized gastric cancer mortality for a selection of 50 countries (Boring *et al.* 1992) during 1986–8. The rank order is based on that for males. The top sextile includes coun-

Table 1.2. Age-adjusted death rates from gastric cancer per 100 000 (1986–8)

Country	Males		Females	
	Rank	Rate	Rate	Rank
South Korea	1	54.6	23.7	1
Costa Rica	2	49.9	23.1	2
USSR	3	38.4	16.5	5
Japan	4	37.9	17.2	4
Chile	5	34.8	14.1	7
China	6	31.2	15.6	6
Ecuador	7	26.8	19.1	3
Poland	8	25.6	9.0	15
Finland	23	14.6	7.7	21
Scotland	24	14.2	6.6	26
Netherlands	25	14.1	5.7	31
England & Wales	26	13.8	5.6	33
Northern Ireland	27	13.7	6.6	27
Ireland	28	13.5	6.4	28
Argentina	29	13.4	5.6	32
Panama	30	12.8	6.8	25
Israel	43	9.2	4.6	42
Denmark	44	9.1	4.7	41
Australia	45	8.5	3.6	47
Canada	46	8.4	3.7	46
Cuba	47	7.6	3.7	45
Kuwait	48	5.5	3.1	48
United States	49	5.3	2.3	49
Thailand	50	1.1	0.6	50

tries in northern Asia, Eastern Europe, and Latin America. Perhaps the most interesting finding is that mortality in Japan is not in the first rank as the incidence data might suggest, reflecting a substantially better survival.

The fourth sextile contains the British Isles, Finland, the Netherlands and two countries in Latin America; the lowest sextile includes countries as diverse as Cuba, Kuwait, Denmark, and the United States and Canada.

Within the European Union there is a band of high and above average mortality which runs from central Italy to the Swiss border. This band of high mortality continues through Bavaria in the south of Germany to almost as far as the Danish border. Within Italy and France rates are low in the southern portions of these countries (Smans *et al.* 1992).

Substantial differences in mortality are seen within many countries. In Japan, standardized mortality ratios are higher in both sexes in the prefectures in the north east of the country, in contrast to liver cancer where the rates are much higher in the west of the country (Kakizoe 1993).

Within Scotland, the city of Glasgow and surrounding regions and the city of Dundee have rates that are double those of largely rural areas.

The relative rank of several European countries has changed over the past 15 years. Greece, which previously had the lowest stomach cancer mortality in Europe, has now been overtaken by France and Denmark which have even lower rates. Stomach cancer mortality in Portugal is now almost twice as high as elsewhere in the European Union and is similar to that seen in Poland, Hungary, former Czechoslovakia, and Romania.

6. RELATIVE FREQUENCY

Table 1.3 presents the relative frequency of gastric cancer, abstracted from Parkin (1986), in a variety of locations throughout the world, by continent. It will be recalled that the relative frequency is the proportion of a given cancer among all cancers, being frequently based on pathological series. Such series often overstate the frequency of the more accessible tumours at the expense of those more difficult of access and it may not be possible to define the population covered. Further, gastric cancers may be diagnosed on radiological grounds, or at surgery, without biopsy confirmation. Frequencies of gastric cancer are thus often higher in a registry covering a given area than in the pathology series emanating from the same region.

It will be noted that many of the entries in Table 1.3 pertain to cancer registries. However, the editors of the *Cancer incidence in five continents* monographs considered that in these areas there was evidence of under-registration or insufficient information on the denominator. On occasion, it may be possible to relate microscopically diagnosed cancers to a defined population as in the cities of Algiers, Oran, and Constantine. This permits the computation of a minimum incidence rate (i.e. whatever the true incidence may be it cannot be less than the minimum rate). When examining Table 1.3, it may be helpful to bear in mind that

Table 1.3.   Relative frequency of gastric cancer (%) world-wide

Continent and Country	Males (%)	Females (%)	Year
AFRICA			
Algeria (Algiers, Oran, Constantine) Histopathology Study	4.4	1.7	1966–75
Kenya National Cancer Registry	4.3	2.4	1968–78
Department of Pathology, Mombassa	3.6	2.8	1981
Liberia Cancer Registry	3.5	1.3	1976–80
Madagascar Pathology Laboratory	1.3	0.5	1979–81
Nigeria Ibadan Cancer Registry	6.0	2.2	1970–6
Zaria Cancer Registry	1.5	1.1	1976–8
Rwanda Department of Pathology, Butare	9.9	6.5	1982–4
The Sudan Cancer Registry	2.7	1.5	1978
Radiation and Isotope Centre, Khartoum	0.6	0.3	1967–84
Swaziland Cancer Registry	2.3	0.3	1979–83
Tunisia Institut Salah-Azaiz	2.1	1.5	1976–80
Uganda Kampala Cancer Registry	2.7	1.6	1971–80
Kuluva Hospital, West Nile District	0.5	–	1961–78
United Republic of Tanzania Muhumbili Medical Centre, Dar es Salaam	1.7	1.5	1980–1
Mwanza Hospital	1.6	0.9	1980–1
Kilimanjaro Cancer Registry	8.6	9.9	1975–9
Zambia The Cancer Registry, Lusaka	5.0	4.9	1981–3
Department of Pathology, Ndola Central Hospital	2.8	1.4	1976–9
Zimbabwe Bulawayo Cancer Registry	4.5	2.6	1973–7
Central Histology Laboratory, Harare	4.6	2.7	1981–2
THE AMERICAS			
Argentina Provincial Cancer Registry, Zona Gran La Plata	6.4	2.6	1978–80
Provincial Cancer Registry, Partido de la Plata	7.2	4.0	1980

Table 1.3.   *(cont'd)*

Continent and Country	Males (%)	Females (%)	Year
Santa Fe Tumour Registry	1.9	1.0	1976–82
Registry of R. Santamarina Hospital, Tandil	6.1	2.5	1977–82
Bolivia			
Cancer Registry, La Paz	13.0	5.0	1978–9
Costa Rica			
National Tumour Registry	23.5	11.5	1979–83
Martinique			
Cancer Registry	11.4	7.3	1981–2
Panama			
Cancer Registry	10.6	4.8	1974–80
Paraguay			
Cancer Registry	11.2	4.5	1975–7
Peru			
Lima Metropolitan Cancer Registry	19.3	10.6	1978
Uruguay			
Department of Pathology, Montevideo	7.7	6.1	1977–81
ASIA			
Burma			
Rangoon Cancer Registry	11.4	8.3	1978–80
India			
Bangalore	10.5	4.6	1982
Madras	13.5	5.2	1982
Chandigarh	3.4	0.7	1982
Dibrugarh	4.8	2.5	1982
Trivandrum	5.2	2.4	1982
Ahmedabad	1.5	1.3	1982
Islamic Republic of Iran			
Register of Iranian Cancer Organization	9.5	3.8	1981–2
Fars Province Cancer Registry	9.4	4.4	1978–81
Kashani Pathology Laboratory, Isfahan	0.2	–	1981–2
Iraq			
Baghdad Cancer Registry	4.4	3.2	1976–82
Kuwait			
Cancer Registry, Kuwaitis	4.4	2.0	1974–8
Cancer Registry, Non-Kuwaitis	4.9	3.8	1974–8
Malaysia (Kuala Lumpur)			
Chinese	7.9	3.2	1980–1
Malaysians	5.7	2.0	1980–1
Indians	9.6	2.6	1980–1
Department of Pathology	5.7	2.0	1980–1

Table 1.3.   *(cont'd)*

Continent and Country	Males (%)	Females (%)	Year
Pakistan			
Karachi, Jinnah Postgraduate Medical Centre	1.9	1.1	1979–83
Hyderabad, Liaquat Medical College, Jamshoro	1.7	0.9	1981–2
Lahore, King Edward College	1.0	0.6	1979–83
Peshawar, Khyber Medical College	1.2	0.7	1979–81
Rawalpindi, Armed Forces Institute of Pathology	2.9	1.8	1979–82
All Centres	1.7	0.9	1981
Philippines			
Central Tumour Registry	6.8	4.2	1977
South Korea			
Central Cancer Registry	29.8	16.9	1982–3
Sri Lanka			
Cancer Registry, Maharagama Cancer Institute, Colombo	1.2	0.6	1977–8
Department of Pathology, University of Peradeniya	3.9	1.6	1976–81
Thailand			
National Register	5.3	2.8	1980
Bangkok, Ramathibodi Hospital Cancer Registry	3.5	2.4	1982–3
Turkey			
National Histopathology Survey	6.4	4.7	1977
Vietnam			
Cancer Hospital, Ho Chi Minh City	0.7	0.2	1976–81
OCEANIA			
Fiji			
Fijians	8.6	1.7	1979–82
Indians	5.8	3.7	1979–82
Cancer Registry of Fiji, Pathology Data	7.1	2.4	1979–82
New Caledonia			
Europeans	3.4	1.7	1977–81
Melanesians	10.7	3.8	1977–81
Registry of New Caledonia	6.4	2.2	1977–81
Papua New Guinea			
Cancer Registry	3.4	1.9	1971–8

in the US White population covered by the SEER programme the relative frequency of gastric cancer was 2.5% in males and 1.6% in females: in contrast, the relative frequencies in Yamagata Prefecture, Japan were 39.9% and 30.0%, respectively.

6.1. Africa

Frequencies in males are, for the most part, in the 2–4% range with the exception of the registries in the Highlands of Tanzania and Rwanda with frequencies of around 9–10%.

6.2. The Americas

Frequencies are low in Argentina. Elsewhere, frequencies are in the 10–20% range tending to be at their highest in Central America (23.5% in males and 11.5% in females in Costa Rica), and second only to those in Japan. In North America frequencies are very low.

6.3. Asia

Frequencies are much higher in South India (Bangalore 10.5% and Madras 13.5% in males) than elsewhere. It is of interest to note that Indians in Malaysia, many of whom migrated from South India, have a frequency (9.6% in males) which is comparable to that of Bangalore and Madras, and higher than those observed in Chinese and Malays. For male Singapore Indians the frequency is 11.8%. The frequencies observed in South Korea are very close to those of Japan.

6.4. Oceania

The highest frequency observed is in Melanesians of New Caledonia (10.7% in males); Europeans dwelling in this Department of France have a much lower frequency (3.4% in males) which is slightly less than in France itself. The repatriation of Europeans to metropolitan France for diagnosis and treatment cannot be excluded.

Although relative frequency data are useful in the absence of incidence or mortality data, these last mentioned sources are to be preferred.

7. TRENDS OVER TIME

Gastric cancer has been a significant public health problem for many years in much of the world. Hoffman (1915) provides crude mortality data for stomach and liver (it was usual to combine these sites in statistical tables at this time) in the US population for each year between 1900 and 1913 with a mean crude rate of 25 per 100 000 in each sex. In Washington DC, the rates in White males and females were 33.4 and 27.1, respectively; corresponding figures for Blacks were 21.3 and 18.1. In Japan during 1909–10 the rate for both sexes combined was 40.0. At this time, rates in Norway (64.1) and Switzerland (70.4) were very high (none of the above rates was age-adjusted).

The records of the Japanese Meiji Life Assurance Company reveal that during 1899–1907, 57.8% of cancer deaths in male assured persons and 36.1% of those in females were caused by stomach cancer.

While it is likely that those insured were not representative of the whole Japanese population, stomach cancer has clearly been a major problem for over a century in Japan. The most remarkable feature in the epidemiology of stomach cancer today is the universal declining trend in both sexes, somewhat more marked in females than males. The decline in incidence and mortality began at different times in different regions of the world. Thus, in US Whites and in Norway, a fall in mortality was observable in the 1930s, a decline which has continued to the present day. In US Blacks, mortality rose until 1950, falling thereafter.

Mortality in Spain only began to decline in the 1960s, later than in many other countries. In Portugal, rates rose in both sexes until about 1970 before beginning to fall; the decline has been among the slowest in Europe. In Chile, another country with very high mortality (Table 1.2), there has been a steady decrease since 1955.

Between 1935 and 1952, mortality in Japan was remarkably stable (Segi *et al.* 1965). Age-standardized rates rose slowly in both sexes until about 1960 and have declined fairly sharply since (Fig. 1.1). The fall in mortality in high incidence Japan has been greater than elsewhere (Tominaga 1987), (Fig. 1.1). Decreasing trends in Norway and Japan, and probably elsewhere, appear to be the result of the dis-

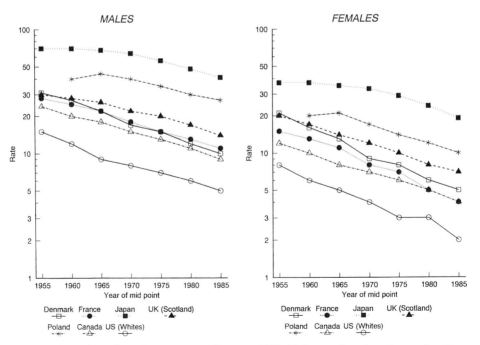

Fig. 1.1. Age-adjusted gastric cancer mortality rates 1953–87, by sex, for selected countries. (From Aoki *et al.* 1992.)

appearance of the 'intestinal' type of this cancer, the variant more subject to international variation, the 'diffuse' type being more constant (see below). The decline may be interrupted. Norwegian rates began to decrease in 1930, stabilized after 1945, and recommenced their decline in 1951 when the deprivation associated with World War II ended.

Incidence and mortality from stomach cancer are lower in European Union (EU) countries than elsewhere in Europe, but a decline has occurred in all areas. Truncated rates (i.e. age 35–64 years) fell by a third to a half in both sexes between 1970 and 1985. The decreases in EU countries are in the range of 10–20% per five-year period: Scotland and Birmingham (England) show even lower rates of 3–4% (Coleman *et al.* 1993).

While such cross-sectional data are of interest, their synoptic nature conceals trends within differing age groups and birth cohorts. The secular decline in mortality has followed a birth cohort pattern, first documented in the United States by Haenszel (1958). In Japan, the declining trend was observed only in cohorts born after 1913. Further, the differences in the rates between successive birth cohorts were less than those observed in England and Wales, Norway, and the United States. Clear birth cohort effects were not seen in Poland and Portugal which Correa and Chen (1994) suggest reflects cross-sectional forces, such as improved diagnosis, rather than true birth cohort effects.

A cohort analysis is given in Fig. 1.2 for gastric cancer incidence in Scotland. On reaching the age of 50–54, successive birth cohorts experienced a lower incidence.

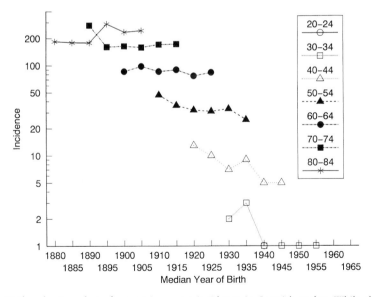

Fig. 1.2. Birth cohort analysis for gastric cancer incidence in Scottish males. While those born between 1880 and 1925 show little change on reaching 60–64 years and above, a fall is seen in subsequent birth cohorts on reaching the age of 55 and below. For clarity, every second age group has been omitted.

Thus, those born in 1935, on attaining this age, had an incidence rate half of that seen in those born around 1910. While this effect is also readily visible for younger age groups it is not seen for ages above 60–64.

From the public health point of view periodic examination of incidence and mortality, for each five-year age group at, say, five-year calendar intervals is worthwhile in that secular changes, in either direction, are first seen in the young (Muir *et al.* 1981; Doll 1990). In the United States, rates in the 40–44 age group have been very close since the 1950s which suggests that most of the fall in mortality may now have occurred.

8. INTRA-COUNTRY VARIATION

In Japan, there appears to be a north/south divide, with stomach cancer mortality and incidence rates higher in the north eastern prefectures (Kakizoe 1993). In Scotland, gastric cancer incidence rates are consistently lower in the rural parts of the north and south with male rates around 10–18; rates between 25 and 30 are concentrated in and around the major cities (Kemp *et al.* 1985). In England and Wales there is again a twofold difference in mortality and incidence rates (OPCS 1994) across the country with lower levels in the south and east and higher levels in the north and west, particularly noticeable in north-west Wales. Mortality is significantly less in rural compared to urban and metropolitan areas (Swerdlow and dos Santos Silva 1993). These differences are considered to be associated with socio-economic and environmental factors. Swerdlow and dos Santos Silva (1993) review some of the other causes suggested to explain the higher levels in Wales. These include zinc: copper ratios in the soil and bracken infestation but these do not correlate any better than socio-economic level. As for several other sites, there are substantial differences in various ethnic groups living in the same country. Rates in Maoris (25.3) are double those in non-Maoris living in New Zealand. Blacks covered by the US SEER registries have rates 50% higher than those in Whites (8.0 and 12.4, respectively), and in Singapore, Chinese incidence rates (34.7) are more than double those in Indians (15.9) (which are identical to those in Madras) and over five times greater than in Singapore Malays (6.4).

Singapore Chinese exhibit substantial differences in risk by language dialect group. Age-standardized incidence rates in 1983–87 for Hokkien, Teochew, Cantonese, Hainanese, and Hakka males were respectively: 39.2, 33.3, 15.2, 18.1, and 20.4. Corresponding rates for females were 17.6, 11.7, 9.8, 10.2, and 8.7 (Lee *et al.* 1992). Such large differences are unlikely to be due to selection or registration bias as a different pattern by dialect group is seen for nasopharynx, oesophagus, and lung cancers.

9. SOCIO-ECONOMIC CLASS AND OCCUPATION

Despite the fall in mortality generally, there appears to be a relationship between stomach cancer and social class. Rates for Whites (5.9) are approximately half those in Blacks (12.2) in Atlanta and a twofold difference in cumulative mortality rates between the highest and lowest socio-economic groups is seen in England and Wales. This risk differential has been maintained since 1911, although mortality has continued to fall over the years in all social strata (Logan 1982). In Scotland, Carstairs and Morris (1991) and Sharp *et al.* (1993) demonstrated a 75% excess risk in incidence in the most deprived compared to the most affluent. Rates are low in social class I (i.e. professional groups) and high in social class V (e.g. unskilled labourers) (Fig. 1.3). While within countries most studies reveal the poor to have more stomach cancer the generally low rates in India must reflect an absence of other risk factors.

Analyses of mortality by occupation in England and Wales (OPCS 1978) show that in the 35–64 age group (i.e. the economically active population), the standardized mortality gastric cancer rate for males in social class V (unskilled manual labourers) was three times greater than that for social class I, the lowest rates being recorded for self-employed professional workers. Among occupations with significantly high proportional mortality ratios were fibre preparers, coal-mine face workers, rubber workers, and unskilled labourers. While it is difficult to separate exposures at work from those associated with the socio-economic group from which these workers are drawn, it is generally considered that occupation *per se* contributes comparatively little to the risk (Fox and Adelstein 1978).

10. MIGRATION

Migration, and in particular, international migration, can lead to a change in risk, as the immigrants, especially second and third generations, adopt the lifestyle and consequently the pattern of incidence of their new abode.

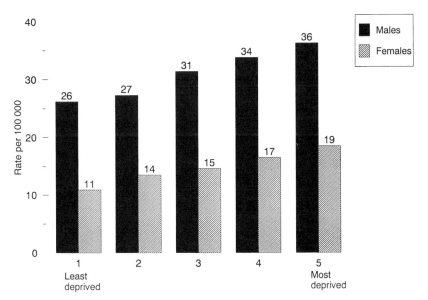

Fig. 1.3. Age-standardized registration rates by deprivation category and sex, Scotland 1981–90. (From Sharp *et al.* 1993.)

The risk of stomach cancer changes slowly in populations moving from high- to low-risk communities. Incidence rates in US (Hawaii) Japanese are 24.3 and 11.1 in males and females, respectively. Although these rates are about one-third of those found in Japan, they are nonetheless approximately three times the rates in US Whites (Fig. 1.4).

Studies of Japanese migrants to the United States confirmed that early exposure to environmental rather than genetic factors have a greater influence on mortality and incidence rates. In subsequent generations born in the United States, the mortality rate declined towards the lower rate of US Whites (Haenszel and Kurihara 1968).

Another large population of Japanese immigrants settled in Brazil, half of whom live in São Paulo state, the remainder in metropolitan São Paulo. During the period 1969–78, stomach cancer was the most common in males and females in Japan-born residents in metropolitan São Paulo (i.e. first-generation Japanese immigrants). The incidence rate from gastric cancer was approximately 1.5 times greater than that of the general population of São Paulo (Fig. 1.4). A significant reduction in incidence was observed in São Paulo Japanese, although the difference was not so pronounced as in Japanese immigrants in the United States (Tsugane *et al.* 1990). This implies a tendency of some immigrants to retain their native eating habits in the new country, such as the Japanese immigrants in Bolivia (Tsugane *et al.* 1985; Tsugane 1989). Oshima and Hanai (1990) also investigated variations between countries and at Japanese migration to other countries and the effects of adopting a Western lifestyle.

These observations on the Japanese are analogous to those for Chinese and Polish migrants to the United States (Muir and Staszewski 1986). Lee *et al.* (1992)

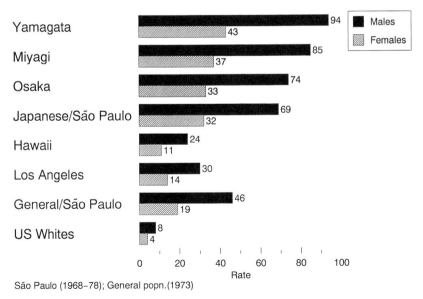

Fig. 1.4. Stomach cancer incidence rates for Japanese populations in various geographic areas: comparison with the general population of São Paulo and US Whites.

observe that there is a statistically significant diminution of risk for Chinese born in Singapore compared with those born elsewhere mainly China.

Within Israel, the risk for Jews born in Israel (9.1) is much less than that seen in Jews born in Europe or America (16.2). The rate for non-Jews in Israel (6.9) is close to that in Kuwaitis (4.1).

Declines in risk with increasing duration of residence have also been observed for some of the European populations migrating to Australia (McMichael et al. 1980). McCredie and Coates (1989) and Armstrong et al. (1983) noted that stomach cancer incidence and mortality were higher in migrants from Wales to Australia than in migrants from England to that country reflecting the situation in the countries of origin.

11. HISTOLOGY

Lauren (1965), advocated categorizing stomach cancer into two histological types, differing in morphology and epidemiological characteristics. Intestinal, or expanding adenocarcinoma, is more usual in males and older age groups. According to Muñoz et al. (1968), this type is prominent in high-risk areas and has been decreasing in relative frequency in the United States and Norway, where mortality rates have been declining. The studies showed that the intestinal-type varies with place and time and is likely to be linked to environmental factors.

The diffuse, or infiltrative type of adenocarcinoma, is equally frequent in both sexes, is more common in younger age groups, and has a worse prognosis than the intestinal type. Hanai et al. (1982), showed that incidence rates of this variant of the disease decreased only slightly for both sexes, compared with a considerable fall in the rates for the intestinal type. Studies have also shown that the intestinal type of cancer prevails in migrants from high-risk populations and the decline in such populations is mainly of this type.

12. SURVIVAL

Survival from stomach cancer is very poor with less than 10% of patients surviving five years after diagnosis. There are remarkable international differences in survival—the five-year relative survival in Japan being very much greater than that in other countries (Figs 1.5, 1.6). This observation is all the more remarkable in the light of the early detection programme available in much of the country.

Oshima and Hanai (1990) reviewed the mass screening programmes undertaken in Japan for gastric cancer. These began in 1957 to detect stomach cancer early and led to a gradual reduction in mortality rates. In 1991, out of a total of nearly 4.2 million people screened, stomach cancer was detected in close to 6000 (0.14%), (Kakizoe 1993). Kogevinas (1990) noted that survival was less favourable in the lower socio-economic strata of England and Wales.

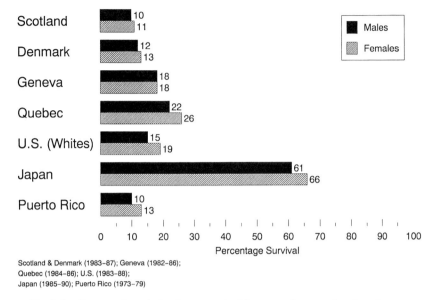

Fig. 1.5.   Comparative relative 5-year survival for stomach cancer in selected areas.

13. COMMENTS

The descriptive epidemiology of gastric cancer uncovers a disease with enormous variation in occurrence throughout the world. These differences are striking at country level and many countries show substantial and significant variations in risk within their boundaries. The increasingly frequent cancer atlas helps to visualize these patterns in a way that no set of tables can (Boyle *et al.* 1989). The universal decline in the disease and the substantial changes in risk in migrant populations all point to the importance of environmental causes.

Yet, the descriptive epidemiology of gastric cancer can only take us so far in elucidation of the aetiology of the disease. The common extension of descriptive data—the correlation or ecological study—can suggest causal hypotheses. A correlation between decreases in mortality and incidence rates has been observed in Osaka, Japan, and the United States. This decline is deemed to be caused by changes in environmental factors, particularly dietary habits, especially the increased intake of Western-style foods compared with a decrease in consumption of traditional Japanese foods.

Tominaga (1987), showed that the death rate decreased along with the diminished intake of rice and salt and an increased intake of milk, milk products, vitamins A and C, and the availability and use of refrigerators in the home. This approach is open to many sources of confounding. Other techniques have to be employed, including the case-control study and prospective investigations which examine risk at the individual rather than the group level. Nonetheless, any causal hypothesis has to be consistent with the observed distribution of the cancer other-

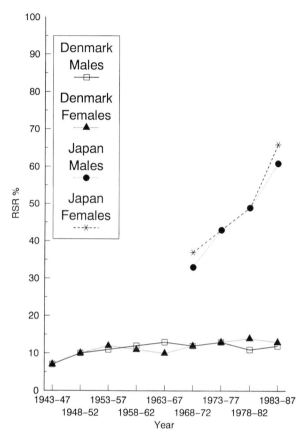

Fig. 1.6. Temporal change in relative 5-year gastric cancer survival (RSR) in Denmark and Japan 1943–7 to 1983–7.

wise it is erroneous or incomplete (Muir 1971). At first glance, the relationship between *Helicobacter pylori* infection, recently classed as a human carcinogen by the International Agency for Research on Cancer and gastric cancer, would appear to match the geographical and social class distribution of the disease (IARC 1994).

REFERENCES

Aoki, K., Kurihara, M., Hayakawa, N., and Suzuki, S. (1992). *Death rates for malignant neoplasms for selected sites and five-year age group in 33 Countries 1953–57 to 1983–87*. University of Nagoya Coop Press.

Armstrong, B.K., Woodings, T.L., Stenhouse, N.S., and McCall, M.G. (1983). *Mortality from cancer in migrants to Australia 1962–1971*. National Health and Medical Research Council, Perth.

Boring, C.C., Squires, T.S., and Tong, T. (1992). *Cancer statistics 1992*. CA, **42**, 19–38.

Boyle, P., Muir, C.S., and Grundmann, E. (ed.) (1989). *Cancer mapping. Recent results in cancer research, No. 114*. Springer, Heidelberg.

Carstairs, V. and Morris, R. (1991). *Deprivation and health in Scotland*. Aberdeen University Press.

Coleman, M., Esteve, J., Damiecki, P., Arslan, A., and Renard, A. (1993). *Trends in cancer incidence and mortality*. IARC Scientific Publications No. 121. International Agency for Research on Cancer, Lyon.

Correa, P. and Chen, V.W. (1994). Gastric cancer. In *Trends in cancer incidence and mortality, Cancer Surveys*, Vols 19/20, (ed. R. Doll,. J.F. Fraumeni, and C.S. Muir) pp. 55–76. Cold Spring Harbour.

Doll, R. (1990). Are we winning the fight against cancer? An epidemiological assessment. *European Journal of Cancer*, **26**, 500–8.

Fox, A.J. and Adelstein, A.M. (1978). Occupational mortality: work or way of life? *Journal of Epidemiology and Community Health*, **32**, 73–8.

Haenszel, W. (1958). Variation in incidence of the mortality from stomach cancer, with particular reference to the United States. *Journal of the National Cancer Institute*, **21**, 213–62.

Heanszel, W. and Kurihara, M. (1968). Mortality from cancer and other diseases among Japanese in the United States. *Journal of the National Cancer Institute*, **40**, 43–68.

Hanai, A., Fujimoto, I., and Taniguchi, H. (1982). Trends of stomach cancer incidence and histologic types in Osaka. In *Trends in cancer incidence*, (ed. K. Magnus), pp. 143–154. Hemisphere, Washington, DC.

Hirsch, A. (1864). *Handbuch der pathologischen und historischen Pathologie*. Berlin.

Hoffman, F. (1915). *The mortality from cancer throughout the world*. The Prudential Press, Newark.

IARC (International Agency for Research on Cancer) (1994). *Schistosomes, liver flukes and Helicobacter pylori. IARC monographs on the evaluation of carcinogenic risk to humans*, Vol. 61. International Agency for Research on Cancer. Lyon.

Kakizoe, T. (ed). (1993). *Figures on cancer in Japan—1993*. Foundation for Promotion of Cancer Research, Tokyo.

Kemp, I.W., Boyle, P., Smans, M., and Muir, C. (1985). *Atlas of cancer in Scotland 1975–1980: Incidence and epidemiological perspective*. IARC Scientific Publications No. 72. International Agency for Research on Cancer, Lyon.

Kogevinas, E. (1990). Longitudinal survey. *Socio-demographic differences in cancer survival 1971–1983. England and Wales*, (Series LS, No. 5). OPCS, London.

Lauren, P. (1965). The two histological main types of gastric carcinoma. Diffuse and so-called intestinal type. *Acta Pathologica Microbiologica Scandinavica*, **64**, 31–49.

Lee, H.P., Chia, K.S., and Shanmugaratnam, K. (1992). *Cancer incidence in Singapore, 1983–1987*. Singapore Cancer Registry.

Logan, W.P.D. (1982). *Cancer mortality by occupation and social class 1851–1971*. IARC Scientific Publications No. 36. International Agency for Research on Cancer, Lyon.

McCredie, M. and Coates, M. (1989). *Cancer incidence in migrants to New South Wales: 1972–1984*. New South Wales Cancer Registry, Sydney.

McMichael, A.J., McCall, M.G., Harstorne, J.M., and Woodings, T.L. (1980). Pattern of gastro-intestinal cancer in European migrants to Australia. The role of dietary change. *International Journal of Cancer*, **25**, 431–7.

Muir, C.S. (1971). Geographical differences in cancer patterns. In *Host environment interaction in the etiology of cancer in Man*, (ed. R. Doll and I. Vodopija), pp. 1–13. IARC Scientific Publications No. 7. International Agency for Research on Cancer, Lyon.

Muir, C.S., Choi, N.W., and Schifflers, E. (1981). Time trends in cancer mortality in some countries. Their possible causes and significance. In *Medical aspects of mortality statistics*, (ed. H. Bostrom and N. Ljungstedt), pp. 269–310. Skandia International Symposia.

Muir, C.S. and Staszewski, J. (1986). Geographical epidemiology and migrant studies. In *Biochemical and molecular epidemiology of cancer*, (ed. C. Harris), pp. 135–48. Liss, New York.

Muñoz, N., Correa, P., Cuello, C., and Duque, E. (1968). Histological types of gastric carcinoma in high- and low-risk areas. *International Journal of Cancer*, **3**, 809–18.

Napalkov, N.P., Tserkovny, Merabishvili, V.M., Parkin, D.M., Smans, M., and Muir, C.S. (1983). *Cancer incidence in the USSR*, (2nd edn, rev.). IARC Scientific Publications No. 48. International Agency for Research on Cancer, Lyon.

OPCS (Office of Population, Census and Surveys) (1978). *Occupational mortality. The Registrar General's decennial supplement for England and Wales, 1970–72*, (Series DS, No. 1). HMSO, London.

OPCS (Office of Population, Census and Surveys) (1994). *1988 Cancer statistics: Registrations in England and Wales 1978*, (Series MB No. 21). HMSO, London.

Oshima, A. and Hanai, A. (1990). *Epidemiology of human stomach cancer*.

Parkin, D.M. (ed.) (1986). *Cancer occurrence in developing countries*. IARC Scientific Publications No. 75. International Agency for Research on Cancer, Lyon.

Parkin, D.M., Muir, C.S., Whelan, S.L., Gao, Y.T., Ferlay, J., and Powell, J. (ed.) (1992). *Cancer incidence in five continents*, Vol. VI. IARC Scientific Publications No. 120. International Agency for Research on Cancer, Lyon.

Parkin, D.M., Pisani, P., and Ferlay, J. (1993). Estimates of the worldwide incidence of eighteen major cancers in 1985. *International Journal of Cancer*, **54**, 594–606.

Segi, M., Kurihara, M., and Matsuyama, T. (1965). *Cancer mortality in Japan 1899–1962*. Sendi, Department of Public Health, Tohoku University School of Medicine.

Sharp, L., Black, R.J., Harkness, E.L., Finlayson, A.R., and Muir, C.S. (1993). *Cancer registration statistics Scotland 1981–1990*. Information and Statistics Division, Edinburgh.

Smans, M., Muir, C.S., and Boyle, P. (1992). *Atlas of cancer mortality in the European Economic Community*. IARC Scientific Publication No. 107. International Agency for Research on Cancer, Lyon.

Swerdlow, A. and dos Santos Silva, A. (1993). *Atlas of cancer incidence in England and Wales 1968–85*. Oxford University Press.

Tominaga, S. (1987). Decreasing trend of stomach cancer in Japan. *Japanese Journal of Cancer Research (Gann)*, **78**, 1–10.

Tsugane, S. (1989). Changes and difference in eating habits of immigrants from Okinawa and those from the Japanese mainland in the Republic of Bolivia. *Japanese Journal of Health, Human Ecology*, **55**, 124–32.

Tsugane, S., Okazaki, I., and Kondo, H. (1985). Life style and health status of Japanese immigrants in Bolivia. *Japanese Journal of Public Health*, **32**, 794.

Tsugane, S., de Souza, J.M.P., Costa, M.L., Mirra, A.P., Gotlieb, S.L.D., Laurenti, R., *et al.* (1990). Cancer incidence rates among Japanese immigrants in the City of São Paulo, Brazil, 1969–78. *Cancer Causes and Control*, **1**, 189–93.

Vigotti, M.A., Cislaghi, C., Balzi, D., Giorgi, D., La Vecchia, C., Marchi, M.I., *et al.* (1988). Cancer mortality in migrant populations within Italy. *Tumori*, **74**, 107–28.

2

Survival of patients with stomach cancer: results from population-based cancer registries

Aya Hanai, Hideaki Tsukuma, Tomohiko Hiyama,
and Isaburo Fujimoto

1. INTRODUCTION

Stomach cancer in Japan still holds the highest incidence (Parkin *et al.* 1992) and mortality (Aoki *et al.* 1992) rates among all countries of the world, though both rates have steadily decreased over an extended period. During the 1950s and 1960s when deaths due to infectious diseases decreased in Japan and cancer became one of the leading causes of death, stomach cancer patients occupied half of the total cancer incidence in this country (JMHW 1963). Early diagnosis and early treatment was the predominant strategy in the fight against cancer in Japan during this time. This is described in Chapter 13. In 1990, the stomach was still the leading site of cancer both in incidence and mortality (RGPCRJ 1993; Kuroishi *et al.* 1993), and it was estimated that this leading position would be maintained until the year 2005–10 (Tsukuma *et al.* 1992).

The survival rate of cancer patients calculated in population-based cancer registries is an important measurement and constitutes a comprehensive and objective index for evaluating cancer control programs in a specified region (Hanai *et al.* 1985; Parkin and Hakulinen 1991).

In Osaka, the Prefectural Government, the Osaka Medical Association, and the Osaka Medical Center for Cancer and Cardiovascular Diseases agreed to start a population-based cancer registration program covering all the Osaka Prefecture with the co-operation of all medical institutions located in the prefecture (Fujimoto *et al.* 1993). Cancer reports and patient prognostic information have been collected from hospitals, general practitioners, and health centers (Hanai *et al.* 1985; OPDH *et al.* 1991).

In this chapter, five-year relative survival rates (Cutler and Ederer 1958; Ederer *et al.* 1961) for stomach cancer patients in Osaka as well as in other registries in Japan are introduced and these figures are compared with the end results from registries in Europe and in North America. Then, time trends of survival rates in Osaka are described along with time trends in the distribution of clinical stage.

2. STOMACH CANCER PATIENTS: FIVE-YEAR SURVIVAL RATES

In Japan, survival rates have been used to evaluate the therapeutic methods of cancer medical care in clinical departments in hospitals. In line with this, department-based site-specific cancer registries have been set up by various academic societies for site-specific cancers, and these have started reporting prognostic data (Tominaga *et al.* 1981). It is, however, difficult to estimate from these data the survival for all cancer cases occurring in the population of a certain region.

As of 1993, 31 population-based cancer registries were operating in Japan. Among them, only three have been conducting periodic follow-up on registered patients and publishing the end-results. Five-year relative survival rates for stomach cancer patients for both sexes from the three registries in Japan: Osaka, Yamagata, and Fukui, ranged from 42% to 51%, as shown in Table 2.1. Fukui showed the highest rate, followed by Yamagata and Osaka (OPDH 1991; Sato *et al.* 1989; FPDH and FMA 1992).

The factors causing differences in survival in these registries, the proportions in incidence of, and 5-year relative survival rates for the screened cases (i.e. those patients who were detected by mass screening programs or health check-ups), are shown in Table 2.1, according to registry. In this table, the same data for other cases (hospital cases) and those patients detected in hospitals or clinics, are also shown. For Yamagata, only crude rates were available. Five-year survival rates for

Table 2.1. Survival rates and proportions of the cases detected by screening programs or health check-ups in three registries in Japan (males and females)

(a) Survival

District	Yr of diagnosis	Relative or crude	Five-year survival rate (%)		
			Total	Cases detected by screening	Others
Osaka	1984–6	Relative	43.0	75.3	41.2
Fukui	1985	Relative	50.9	94.0	43.9
Yamagata	1974–82	Crude	42.2	78.6	33.8

(b) Proportion of cases

District	Yr of diagnosis	Total number of cases	Proportion of cases (%)		
			Total	Cases detected by screening	Others
Osaka	1984–6	8233	100	6.0	94.0
Fukui	1985	757	100	14.0	86.0
Yamagata	1974–82	5621	100	19.1	80.9

screened cases ranged from 75% to 94%, which was a little more than twice the survival of 34–44% for hospital cases in these registries.

The proportion of screened cases was smallest in Osaka, and those in Fukui and in Yamagata were twice and three times higher than that in Osaka, respectively. It was revealed that both the higher proportion and higher survival rate for screened cases in a region influenced to some extent the survival rates for the total cases occurring in a region.

Survival rates for hospital cases also differed among registries. These differences seemed to be caused by differences in the distribution of clinical stage and the proportion of surgically treated cases. Survival rates according to clinical stage were, however, available only in Osaka, and the comparison among registries could not be performed.

3. STOMACH CANCER SURVIVAL: INTERNATIONAL COMPARISONS

There are many difficulties in carrying out periodic follow-up surveys for all registered cancer patients. Only a small number of registries in the world have published their own patient prognostic results. In Table 2.2, five-year relative survival rates for stomach cancer patients in three registries in Japan are shown in the upper half, and those of the SEER Program in the United States (Ries *et al.* 1990), Saskatchewan, Canada (Tan and Robson 1991), Geneva, Switzerland RGT 1988), Denmark (Carstensen *et al.* 1993), and Scotland (Black *et al.* 1993) are shown in the lower half. When comparing these prognostic results, survival rates were observed to be higher in registries in Japan and lower in those of other countries. No standard errors were available for registries other than Osaka and Scotland. The difference in the survival rates between these two registries was statistically significant. Differences between any of the Japanese registries and those of other

Table 2.2. Comparison of 5-year relative survival rates in six countries (males and females)

Country	District or ethnic group	Yr of diagnosis	No. of cases observed	5-year RSR (%)	
Japan	Osaka	1984–6	8 519	43.0	(SE:0.6)
	Yamagata	1974–82	7 378	46.7	
	Fukui	1984–5	1 467	50.9	
US (SEER)	Whites	1981–6	17 692	15	
	Blacks	1981–6	2 417	17	
Canada	Saskatchewan	1980–6	670	17.4	
Switzerland	Geneva	1978–82	286	21.5	
Denmark		1983–7	3 843	12.2	
Scotland		1983–7	5 146	10.6	(SE:1.3)

RSR, relative survival rate; SE, standard error.

countries would undoubtedly be significant if their standard errors were available. Methods for registration, reporting rate, methods for following-up, rate of lost cases, patient selection in survival calculation, expected survival rates, etc., would, of course, be different among registries in different countries (Austin 1983; Hanai and Fujimoto 1985). However, distinct differences in survival between Japan and other countries cannot be explained by methodological differences among registries alone.

Distribution of clinical stage and the survival rates by clinical stage were only available for three registries; Osaka in Japan (OPDH *et al.* 1991), the SEER Program in the United States (Ries *et al.* 1990), and Denmark (Carstensen *et al.* 1993). The classification scheme for the clinical stage used in two registries; Osaka and Denmark, was partly modified from 'extent of disease' developed by the SEER Program (SEER 1993).

Five-year relative survival rates according to clinical stage for stomach cancer patients registered into the three registries are shown in Table 2.3. Survival rates for localized cases and for cases with regional extension were as high as 86% and 32%, respectively in Osaka, which were about 1.5–1.6 times higher than those in the SEER Program. Survivals in Denmark stayed below two-thirds of those in the SEER Program.

As shown in Table 2.4, the proportion of localized cases was largest in Osaka. The proportions in the SEER Program and Denmark were one-half and two-thirds of those of Osaka, respectively. No difference was observed among registries in the proportion of cases with regional extension, except for Blacks in the United States. The proportion of cases with remote metastasis was smaller in Osaka and larger in other registries. Stage-unknown cases existed in roughly the same proportion for all three registries.

From these results, it was found that differences in the proportion of cases with localized stage and also differences in the survival rates of those cases produced the difference in survival rates for all cancer cases. It was also revealed that these were

Table 2.3. Comparison of 5-year survival rates according to extent of disease: Japan, United States, and Denmark

Country	District or ethnic group	Yr of diagnosis	Sex	5-year survival rate (%)				
				All cases	Localized	Regional	Remote	Unknown
Japan[a]	Osaka	1984–6	M&F	43.0	85.7	32.0	2.1	22.2
US (SEER)[a]	Whites	1981–6	M&F	15	54	15	2	9
	Blacks		M&F	17	52	16	2	14
Denmark[b]		1978–87	M	8.4	25.6	5.7	0.4	6.1
			F	10.4	34.2	6.8	0.9	7.6

[a] Relative survival rate. [b] Crude survival rate.
The data from SEER is rounded to the nearest whole number.

Table 2.4.   Comparison of distribution of extent of disease: Japan, United States and Denmark

Country	District or ethnic group	Yr of diagnosis	Sex	No. of cases observed	Proportion of cases (%)			
					Localized	Regional	Remote	Unknown
Japan	Osaka	1984–6	M&F	8519	32.8	35.6	18.5	13.0
US (SEER)	Whites	1981–6	M&F	17 692	16	35	36	13
	Blacks		M&F	2417	18	29	40	13
Denmark		1978–87	M	5083	21.6	33.8	30.6	14.0
			F	3173	20.0	32.6	31.5	16.4

The data from SEER is rounded to the nearest whole number.

mainly caused by the increased popularity of both the stomach cancer screening programs and the well-developed diagnostic techniques available in regional hospitals. Furthermore, it may be that clinical doctors in Japan are somewhat more conscious of finding stomach cancer in an earlier stage than in other countries, because of the high incidence of stomach cancer in this country.

Differences also existed in the survival rates in every other category of clinical stage except for cases with remote metastasis. In a comparative study with the US SEER Program, to clarify the reasons for the differences in survival for stomach cancer patients, Hanai *et al.* (1985) reported that the proportion of so-called Lauren's intestinal-type of carcinoma was higher in patients from Japanese populations (58% among Japanese in Osaka and 57% among Japanese in Hawaii) than in the White population (40%) from the US SEER Program. However, when comparing patient groups of intestinal-type and diffuse-type of carcinoma, almost the same survival rate was observed under the same conditions as receiving curative surgical treatment at the localized stage. They also reported that the most important factor influencing the survival differences seemed to be the difference in the proportion of surgically operated cases. It was higher in the Japanese population (64% for Japanese in Osaka and 67% for Japanese in Hawaii) than in the US White population (51%).

4. STOMACH CANCER IN JAPAN: IMPROVEMENT IN PROGNOSIS

Five-year relative survival rates for stomach cancer patients in Osaka from 1975 to 1986 are shown in Fig. 2.1 with those for other sites of cancer (Hanai *et al.* 1993). Stomach cancer showed a survival rate slightly above the average of all other sites of cancer. Survival for stomach cancer rose 14% during the period from 1975–7 to 1984–6. Meanwhile, the average rate of all sites of cancer was improved by 6%.

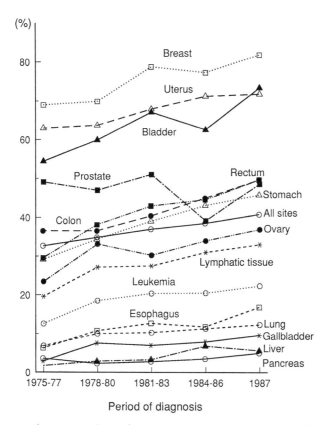

Fig. 2.1. Five-year relative survival rates for cancer by site (both sexes included) (Osaka, 1975–86).

A modified clinical stage used in the Osaka Cancer Registry consisted of four categories: (1) localized; (2) regional lymph node involvement; (3) direct invasion to adjacent organs; and (4) remote metastasis.

Changes in five-year relative survival rates over years are shown according to clinical stage in Table 2.5. In 1984–6, the survival rate for group (1) in Osaka was as high as 86%. Groups (2) and (3) showed 44% and 15%, respectively. Group (4) showed only 2% in Osaka.

A great improvement was observed in the survival rate for group (1) with an 18% rise from 1975–7 to 1984–6, and a substantial improvement was seen for groups (2) and (3). The survival rate for group (4) maintained a low rate.

Change over time in the distribution of extent of disease in Osaka is shown in Table 2.6. The proportion of stage-unknown cases decreased from 31% to 13% during the observation period. The proportion for group (1) has increased, and those for groups (2) and (3) have decreased. These results suggest that cases diagnosed in more advanced stages in the earlier period were diagnosed in the localized stage in the later period with an improvement in diagnostic techniques (OPDH *et al.* 1991).

Table 2.5.   Time trends of 5-year survival rates (%) by extent of disease; Osaka
(1975–86, males and females)

| Yr of diagnosis | All reported cases | Localized | | Regional | | Remote | Stage unknown |
		Overall	*with curative resection*	Lymph node involvement	Direct extension		
1975–7	29.1	67.6	85.8	38.7	6.4	2.2	28.0
1978–80	34.3	79.1	87.7	38.9	9.3	2.2	29.3
1981–3	39.0	85.1	91.2	46.3	10.9	1.9	21.4
1984–6	43.0	85.7	90.0	43.7	15.4	2.1	22.2

Table 2.6.   Time trends of distribution (%) of extent of disease; Osaka (1975–86,
males and females)

| Yr of diagnosis | Localized | | Regional | | Remote metastasis | Stage unknown |
	Overall	*with curative resection*	Lymph node involvement	Direct extension		
1975–7	25.1	16.6	28.5	26.6	19.9	31.0
1978–80	28.6	22.2	27.0	21.7	22.7	22.1
1981–3	31.2	26.8	27.6	20.2	20.9	17.1
1984–6	37.7	33.1	23.8	17.2	21.3	13.0

Patients who were detected in the localized stage and received curative resection
should currently have the highest survival rate. They showed a high survival rate
of 86% even in 1975–7 with a certain improvement up to 1984–6, as shown in
Table 2.5. The proportion of cases with such favorable conditions increased twice
during the observation period, as shown in Table 2.6. From these results, treatment
for localized cases can be considered to be well established in Japan.

When evaluating the progress of medical care for cancer patients based on the
time trends of survival rates, it is necessary to confirm whether or not an improvement in survival is valid. Bailer and Smith (1986) have asserted that the age-
standardized mortality rate is only one of the effective indices for evaluating cancer
control programs. To examine whether or not an observed improvement in the survival rates for cancer patients in Osaka resulted in a decrease in cancer mortality,
the relative decrease in mortality to incidence must be observed.

In Osaka, trends in stomach cancer age-standardized incidence rates and in age-
standardized mortality rates decreased in parallel from 1963 to 1975. However, after
that, the mortality rate decreased more rapidly than the incidence rate and the difference between these two rates gradually became larger. This suggested that in Osaka
an improvement in survival has promoted a decrease in mortality (Fujimoto *et al.*
1990; Hanai and Fujimoto 1992). It may be difficult to avoid the influence of lead

time bias as well as over diagnosis bias in this situation in Japan, where early diagnosis has been encouraged. Longer, more extensive observation of the trends of both incidence and mortality rates may be necessary to assess effectively this situation.

From the above comparison between Japan and other countries of the survival rates for stomach cancer patients at population-based cancer registries, the following can been concluded. (1) survivals in Japan were significantly higher than those in other countries. (2) Survivals were improved in 1975–1986 in Osaka. (3) Two factors contributed to this survival improvement in Japan: (a) an increase in the number of patients diagnosed in an earlier stage, and (b) an increase in the number of patients receiving curative resection during the first course of treatment for stomach cancer.

REFERENCES

Aoki, K., Kurihara, M., Hayakawa, N., and Suzuki, S., (ed.) (1992). *Death rates for malignant neoplasms for selected sites by sex and five-year age group in 33 countries, 1953–57 to 1983–87*. Nagoya, University of Nagoya Co-operative Press.

Austin, D.F. (1983). Cancer Registries: A tool in epidemiology. In: Lilienfeld, A.M. (ed.), *Review of cancer epidemiology*, Vol. 2, pp. 118–40. Elsevier, New York.

Bailer III, J.C. and Smith, E.M. (1986). Progress against cancer? *N. Engl. J. Med.*, **314**, 1226–32.

Black, R.J., Sharp, L., and Kendrick, S.W. (ed.) (1993). *Trends in cancer survival in Scotland, 1968–1990*. pp. 22–3. National Health Service in Scotland, Edinburgh.

Carstensen, B., Storm, H.H., and Schou, G. (1993). Survival of Danish cancer patients, 1943–1987. *APMIS Supplementum*, No. 33, **101**, 41–5.

Cutler, S.J. and Ederer, F. (1958). Maximum utilization of the life table method in analyzing survival. *J. Chronic Dis.*, 8, 699–712.

Ederer, F., Axtell, L.M., and Cutler, S.J. (1961). *The relative survival rate: a statistical methodology*. National Cancer Institute Monograph No. 6, Cancer: End results and mortality trends in cancer, pp. 101–21. Public Health Service, Washington, DC.

Fujimoto, I., Hanai, A., Kitagawa, T., Morinaga, K., and Ominato, S. (1990). Regional cancer registry. *Taisya*, **27**, 361–9. (In Japanese)

Fujimoto, I., Hanai, A., Hiyama, T., Tsukuma, H., Takasugi, Y., and Sugaya, T. (ed.) (1993). *Cancer incidence and mortality in Osaka, 1963–1989*, pp. 226–35. Osaka, Osaka Foundation for Prevention of Cancer and Circulatory Diseases.

FPDH (Fukui Prefectural Department of Health) and FMA (Fukui Medical Association) (1992). *Cancer incidence in Fukui Prefecture in 1989*, pp. 19. Fukui Prefectural Government.

Hanai, A. and Fujimoto, I. (1985). Survival rate as an index in evaluating cancer control. In: Parkin, D.M., *et al.* (ed.), *The role of the registry in cancer control*, pp. 87–107. IARC Scientific Publications No. 66. IARC, Lyon.

Hanai, A. and Fujimoto, I. (1992). Evaluation of cancer care by the measure of survival for cancer patients. In: Suemasu *et al.* (ed.), *Clinical epidemiology on cancer*, pp. 83–92. Progress in Cancer Clinics No. 36. Medical View, Tokyo. (In Japanese)

Hanai, A., Ries, L.G., Young, J.L., and Fujimoto, I. (1985). *Difference in stomach cancer survival between whites and Japanese*. Proceedings of the 1985 Annual Meeting of SEER Program.

Hanai, A., Tsukuma, H., Hiyama, T., and Fujimoto, I. (1993). Five-year relative survival rates for cancer patients in Osaka. In: Tominaga *et al.* (ed.), *Cancer statistics—Incidence, mortality, prognosis*, pp. 145–52. Shinohara-Shuppan, Tokyo. (In Japanese)

JMHW (Japanese Ministry of Health and Welfare) (1963). *Age-adjusted mortality rates by cause of death: 1960*. A special report of vital statistics HWSA (Health and Welfare Statistics Association), Tokyo. (In Japanese)

Kuroishi T., Hirose, K., Tajima, K., and Tominaga, S. (1993). Cancer mortality in Japan. In: Tominaga, S., *et al.* (ed.) *Cancer statistics—Incidence, mortality, prognosis*; pp. 1–106. Shinohara-Shuppan. Tokyo. (In Japanese)

OPDH (Osaka Prefectural Department of Health), *et al.* (1991). *Five-year relative survival rates for cancer patients in Osaka and the trends, 1975–1983*. Cancer in Osaka, No. 49. Osaka Prefectural Government.

Parkin, D.M. and Hakulinen, T. (1991). Analysis of survival. In: Jensen, O.M., *et al.* (ed.), *Cancer registration principles* and methods, pp. 159–76. IARC Scientific Publication No. 95. IARC, Lyon.

Parkin, D.M., Muir, C.S., Whelan, S.L., Gao Y.T., Ferlay, J., and Powell, J. (ed.), (1992). *Cancer incidence in five continents*, Vol. VI. IARC Scientific Publications No. 120. IARC, Lyon.

RGT (Registre Genèvois des Tumeurs) (1988). *Cancer a Genève, incidence mortalité survie, 1970–1986*, p. 62. Geneva.

RGPCRJ (Research Group for Population-based Cancer Registration in Japan). (1993). Cancer incidence in Japan. In: Tominaga, S., *et al.* (ed.), *Cancer statistics—Incidence, mortality, prognosis*, pp. 107–44. Shinohara-Shuppan. Tokyo. (In Japanese)

Ries, L.G., Hankey, B.F., and Edwards, B.K. (ed.) (1990). *Cancer statistics review, 1973–1987*, pp. IV. 8–IV. 15. National Cancer Institutes of Health, Bethesda.

Sato, Y., Higuchi, M., Sato, H., Fukase, Y., and Ogasawara, M. (1989). Survivals for cancer patients registred in Yamagata Cancer Registry. In: Fujimoto, I. (ed.), *Annual Report of the research group for population-based Cancer Registries, 1988*, pp. 57–67. The Research Group, Osaka.

SEER. (1993). *Comparative staging guide for cancer*. NIH Pub. No. 93–3540. Version 1.1, NIH, Bethesda.

Tan, L.K. and Robson, D.L. (ed.) (1991). *Trends in cancer survival in Saskatchewan, 1967 to 1986*, pp. 12–15. Saskatchewan Cancer Foundation Research Committee, Regina.

Tominaga, S., Fujimoto, I., Fukushima, N., Aoki, K., and Hirayama, T. (ed.) (1981). Cancer statistics—Incidence, mortality, prognosis. *Jpn. J. Cancer Clin.*, **27**, 539–88. (In Japanese)

Tsukuma, H., Kitagawa, T., Hanai, A., Fujimoto, I., Kuroishi T., and Tominaga, S. (1992). Incidence of cancer predictions in Japan up to the year 2015. *Jpn. J. Cancer Clin.*, **38**, 1–10. (In Japanese).

Part II: Etiology

3

Etiology

Shaw Watanabe, Shoichiro Tsugane, and Naohito Yamaguchi

1. INTRODUCTION

Both incidence and mortality rates of gastric cancer have been declining in recent decades. However, it still remains a serious problem in many countries, such as Japan, China, eastern and northern European countries, and mid and south American countries (Aoki *et al.* 1992; Coleman *et al.* 1993). In Japan, falling mortality rates are a reflection of declining incidence rates, although the mass screening program contributes to it.

Because of the increase of an ageing population, the absolute number of gastric cancer patients has been increasing. The decline of gastric carcinoma was mainly due to the decline of well-differentiated tubular/papillary adenocarcinoma in the antrum (Inoue *et al.* 1993). Recently, the increasing trend of gastric cancer localized in the cardia is recognized, by several cancer registries, in White males in the United States and Western Europe (Blot *et al.* 1991; Zheng *et al.* 1993). These changes need new etiological research on gastric cancer.

Although a number of epidemiological studies on gastric cancer have been done, most of them have not given sufficient consideration to the long development period of cancer, which may have been influenced by many risk factors, as well as preventive factors. In this chapter, characteristics of gastric cancer for an etiological study are summarized, and various epidemiological findings are interpreted concerning the mechanisms of gastric cancer development.

2. ETIOLOGICAL CHARACTERISTICS OF GASTRIC CANCER

2.1. Histological variation of gastric cancer and genetic changes

Gastric cancers show different biological characteristics according to their histological type and tumor site. Tubular, mucinous, and papillary carcinomas in the World Health Organization (WHO) classification can be roughly transcribed to the intestinal-type group (Lauren's classification), and signet-ring and more than half of undifferentiated carcinomas into the diffuse-type group. Generally, Lauren's classification has been the one most used for epidemiologists.

Very rarely, choriocarcinoma occurs in the stomach. Other types of gastric neoplasms comprise malignant lymphoma, plasmacytoma, carcinoid tumor, and stromal cell tumors (Basson *et al.* 1992). Sometimes, carcinoid tumors occur in

Zollinger–Ellison syndrome patients. Chronic inflammation may have a relationship with the occurrence of malignant lymphoma.

Accumulation of genetic changes in both oncogenes and tumor-suppressor genes are observed in stomach cancer. Genetic alterations appear to differ in the intestinal and diffuse-type (Tahara 1993). Inactivation of the p53 gene and activation of the c-*met* gene were most commonly implicated in both well-differentiated adenocarcinoma and poorly differentiated adenocarcinoma at an early stage of stomach cancer. Alteration of APC, DCC and *bcl*-2 genes are frequently associated with well-differentiated adenocarcinoma. The latter is also overexpressed in poorly differentiated adenocarcinoma or signet-ring cell carcinoma (Nakatsuru *et al.* 1992). However, the K-*sam* gene is amplified preferentially in scirrhous-type poorly differentiated adenocarcinoma (Tahara 1993; Terada *et al.* 1991). The occurrence of *p53* and K-*ras* mutations or *tpr-met* rearrangement at the stage of intestinal metaplasia and adenoma of the stomach supports the hypothesis of stepwise development of gastric cancer (Tahara 1993).

These genetic changes are thought to occur by stochastic probability over a long period. Some factors that induce these genetic alterations have been obtained by experimental carcinogenesis, but the relationship between genetic changes and life style has not yet been investigated in human gastric cancer.

2.2.   Growth rates

Fujita (1981) estimated the growth curve of gastric cancer by calculating tumor doubling time from human gastric cancer, and recognized three different stages, see Fig. 3.1. It is generally accepted that the development of cancer takes 20–30 years from onset to the clinical stage.

Our mathematical model (Yamaguchi *et al.* 1990), incorporated the processes of both cancer induction and subsequent tumor growth. Exponential growth was assumed and clinical appearance (surfacing) was formulated as a stochastic process and related to tumor diameter. The number of stages in cancer induction and tumor growth rate were simultaneously estimated for each histological subtype, using the maximum likelihood procedure. Risk factors in signet-ring cell carcinoma, mucinous carcinoma, and poorly differentiated adenocarcinoma are suggested to be operating in earlier life at the same magnitude for both males and females. However, in papillary adenocarcinoma and well-and moderately differentiated adenocarcinoma, risk factors operate at higher magnitudes for males at all ages (Fig. 3.2). It can be postulated that some host factors, such as genetic predisposition, play a role in the former types, whereas environmental factors, such as diet and lifestyle, have an effect in the latter types. This model fitted better than that of the Amirtage–Doll model, except for well-differentiated adenocarcinoma.

2.3.   Precancerous lesions

Classification of precancerous lesions is important both for etiological and intervention studies. In instences of papillary and tubular adenocarcinoma, serial

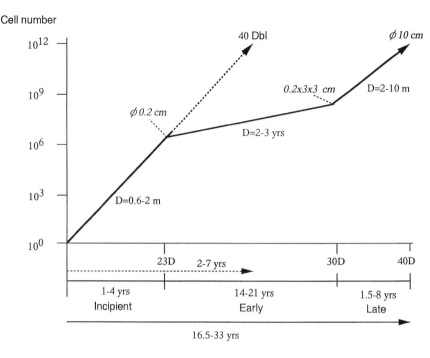

Fig. 3.1. The growth curve of human gastric cancer. Growth of human gastric cancer estimated from tumour doubling time (D). When the tumour becomes 10 cm in dimension, number of tumour cells would be 10^{12} and most patients die. Most cancers have three different growth rates, but some develop rapidly (dotted line) and reach 10^{12} cells after 40 divisions (Dbl). Modified from Fujita (1981).

changes have been identified from superficial gastritis, chronic atrophic gastritis, and colonic metaplasia to dysplasia (Correa *et al.* 1975; Correa 1992). Since serum diagnosis for chronic atrophic gastritis has been developed by measuring pepsinogen I/II (Miki *et al.* 1984), the correlation between the prevalence rates for chronic atrophic gastritis and the standardized mortality ratio for gastric cancer has been studied extensively, and has strongly supported the hypothesis that chronic atrophic gastritis might be a precancerous lesion (Fukao *et al.* 1993).

Areas of high gastric cancer incidence also usually show a high prevalence of chronic atrophic gastritis. In China, intestinal metaplasia was found in 33% of the population in a high prevalence area of stomach cancer; and dysplasia, common in the lesser curvature of the body and in the angulus, in 20% (You *et al.* 1993).

Follow-up data from mass screening by endoscopy helped to clarify the natural history of gastritis. Kato *et al.* (1992*b*) found that, if the baseline endoscopic findings indicated the presence of atrophic gastritis, the risk of developing stomach cancer during 4.4 years of the average follow-up period was increased 5.70-fold, compared with no indication at the baseline. Tatsuta *et al.* (1993) reported a similar risk (5.76-fold) in patients with severe fundal atrophic gastritis diagnosed by the endoscopic Congo red test.

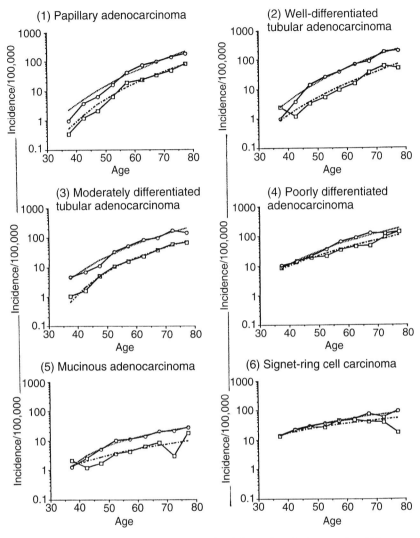

Fig. 3.2. Observed and fitted age-incidence curves for different histologic types. Sex difference and the slope of curves are similar in papillary, well differentiated, and moderately differentiated adenocarcinoma, but different in poorly differentiated and signet-ring cell carcinoma. Mucinous adenocarcinoma also shows different curve. Male observed (–○–), female observed (–□–), male fitted (––––), and female fitted (–·–·–).

Regenerated epithelial cells often become metaplastic or dysplastic mucosa. The incomplete type (colonic type) tends to progress more frequently to carcinoma compared to complete-type (intestinal-type) metaplasia. Repeated observation of dysplasia by the Interdisciplinary Group on Gastric Epithelial Dysplasia (Fertitta *et al.* 1993) showed that cancer was associated with 36% of moderate dysplasia cases and with 80% of severe cases. Dysplastic changes were no longer detectable at follow-up in 27% of the moderate cases and in 10% of the severe cases. The relative risks for the two lesions being associated with or developing into gastric cancer were 26 and 132, respectively. In the former report by Rugge *et al.* (1991), diagnosis of cancer was reached within the first year of follow-up in 14 cases and after one year in 7 cases (13–39 months). Although the surgical diagnosis was dysplasia, by taking into consideration the growth rate, these lesions might have been malignant.

In a case-control study by Kato *et al.* (1992*a*), the relative risk (RR) of stomach cancer was 5.13 if a patient had any type of atrophic gastritis. RR associated with severe atrophy was 7.73. A clear difference in risk appeared in the analyses by histological type of cancer. The RR associated with atrophic gastritis was 24.71 for the intestinal-type and 3.49 for the diffuse-type.

Precancerous lesions of diffuse-type carcinoma, especially of signet-ring cell carcinoma, have not yet been well identified. A rare condition of gastritis, gastritis cystica profunda, is known to be highly associated with the later development of gastric cancer (Watanabe 1979).

2.4. Multiple primary cancer

Early occurrence of cancer and multiple primary cancer often provide clues to cancer etiology, because they may be a result of high exposure to carcinogens or a predisposition to cancer. Gastric cancer showed a significantly higher association with upper gastrointestinal cancer, such as oropharynx and esophagus, than with colon and rectum cancer (Watanabe *et al.* 1985). These findings suggested the presence of common, but separate carcinogenic effects on the upper and lower alimentary canal. To date, no specific factors have been identified for multiple gastric cancer.

A case-control study on single and multiple gastric cancer in relation to dietary, smoking, and drinking habits was carried out in Saitama Prefecture, Japan (Hoshiyama and Sasaba, 1992). Significant dose–response relationships were observed: salty foods, miso fermented soya bean paste soup, boiled fish, pickled vegetables, were risk factors; and nuts, raw vegetables, and seaweed, were protective factors in single gastric cancer cases. In addition, miso soup, fruits, and seaweed were common protective factors in multiple cancer cases, and no specific factors were found to be a risk for multiple primary cancer.

3. DIETARY FACTORS

In a human model of gastric carcinogenesis, chronic atrophic gastritis is a key lesion in the intestinal-type. This gastritis has been linked to excessive salt intake and infection with *Helicobacter pylori* (Tsugane *et al.* 1993). Nitrosating agents are candidate carcinogens as the initiator, and could originate in the gastric cavity or in the inflammatory infiltrate (Correa 1992; Bartsch *et al.* 1992).

Dietary habits may influence gastric carcinogenesis, but it is very difficult to measure accurately food consumption and its effects. It might be possible to determine risk factors associated with diet by using data obtained when diet is altered—following gastric disease.

3.1. Salt

Salt can wash out the mucous layer on the epithelium, causing gastric irritation, and may induce superficial atrophic gastritis. In our ecological study in five different areas in Japan, a significant correlation was found between the amount of salt excreted in urine over 24 hours, and stomach cancer mortality in both men and women (Tsugane *et al.* 1993). Salt intake, estimated from the consumption of salty foods, especially of highly salted foods, was associated with stomach cancer mortality (Kono *et al.* 1988). Such positive association was also recognized in China. Multivariate regression analysis on stomach cancer mortality data and dietary and biochemical data from 65 chinese counties showed significant positive associations with consumption of salted vegetables (Kneller *et al.* 1992). Odds ratios of salted foods in several case-control studies were around 2.0 (Tajima and Tominaga, 1985; You *et al.* 1988; Demirer *et al.* 1990; Ramon *et al.* 1993).

Experimentally, administration of salt together with N-methyl-N'-nitro-nitrosoguanidine (MNNG) enhanced the incidence of stomach cancer in rats (Tatematsu *et al.* 1975). As salt administration did not enhance carcinogenesis after MNNG treatment, earlier mucosal cell damage was considered to enhance the chance of initiation by MNNG.

3.2. Nitrosoamines

Chemical carcinogens in the diet have been investigated over a long period. N-nitroso compounds (NOC) are the most likely carcinogens in both human and animals (Sugimura and Fujimura 1967; Mirvish 1983; Miller and Miller 1986; Bartsch *et al.* 1992). Sensitive procedures have been developed to estimate the effect of NOC exposure on humans, and applied in ecological and cross-sectional studies. Kamiyama *et al.* (1986) showed that inhabitants in high-risk areas for stomach cancer had significantly higher exposure to endogenous NOC.

Humans are not only exposed to preformed NOCs but also to a wide range of precursors and nitrosating agents which can react, *in vivo*, to form potentially carcinogenic NOC and diazo compounds (Bartsch *et al.* 1992). The presence of large numbers of bacteria may convert nitrate to nitrite and subsequent nitrosation *in vivo*. Nitrite, nitrate, and nitrosating agents can also be synthesized endogenously in enzymic reactions mediated by activated macrophages and neutrophils, via the enzyme, nitric oxide synthase. Nitric oxide has recently been shown to be formed from L-arginine by nitric oxide synthase in various tissues (Bartsch *et al.* 1992).

In our cross-sectional study, the excreted amount of N-nitrosothioproline (NTPRO) and N-nitrosomethylthioproline (NMTPRO) in 24-hour urine, correlated with stomach cancer rates (Tsugane *et al.* 1992*b*). The low excretion levels of NTPRO and NMTPRO in the lowest risk area for stomach cancer were noteworthy, regardless of the high level of nitrate excretion in the same area. The precise role of bacterial overgrowth in NOC synthesis and/or inducing oxidative stress in stomach mucosa remains to be clarified.

An analysis of 178 samples of drinking water for nitrates and nitrites was carried out, to examine the relationship between gastric cancer and quality of different types of drinking water and nitrate intake via water. It showed that the nitrate content in the local drinking water was generally very high (a mean 109.6 mg/l) in high prevalence areas (Xu *et al.* 1992).

Kumar *et al.* (1992) suggested that the nitrosation of caffeidine produced mononitrosocaffeidine and dinitrosocaffeidine. In view of the well-known structure–activity relationships of these NOCs, their possible endogenous formation due to high consumption of salted tea may be a critical risk factor for the common occurrence of esophageal and gastric cancers in Kashmir.

DNA-adduct formation by NOCs was inhibited by vitamin C. Sobala *et al.* (1993) investigated, simultaneously, concentrations of gastric juice ascorbic acid, total vitamin C, nitrites and NOCs with fasting gastric juice, and found that low ascorbic acid levels were present in chronic atrophic gastritis patients. This suggests a lowered antioxidant defense state and reduced nitrite-scavenging capacity of the stomach in these patients. Ascorbic acid depletion may occur by reactions with nitrite, which is produced by nitrate-reducing bacteria in the achlorhydric stomach, or by reactive oxygen resulting from chronic *Helicobacler pylori* infection in the gastric mucosa (Mai *et al.* 1991).

3.3. Other carcinogens

Tumor development was induced in the rat glandular stomach by adding N-methyl-N'-nitro-N-nitrosoguanidine (MNNG) to the drinking water (Sugimura and Fujimura 1967). 4-Nitroquinoline 1-oxide or 4-hydroxyaminoquinoline 1-oxide in drinking water also induced adenocarcinoma in the mouse glandular stomach, but cancer incidence was low, despite the high mortality rate (Mori 1967; Mori *et al.* 1969). N-methyl-N-nitrosourea (MNU) in drinking water yielded well- and poorly differentiated adenocarcinoma and signet-ring cell carcinoma (Tatematsu *et al.* 1992). These chemical carcinogens are useful when studying mechanisms and morphological changes during carcinogenesis.

Extraction and purification of carcinogenic substances from cooked foods have been carried out extensively, and more than 20 heterocyclic amines have been identified in broiled meat and fish (Sugimura and Sato 1983; Sugimura 1985). These substances cause cancer in various organs, but not so far, in the stomach in experimental animals. In some case-control studies, frying and broiling of meat, which may include heterocyclic amines, was associated with an increased risk of stomach cancer compared to boiling of meat (RR = 1.7–2.1) (Ikeda *et al.* 1983; Jedrychowski *et al.* 1992).

3.4. Preventive factors

Dietary intake of fresh vegetables and fruits has consistently showed an inverse association with stomach cancer risk (Correa *et al.* 1985; Risch *et al.* 1985; La Vecchia *et al.* 1987; You *et al.* 1988; Coggan *et al.* 1989; Kato *et al.* 1990; Graham *et al.* 1990; Boeing *et al.* 1991; Buiatti *et al.* 1990; Gonzales *et al.* 1991). Hirayama (1990) reported, in their population-based prospective study, that the intake of green-yellow vegetables, such as carrots, spinach, etc., may suppress gastric cancer mortality.

Vitamin C in these vegetables and fruits is known to inhibit the formation of NOCs (Mirvish 1983); they also contain beta-carotene which is a potent antioxidant.

In our ecological study, the samples from five different areas in Japan were analysed for micronutrient levels of vitamins A, C, and E, beta-carotene, and lycopene in plasma. No protective effect of micronutrients was suggested in this correlation study. However, a inverse correlation between plasma lycopene level and stomach cancer mortality was observed (Tsugane *et al.* 1992*b*). A preventive dose–response relationship was observed between serum beta-carotene and pre-valence of chronic atrophic gastritis (Tsugane *et al.* 1993). A significant inverse association with intake of green vegetables and levels of plasma selenium and beta-carotene was observed by the cross-sectional study in China (Kneller *et al.* 1992).

Recent case-control studies by Ramon *et al.* (1993) and Buiatti *et al.* (1990) indi-cated that intake of fruits, fresh vegetables, and olive oil appeared to decrease the odds ratio to 0.4–0.5. These foods are rich in vitamins C and/or E. Indeed, on the whole, the intake of cereals, rice, vegetables, and fruits was not associated with gastric cancer risk. The consumption of mainly whole meal bread showed a relative risk (RR) of 0.18 (95%, CI 0.07–0.44) compared with a consumption of mainly white bread (Jedrychowski *et al.* 1992). In a prospective study of Japanese–Americans in Hawaii, serum beta-carotene levels at baseline were lower in men who developed stomach cancer than in controls (Nomura *et al.* 1985).

Green-yellow vegetables contain other preventive substances, such as indole compounds, ellagic acids, isoflavonoids, etc. (other, so far unknown, chemicals may also exist that prevent cancer.) Green tea may also contain protective factors against stomach cancer (Tajima and Tominaga 1985; Kono *et al.* 1988). Indi-viduals living in green tea harvesting areas usually show low stomach cancer mor-tality. Tannic acid in the green tea, or (-)-epigallocatechin gallate extracted from green tea, showed strong antipromoter effects (Fujiki *et al.* 1992). Consumption of garlic decreases stomach cancer risk, as shown in case-control studies in China and Italy (You *et al.* 1989; Buiatti *et al.* 1990). Garlic oil and its extracts, diallyl sulfide, indicated antipromoter activity (Belman 1983; Wargovich 1987).

Selenium is a core metal of glutathione-*S*-transferase. Selenium data from the toe-nails were analysed in a nested case-control study in Denmark. In a multivari-ate analysis of 104 patients with stomach cancer, the relative risk of stomach cancer for subjects in highest quintiles of toe-nail selenium level was 0.64, and an inverse association was present between toe-nail selenium levels and stomach cancer in men, but not in women (van den Brandt *et al.* 1993).

4. TOBACCO AND ALCOHOL

The association between smoking and gastric cancer was well reviewed in 1982 by the Surgeon General of the United States. In Hirayama's prospective cohort, the rela-tive risk of smoking was 1.6, 1.7, 1.4, and 1.3 in four successive periods from 1966 to

1981. From this data, promoter effects of tobacco smoke seems to be more certain. The smoking habit is especially related to carcinoma in the cardia, so if the location of stomach cancer is limited to the cardia, the relative risk of smoking should increase.

In a case-control study by Kato *et al.* (1992*b*), stomach cancer patients tended to consume more cigarettes and alcohol. Another case-control study by Nomura *et al.* (1990) showed increased relative risk of smoking as one of the major risk factors for gastric cancer. In recent US studies, the relative risk of current smokers becomes 2.3–2.6 (Kabat *et al.* 1993; Kneller *et al.* 1992).

Smoking-related DNA adducts in human gastric cancer is direct evidence of tobacco carcinogenesis (Dyke *et al.* 1992). The analysis of histologically confirmed gastric cancer in Oxfordshire, UK, in two five-year periods from 1960–4 to 1984–8 showed that the incidence of cardia cancer increased from 2.8 to 5.2/100 000 (Rios-Castellanos *et al.* 1992). There was a marked association between smoking and cardia cancer (RR = 4.5), thus the effects of smoking in Japan may appear more clearly in the future.

Risk from alcohol consumption for stomach cancer was indicated in a 1988 IARC monograph, but the causal relationship has not yet been established.

5. INFLAMMATION

5.1. Markers for chronic inflammation

Chronic atrophic gastritis has now been established as being a precancerous lesion for intestinal-type gastric cancer. The disease causes various local responses including cell proliferation, and many biomarkers are now available (Correa 1991). Pepsinogens I and II, ferritin, and transferin, and others are examples (Palli *et al.* 1991; Kabuto *et al.* 1993). Recently, *Helicobacter pylori* infection is considered to have a potential for carcinogenesis, as bacteriotoxins can directly transform the mucosa. Chronic inflammation causes cell proliferation for regeneration, and inflammatory cells produce free radicals which damage the DNA of mucosal cells. Cytokines from lymphocytes induce epidermal growth factor which stimulates mucosal cells to proliferate. Proliferation itself increases the possibility of mutation in cellular DNA. Replicating single strands of DNA are more susceptible to genotoxic effects of exogeneous mutagens.

In our ecological study, the serum ferritin level was inversely related to gastric cancer mortality (Kabuto *et al.* 1993). Nomura *et al.* (1992) examined sera of gastric cancer patients which had been stored between 1967 and 1970 in a cancer-free state. The inverse association with serum ferritin was stronger for the 21 cases diagnosed within 15 years of examination ($P = 0.02$) than for the 25 cases diagnosed after 15 years ($P = 0.15$).

5.2. Helicobacter pylori

Helicobacter pylori infection has been an important topic in cancer epidemiology in recent years. A positive association between helicobacter infection and stomach cancer has been consistent in both cross-sectional and case-control studies (Forman *et al.* 1991; Parsonnet *et al.* 1991, 1993; Nomura *et al.* 1991; Fukao *et al.* 1993; Palli *et al.* 1993 Fukuda *et al.* 1995. The association between the prevalence of *H. pylori* infection and gastric cancer rates was studied in 17 populations from 13 countries, chosen to reflect the global range of gastric cancer incidence (EUROGUST 1993). A statistically significant association was present between the prevalence of seropositivity and cumulative rates for both gastric cancer incidence and mortality, with regression coefficients of 2.68 ($P = 0.001$) and 1.79 ($P = 0.002$), respectively. The findings are consistent with an approximately sixfold increased risk of gastric cancer in populations with 100% *H. pylori* infection, compared with populations with no infection.

However, *Helicobacter pylori* infection is not considered as having a causal relationship to gastric cancer. Prevalence of helicobacter infection is 70–80% in most areas in Japan, and *H. pylori*-associated gastritis, predominantly of antral localization, is often common in low-risk areas of gastric cancer (Sierra *et al.* 1992). Some case-control studies found that the prevalence of *H. pylori* infection in gastric cancer patients was the same between cases and controls (77% vs. 79%) (Kuipers *et al.* 1993).

From current evidence, it seems premature to carry out *H. pylori* eradication therapy for large-scale primary prevention of gastric cancer.

5.3.   Epstein–Barr Virus

Involvement of Epstein–Barr virus (EBV) has been reported in gastric cancer cells with lymphoepithelioid features (Burke *et al.* 1990; Shibata *et al.* 1993; Min *et al.* 1991). Tokunaga *et al.* (1993) examined more than 1800 surgically resected gastric cancers by *in situ* hybridization and polymerase chain reaction, and found that younger cases (25.0% in males, 17–34 years of age), cardial location (10.5%), and stump carcinoma (26.1%), showed the presence of EBV genome in cancer cells. Histologically, lymphoepithelioid-type showed 100% positivity in males and 67% in females, 16% positivity in male solid-type poorly differentiated type, 9.5% in male moderately differentiated adenocarcinoma, and 2–3% in other types (Tokunaga *et al.* 1993). The frequency of EBV-related gastric carcinoma in Japan may be about three times higher than in the North American population.

Shibata *et al.* (1993) showed that the EBV-associated gastric cancer among Japanese–American men and women living in Hawaii were 14.3% in men and 5.7% in women. The relatively high incidence of gastric cancer compared to other EBV-associated tumors makes EBV-associated gastric cancer potentially one of the most common EBV-related tumors.

5.4.   Surgery

Gastric surgery causes neutralization of gastric acidity and increases luminal bacterial flora (Greenlee *et al.* 1974). Persistent reflux of secondary bile after gastric surgery promotes chronic gastritis with resultant metaplasia. These conditions may increase the incidence of stomach cancer. The anaerobic bacteria converting nitrates consumed in the diet to nitrites is an additional attributable risk.

Fisher *et al.* (1993) analysed data from a 15 983 cohort from medical admission records in the US Department of Veterans, of military veterans hospitalized during 1970–1. A statistically significant increase in risk of stomach cancer was demonstrated among males during the 20 years following gastric surgery (RR = 1.9). Also, the risk of developing gastric cancer was greatest among those treated by gastrectomy for any type of ulcer (RR = 2.6) or gastric ulcer (RR = 2.9). Many cohort studies found an increased gastric cancer risk 15 or more years after gastric surgery. Rates of stomach cancer seemed to be higher following the Billroth II gastrectomy than after treatment with a Billroth I procedure, probably due to continuous bathing of the gastric stump anastomosis with secondary bile acids (Fischer *et al.* 1983). The hypoacidity resulting from vagotomy also yields an overgrowth of bacteria, but the absence of gastric atrophy appears to decrease the likelihood of a carcinogenic process, at least within the first 20 years of follow-up.

However, Tokudome *et al.* (1984) reported the results of prospective study on 3827 Japanese patients who had undergone partial gastrectomy for benign disease during 1948 and 1970. The number of observed and expected deaths from stomach cancer in 1981 were 11 and 52.9, respectively, the ratio being 0.21 ($P < 0.01$). The high prevalence of gastric cancer in Japan may hide the gastrectomy risk.

6. HORMONES

The influence of hormones on gastric cancer development has not been investigated fully. Estrogen receptors (ER) were present in 50% cases of Chinese patients with gastric cancers (Wu *et al.* 1992). Dehydroepiandrosterone prevents a variety of spontaneous and chemically induced tumors in experimental carcinogenesis. The association between circulating levels of dehydroepiandrosterone and dehydroepiandrosterone sulfate and the development of gastric cancer was examined by measuring the serum levels of these steroids in 13 gastric cancer patients, who had donated serum to the Washington County Maryland serum bank in 1974, and in 52 matched controls (Gordon *et al.* 1993). Prediagnostic serum levels of dehydroepiandrosterone were 38% lower in cases as compared to controls ($P = 0.09$). The risk of developing gastric cancer increased with decreasing levels of both steroids. These results suggest that these steroids play a role in the prevention of gastric cancer.

7. PREDISPOSITION

Gastric cancer often accumulates in a family pedigree. Family members with similar dietary habits may be exposed to the same carcinogen which presumes familial aggregation by genetic predisposition. However, the presence of genetic burden in diffuse carcinoma has seldom been reported. Diffuse-type carcinoma develops in relatively young people, and the presence of predisposition was considered. Horio *et al.* (1994) reported a family with a germline antisense mutation in the p53 gene, and in which younger onset of stomach cancer (signet-ring type) was frequent.

Gastric cancer has been recognized as being an extracolonic manifestation in patients with familial adenomatous polyposis (FAP). Among FAP patients, about 5% of cases were found to have associated gastric cancer. In Koreans, the incidence of gastric cancer is much higher than reports from Japan and other countries, and the relative risk becomes 6.9 (Park *et al.* 1992)

There has been a debate whether or not individuals with blood type A tend to be prove to gastric cancer (Demirer *et al.* 1990). David *et al.* (1993) found that single nucleotide deletion had occurred at position 261 in the O allele in so-called 'incompatible histo-blood group A antigen' of gastric cancer in blood group O patients. Rejection of cancer cells by the natural occurrence of antibodies to non-self blood group antigens may result in the well-known lower incidence of gastric cancer among type O individuals in contrast to type A person.

Dickey *et al.* (1993) examined the Lewis blood group phenotype in 101 patients with symptoms of dyspepsia; 32% were non-secretors, 36% had antral gastritis, gastric ulcer, erosive duodenitis, duodenal ulcer, or some combination; and 58% had *H. pylori* infection. Overall, the relative risk of gastroduodenal disease for non-secretors compared with secretors was 1.9.

Patients with late-onset hypogamma-globulinemia have a very high risk of developing gastric cancer. The high frequency of gastric mucosa atrophy in these patients is attributable to the low gastrin content of the antral mucosa, low serum pepsinogen A level and pepsinogen A/C ratio, and reduced serum gastrin secretion in response to bombesin stimulation. As X-linked agamma-globulinemia does not show increased frequency of gastric cancer, it is unlikely that the immunoglobulin deficiency *per se* is responsible for the development of gastritis (den Hartog *et al.* 1992).

A retrospective cohort study on 2021 male and 2496 female pernicious anemia patients was carried out to follow-up for more than 20 years for a subsequent risk of cancer. Cancer of the stomach (SIR = 2.9) was the most prominent, then esophagus (SIR = 3.2), pancreas (SIR = 1.7), myeloid leukemia in men (SIR = 4.4), and multiple myeloma in women (SIR = 2.5). An excess of gastric carcinoid tumors was also high. The risk of stomach cancer was highest in the first year after diagnosis of pernicious anemia (SIR = 7.4) probably due to the inclusion of prevalent cases, but an increased risk persisted throughout the follow-up period (Hsing *et al.* 1993).

The Zollinger–Ellison syndrome (ZES) is characterized by hyperchlorhydria due to sustained hypergastrinemia of tumoral origin. In patients with ZES, fundic argyrophil carcinoids develop only in those who have multiple endocrine neoplasia type 1 (Cadiot *et al.* 1993).

Iodide-deficient individuals with goitre have shown more atrophic gastritis than normal subjects (Venturi *et al.* 1993). These data allows us to hypothesize that iodide deficit or iodide excess might constitute a new risk factor for gastric cancer.

Familial lymphoma is uncommon and is usually associated with various forms of hereditary immunodeficiencies. Primary gastric lymphomas seldom occur in these families (Hayoz *et al.* 1993).

8. SUMMARY

Stomach cancer is still a leading cause of cancer death in many countries. Cumulative alteration of oncogenes and tumor-suppressor genes has clarified the difference between intestinal-and diffuse-type gastric cancer. Multiple factors influence the initiation, promotion, and progression of gastric cancer over long periods (Fig. 3.3). So far, risk and protective factors at each stage have not been well clarified, but dietary factors undoubtedly affect cancer development, for example, salt consumption is a consistent risk factor. Japanese–Americans show a decrease in the incidence of gastric cancer to one-third of that in Japan (Haenszel and Kurihara 1968). Changes of lifestyle could prevent at least half the gastric cancers in high prevalence areas. In addition to secondary prevention, strategies for primary prevention become increasingly more important.

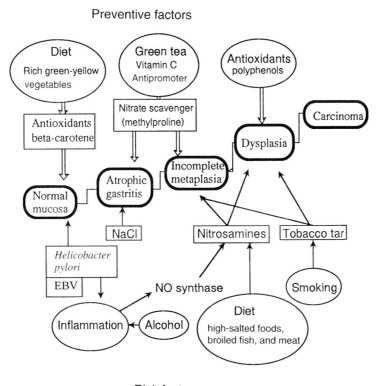

Fig. 3.3. Preventive factors and risk factors for gastric cancer. The stepwise development of cancer is influenced by various risk factors and preventive factors. Inflammation shortens the cell proliferation cycle and infiltrated inflammatory cells contribute to deliver NO synthase to form nitrosamines. Helicobacter pylori infection and NaCl cause chronic atrophic gastritis. Tobacco tar is more related to cardiac cancer. Most antioxidants are known to prevent gastric cancer, but the precise mechanism is still unknown.

REFERENCES

Aoki, K., Kurihara, M., Hayakawa, N.N., and Suzuki, S. (1992). *Death rates of malignant neoplasms for selected sites by sex and five-year age group in 33 countries 1953–57 to 1983–87.* University of Nagoya Coop Press, Nagoya.

Bartsch, H., Ohshima, H., Pignatelli, B., and Calmels, S. (1992). Endogenously formed N-nitroso compounds and nitrosating agents in human cancer etiology. *Pharmacogenetics*, **2**, 272–7.

Basson, MD., Modlin, IM., and Flynn, S.D. (1992). Current clinical and pathologic perspectives on gastric stromal tumors. *Surg. Gynecol. Obstet.*, **175**, 477–89.

Belman, S. (1983). Onion and garlic oil inhibit tumor promotion. *Carcinogenesis*, **8**, 1063–5.

Blot, W.J., Susan, S.D., Kneller, R.W., and Fraumeni, J.F. Jr. (1991). Rising incidence of adenocarcinoma of the esophagus and gastric cardia. *JAMA*, **265**, 1287–9.

Boeing, H., Jedrychowski, W., and Wahrendorf, J. (1991). Dietary risk factors in intestinal and diffuse types of stomach cancer: a multicenter case-control study in Poland. *Cancer Causes Control*, **2**, 227–33.

Buiatti, E., Palli, D., Decarli, A., *et al.* (1990). A case-control study of gastric cancer and diet in Italy. II. Association with nutrients. *Int. J. Cancer*, **45** 896–901.

Burke, A.P., Yen, B., Shekitka, K.M., and Sobin, L.H. (1990). Lymphoepithelial carcinoma of the stomach with Epstein–Barr virus demonstrated by polymerase chain reaction. *Mod. Pathol.*, **3**, 377–80.

Cadiot, G., Lehy, T., and Mignon, M. (1993). Gastric endocrine cell proliferation and fundic argyrophil carcinoid tumors in patients with the Zollinger–Ellison syndrome. *Acta Oncol.*, **32**, 135–40.

Coggon, D., Barker, D.J.P., Cole, R.B. and Nelson, M. (1984). Stomach cancer and food storage. *J. Natl. Cancer. Inst.*, **815**, 1178–82.

Coleman, M.P., Esteve, J., Damiecki, P., Arslan, A., and Renard H. (1993). *Trends in cancer incidence and mortality*, Vol. 121. IARC, Lyon.

Correa, P. (1991). The new era of cancer epidemiology. *Cancer Epidemiol. Biomarkers and Prev.*, **1**, 5–11.

Correa, P., Haenszel, W., Cuello, C., Arder M., and Tannenbaum, S.R. (1975). A model for gastric cancer epidemiology. *Lancet*, **2**, 58–60.

Correa, P., Fontham, E., Pickle, L.W., Chen, V., Lin, Y., and Haentzel, E. (1985). Dietary determinants of gastric cancer in South Louisiana inhabitants. *J. Natl. Cancer Inst.*, **75**, 645–54.

Correa. P. (1992) Human gastric carcinogenesis: a multistep and multifactorial process—First American Cancer Society Award Lecture on Cancer Epidemiology and Prevention. *Cancer Res.*, **52**, 6735–40.

David, L., *et al.* (1993). Biosynthetic basis of incompatible histo-blood group A antigen expression: Anti-A transferase antibodies reactive with gastric cancer tissue of type O individuals. *Cancer Res.*, **53**, 5494–500.

Demirer, T., Icli, F., Uzunalimoglu, O., and Kucuk, O. (1990). Diet and stomach cancer incidence. A case-control study in Turkey. *Cancer*, **65**, 2344–8.

den Hartog, G., Jansen, J.B., van der Meer, J.W., and Lamers, C.B. (1992). Gastric abnormalities in humoral immune deficiency syndromes. *Scand. J. Gastroenterol.*, **194**, (suppl), 38–40.

Dickey, W., Collins, J.S., Watson, R.G., Sloan, J.M., and Porter, K.G. (1993). Secretor status and *Helicobacter pylori* infection are independent risk factors for gastroduodenal disease. *Gut*, **34**, 351–3.

Dyke, G.W., Craven, J.L., Hall, R., and Garner, R.C. (1992). Smoking-related DNA adducts in human gastric cancers. *Int. J. Cancer*, **52**, 847–50.

Fertitta, A.M., Comin, U., Terruzzi, V., *et al.* (1993). Clinical significance of gastric dysplasia: a multicenter follow-up study. *Endoscopy*, **25**, 265–8.

Fischer, A.B., Graem, N., and Jensen, O.M., (1983). Risk of gastric cancer after Billroth II resection for duodenal ulcer. *Br. J. Surg.*, **70**, 552–4.

Fisher, S.G., Davis, F., Nelson, R., Weber, L., Goldber, J., and Haenszel, W. (1993). A cohort study of stomach cancer risk in men after gastric surgery for benign disease. *J. Nat. Cancer Inst.*, **85**, 1303–10.

Forman, D., Newell, D.G., and Fullerton, F. (1991). Association between infection with *Helicobacter pylori* and risk of gastric cancer: Evidence from a prospective investigation. *BMJ*, **302**, 1302.

Fujiki, H., Yoshizawa, S., and Horiuchi, T. (1992). Anticarcinogenic effects of (-)- epigallocatechin gallate. *Prev. Med.*, **21**, 503–9.

Fujita, S. (1981). Occurrence and development of gastric cancer by cell kinetics. *Proc. Japan Pathol. Society*, **1981**, 70, 23–54.

Fukao, A., Komatsy, S., and Tsubono, Y. (1993). *Helicobacter pylori* infection and chronic atrophic gastritis among Japanese blood donors: a cross-sectional study. *Cancer Causes Control*, **4**, 307–12.

Fukuda, H., Saito, D., Hayashi, S., *et al.* (1995). *Helicobacter pylori* infection, serum pepsinogen level and gastric cancer: A case-control study in Japan. Jpn. J. *Cancer Res.*, **86**, 64–71.

Gonzales, C.A., Sanz, J.M., and Marcos, G. (1991). Dietary factors and stomach cancer in Spain: a multi-center case-control study. *Int. J. Cancer*, **49**, 513–19.

Gordon, G.B., Helzlsouer, K.J., Alberg, A.J., and Comstock, G.W. (1993). Serum levels of dehydroepiandrosterone and dehydroepiandrosterone sulfate and the risk of developing gastric cancer. *Cancer Epidemiol. Biomarkers Prev.*, **2**, 33–5.

Graham., S., Haughey, B., and Marshall, J. (1990). Diet in the epidemiology of gastric cancer. *Nutr. Cancer*, **13**, 19–34.

Greenlee, H.B., Bibit, R., and Paez, H. (1974). Bacterial flora of the jejunum following peptic ulcer surgery. *Arch. Surg.*, **102**, 260–5.

Haenszel, W. and Kurihara, M. (1968). Studies of Japanese migrants. I. Mortality from cancer and other diseases among Japanese in the United States. *J. Natl. Cancer Inst.*, **40**, 43–68.

Hayoz, D., Extermann, M., Odermatt, B.F., Pugin, P., Regamey, C., and Knecht, H. (1993). Familial primary gastric lymphoma. *Gut*, **34**, 136–40.

Hirayama. T. (1990). *Lifestyle and mortality. A large-scale census-Based cohort study in Japan*. Karger, Basel.

Horio, Y., Suzuki, H., Ueda, R., *et al.* (1994). Predominantly tumor-limited expression of a mutant allele in a Japanese family carrying a germline p53 mutation. *Oncogene*, **9**, 1231–5.

Hoshiyama, Y. and Sasaba, T. (1992). A case-control study of single and multiple stomach cancers in Saitama Prefecture, Japan. *Jpn. J. Cancer Res.*, **83**, 937–43.

Hsing, A.W., Hansson, L.E., and McLaughlin, J.K. (1993). Pernicious anemia and subsequent cancer. A population-based cohort study. *Cancer*, **71**, 745–50.

IARC (1988). Alcohol drinking. *IARC Monogr. Eval. Carcinogenic Risks Hum.*, **44**, 194–207.

Ikeda, M., Yoshimoto, K., and Yoshimoto, T. (1983). A cohort study on the possible association between broiled fish intake and cancer. *Jpn. J. Cancer Res.*, **74**, 640–8.

Inoue, M., Tajima, K., Kitoh, T., *et al.* (1993). Changes in histopathological features of gastric carcinoma over a 26-year period (1965–1990). *J. Surg. Oncol.*, **53**, 255–60.

Jedrychowski, W., Boeing, H., Popiela, T., Wahrendorf, J., Tobiasz-Adamczyk, B., and Kulig, J. (1992). Dietary practices in households as risk factors for stomach cancer: a familial study in Poland. *Eur. J. Cancer Prev.*, **1**, 297–304.

Kabat, G.C., Ng, S.K., and Wynder, E.L. (1993). Tobacco, alcohol intake, and diet in relation to adenocarcinoam of the esophagus and gastric cardia. *Cancer Causes Control*, **4**, 123–32.

Kabuto, M., Imai, H., Tsugane, S., and Watanabe, S. (1993). Does high gastric cancer risk associated with low serum ferritin level reflect achlorohydria? An examination via cross-sectional study. *Jpn. J. Cancer Res.*, **84**, 844–51.

Kamiyama, S., Michioka, O., Simada, A., and Miura, K. (1986). Mutagenic components of diet and epidemiology of stomach cancer. *Gan-no-Rinsho*, **32**, 699–706.

Kato. I., Tominaga, S., Ito, Y., *et al.* (1990). A comparative case-control analysis of stomach cancer and atrophic gastritis. *Cancer Res.*, **50**, 6559–64.

Kato, I., Tominaga, S., Ito, Y., *et al.*, (1992*a*). Atrophic gastritis and stomach cancer risk: cross-sectional analyses. *Jpn. J. Cancer Res.*, **83**, 1041–6.

Kato, I., Tominaga, S., Ito, Y., *et al.* (1992*b*). A prospective study of atrophic gastritis and stomach cancer risk. *Jpn. J. Cancer*, **83**, 1137–42.

Kneller, R.W., McLaughlin, J.K., Bjelke, E., *et al.*, (1991). A cohort study of stomach cancer in a high-risk American population. *Cancer*, **68**, 672–8.

Kneller, R.W., Guo, W.D., and Hsing, A.W. (1992). Risk factors for stomach cancer in sixty-five Chinese counties. *Cancer Epidemiol. Biomarkers Prev.*, **1**, 113–18.

Kono, S., Ikeda, M., Tokudeome, S., and Kuratsune, M. (1988). A case-control study of gastric cancer and diet in northern Kyushu, Japan. *Jpn. J. Cancer Res.*, **79**, 1067–74.

Kuipers, E.J., Gracia-Casanova, M., Pena, A.S., *et al.* (1993). *Helicobacter pylori* serology in patients with gastric carcinoma. *Scand. J. Gastroenterol.*, **28**, 433–7.

Kumar, R., Mende, P., Wacker, C.D., Spigelhalder, B., Preussmann, R., Siddiqi, M. (1992). Caffeine-derived *N*-nitroso compounds. I: Nitrosable precursors from caffeine and their potential relevance in the etiology of oesophageal and gastric cancers in Kashmir, India. *Carcinogenesis*, **13**, 2179–82.

La Vecchia, C., Negiri, E., Decarli, A., D' Avanzo, B., and Franceshi, S. (1987). A case-control study of diet and gastric cancer in northern Italy. *Int. J. Cancer*, **40**, 484–9.

Lauren, P.A. and Nevalainen, T.J. (1993). Epidemiology of intestinal and diffuse types of gastric carcinoma. A time-trend study in Finland with a comparison between studies from high-and low-risk areas. *Cancer*, **71**, 2926–33.

Mai, V.E., ???Peres-Peres???, G.I., Wahl, L.M., Wahl, S.M., Blaser, H.J., and Smith, P.D. (1991). Soluble surface proteins from *Helicobacter pylori* activate monocytes/macrophages by lipopolysacharide-independent mechanism. *J. Clin. Invest.*, **82**, 894–900.

Miki, K., Ichinose, M., Kawamura, N., and Matsuchima, M. (1984). The significance of low pepsinogen levels to detect stomach cancer associated with extensive chronic gastritis in Japanese subjects. *Jpn. J. Cancer Res.*, **80**, 111–14.

Miller, E.C. and Miller, J.A. (1986). Carcinogens and mutagens that may occur in foods. *Cancer*, **15**, (suppl.), 1795–803.

Min, K-W., Holmquist, S., and Peiper, S.C. (1991). Poorly differentiated adenocarcinoma with lymphoid stroma (lymphoepithelioma-like carcinoma) of the stomach: report of three cases with Epstein–Barr virus genome demonstrated by the polymerase chain reaction. *Am. J. Clin. Pathol.*, **96**, 219–27.

Mirvish. S.S. (1983). The etiology of gastric cancer: intragastric nitrosamide formation and other theories. *J. Natl. Cancer Inst.*, **71**, 629–47.

Mori, K. (1967). Carcinoma of the glandlar stomach of mice by instillation of 4-nitroquino-line 1-oxide. *Gann*, **58**, 389–93.

Mori, K., Ohta, A., Murakami, T., Tamura, M., and Kondo, M. (1969). Carcinoma of the glandular stomach of mice induced by 4-hydroxyaminoquinoline 1-oxide hydrochloride. *Gann*, **60**, 151–4.

Muir, C.S., Waterhouse, J., Mack, T., Powell, J., and Whelan, S. (1987). *Cancer incidence in five continents*, Vol. 5. IARC, Lyon.

Nakatsuru, S., Yanagisawa, A., Ichii, S., *et al.*, (1992). Somatic mutation of the APC gene in gastric cancer: frequent mutations in very well differentiated adenocarcinoma and signet-ring cell carcinoma. *Hum. Mol. Genet.*, **1**, 559–63.

Nomura, A.M.Y., Stemmermann, G.N., Heheilbrun, L.K., Salkeld, R.M., and Vuileumier, J.P. (1985). Serum vitamin levels and the risk of cancer of specific sites in men of Japanese ancestry in Hawaii. *Cancer Res.*, **45**, 2369–72.

Nomura, A., Grove, J.S., Stemmermann, G.N., and Severson, R.K. (1990). A prospective study of stomach cancer and its relation to diet, cigarettes, and alcohol consumption. *Cancer Res.*, **50**, 627–31.

Nomura, A., Stemmermann, G.N., and Chyou, P. (1991). *Helicobacter pylori* infection and gastric carcinoma in a population of Japanese–Americans in Hawaii. *N. Engl. J. Med.*, **325**, 1132.

Nomura, A., Chyou, P.H., and Stemmermann, G.N. (1992). Association of serum ferritin levels with the risk of stomach cancer. *Cancer Epidemiol. Biomarkers Prev.*, **1**, 547–50.

Ohshima, H. and Bartsch, H. (1981). Quantitative estimation of endogenous nitrosation in humans by monitoring N-nitrosoproline excreted in the urine. *Cancer Res.*, **41**, 3658–62.

Palli, D., Decarli, A., Cipriani, F., *et al.* (1991). Plasma pepsinogens, nutrients, and diet in areas of Italy at varying gastric cancer risk. *Cancer Epidemiol. Biomarkers Prev.*, **1**, 45–50.

Palli, D., Decarli, A., Cipriani, F., *et al.* (1993). *Heliocobacter pylori* antibodies in areas of Italy at varying gastric cancer risk. *Cancer Epidemiol. Biomarkers Prev.*, **2**, 37–40.

Park, J.G., Park, K.J., Ahn, Y.O., *et al.* (1992). Risk of gastric cancer among Korean familial adenomatous polyposis patients. Report of three cases. *Dis. Colon Rectum*, **35**, 996–8.

Parsonnet, J., Friedman, G.C., and Vandersteen, D.P. (1991). *Helicobacter pylori* infection and risk for gastric cancer. *N. Engl. J. Med.*, **325**, 1127.

Parsonnet, J., Samloff, I.M., Nelson, L.M., *et al.* (1993). *Helicobacter pylori*, pepsinogen, and risk for gastric adenocarcinoma. *Cancer Epidemiol. Biomarker Prev.*, **2**, 461–6.

Ramon, J.M., Serra, L., Cerdo, C., and Oromi, J. (1993). Dietary factors and gastric cancer risk. A case-control study in Spain. *Cancer*, **71**, 1731–5.

Rios-Castellanos, E., Sitas, F., Shepherd, N.A., and Jewell, D.P. (1992). changing pattern of gastric cancer in Oxfordshire. *gut*, **33**, 1312–7.

Risch, H.A., Jain, M., and Choi, N.W. (1985). Dietary factors and the incidence of cancer of the stomach. *Am. J. Epidemiol.*, **122**, 947–59.

Rugge, M., Farinati, F., Di Mario, F., Baffa, R., Valiante, F., and Cardin, F. (1991). Gastric epithelial dysplasia: a prospective multicenter follow-up study from the Interdisciplinary Group on Gastric Epithelial Dysplasia. *Hum. Pathol.*, **22**, 1002–8.

Shibata, D., Hawes, D., Stemmermann, G.N., and Weiss, L.M. (1993). Epstein–Barr virus-associated gastric adenocarcinoma among Japanese Americans in Hawaii. *Cancer Epidemiol. Biomarkers Prev.*, **21**, 213–7.

Sierra, R., Munoz, N., Pena, A.S., *et al.* (1992). Antibodies to *Helicobacter pylori* and pepsinogen levels in children from Costa Rica: comparison of two areas with different risks for stomach cancer. *Cancer Epidemiol. Biomarkers Prev.*, **1**, 449–54.

Sobala, G.M., Schorah, C.J., Pignatelli, B., *et al.* (1993). High gastric juice ascorbic acid concentrations in members of a gastric cancer family. *Carcinogenesis*, **14**, 291–2.

Sugimura, T. and Fujimura, S. (1967). Tumor production in glandular stomach of rat by N-methyl-N′-nitro-N-nitrosoguanidine. *Nature*, **216**, 943–4.

Sugimura, T. and Sato, S. (1983). Mutagens-carcinogens in foods. *Cancer Res.*, 43 (suppl.), 2415s–21s.

Sugimura, T. (1985). Carcinogenicity of mutagenic heterocyclic amines formed during the cooking process. *Mutation Res.*, **150**, 33–41.

Surgeon General of the United States (1982) *The health consequences of smoking. United States Public Health Service, Rockville.*

Tahara, E. (1993). Molecular mechanism of stomach carcinogenesis (Editorial). *J. Cancer Res. Clin. Oncol.*, **119**, 265–72.

Tajima, K. and Tominaga, S. (1985). Dietary habits and gastro-intestinal cancers: a comparative case-control study of stomach and large intestinal cancers in Nagoya. *Jpn. J. Cancer Res.*, **76**, 705–16.

Tatematsu, M., Takahashi, M., Fukushima, S., Hananouchi, M., and Shirai, T. (1975). Effects in ras of sodium chloride on experimental gastric cancers induced by N-methyl-N′-nitro-N-nitrosoguanidine or 4-nitroquinoline-1-oxide. *J. Natl. Cancer Inst.*, **55**, 101–6.

Tatematsu, M., Ogawa, K., Hoshiya T., *et al.* (1992). Induction of adenocarcinoma in the glandular stomach of BALB/C Mice treated with N-methyl-N-nitrosourea. *Jpn. J. Cancer Res.*, **83**, 915–18.

Tatsuta, M., Iishi, H., Nakaizumi, A., *et al.* (1993). Fundal atrophic gastritis as a risk factor for gastric cancer. *Int. J. Cancer*, **53**, 70–4.

Terada, M., Sakamoto, H., Ohmura, Y., *et al.* (1991). Biological significance of gene amplification in carcinogenesis. In *Multistage carcinogenesis*, (ed. C.C. Harris *et al.*), pp. 371–80. Japan Scientific Societies Press, CRC Press, Tokyo, London.

EUROGAST Study Group (1993). An international association between *Helicobacter pylori* infection and gastric cancer. *Lancet*, **34**, 1359–62.

Tokudome, S., Kono, S., and Ikeda, M. (1984). A prospective study on primary gastric stump cancer following partial gastric surgery for benign gastroduodenal diseases. *Cancer Res.*, **44**, 2208–12.

Tokunaga, M., Uemura, Y., Tokudome, T., *et al.* (1993). Epstein–Barr virus related gastric cancer in Japan: A molecular patho-epidemiological study. *Acta Pathol. Jpn.*, **43**, 574–81.

Tsugane, S., Gey, F., Ichinowatari, Y. *et al.*, (1992a). Cross-sectional epidemiological study for assessing cancer risks at the population level-correlation analyses with mortality. *J. Epidemiol.*, **2**, 83–9.

Tsugane, S., Tsuda., M., Gey, F., and Watanabe, S. (1992b). Cross-sectional study with multiple measurements of biological markers for assessing stomach cancer risk at the population level. *Environ. Health Perspect.*, **98**, 207–10.

Tsugane, S., Kabuto, M., Imai, H., *et al.*, (1993). *Helicobacter pylori*, dietary factors and atrophic gastritis in five Japanese populations with different gastric cancer mortality. *Cancer Causes Control*, **4**, 297–305.

van den Brandt, P.A., Goldbohm, R.A. and van't Veer, P. (1993). A prospective cohort study on toenail selenium levels and risk of gastrointestinal cancer. *J. Natl. Cancer Inst.*, **85**, 224–9.

Venturi, S., Venturi, A., Climini, D., Arduini, C., Venturi, M., and Guidi, A. (1993). A new hypothesis: Iodine and gastric cancer. *Eur J. Cancer Prev.*, **2**, 17–23.

Wargovich, M.J. (1987). Dialyl sulfide, a flavor component of garlic (*Allium sativum*) inhibits dimethylhydrazine-induced colon cancer. *Carcinogenesis*, **8**, 487–9.

Watanabe, S. (1979). Gastritis cystica profunda. Histopathological study of nine cases. *Jpn. J. Clin. Oncol.*, **9**, 79–86.

Watanabe, S., Kodama, T., Shimosato, Y., and Arimoto, H. (1985). Second primary cancers in patients with gastrointestinal cancers. *Jpn. J. Clin. Oncol.*, **15** (suppl.), 171–182.

WU, C.W., Lui, W.Y., P'eng F.K., and Chi, C.W. (1992). Hormonal therapy for stomach cancer. *Med. Hypotheses*, **39**, 137–9.

Xu, G., Song, P., and Reed, P.l. (1992). The relationship between gastric mucosal changes and nitrate intake via drinking water in a high-risk population for gastric cancer in Moping county, China. *Eur. J. Cancer Prev.*, **1**, 437–43.

Yamaguchi, N., Watanabe, S., Maruyama, K., and Okubo, T. (1990). Analysis of stomach cancer incidence by histologic subtypes based on a mathematical model of multistage cancer induction and exponential growth. *Jpn. J. Cancer Res.*, **81**, 1109–17.

You, W.C., Blot, W.J., Chang, Y.S., *et al.*, (1988). Diet and high risk of stomach cancer in Shandong, China. *Cancer Res.*, **48**, 3518–23.

You, W.C., Blot, W.J., and Chang, Y.S. (1989). Allium vegetables and reduced risk of stomach cancer. *J. Natl. Cancer Inst.*, **81**, 162–4.

You, W.C., Blot, W.J., and Li, J.Y. (1993). Precancerous gastric lesions in a population at high risk of stomach cancer. *Cancer Res.*, **53**, 1317–21.

Zheng, T., Mayne, S.T., and Holford, T.R. (1989). The time trend and age-period-cohort effects on incidence of adenocarcinoma of the stomach in Connecticut from 1955–1989. *Cancer*, **72**, 330–40.

4

Pathology

Eiichi Tahara

1. CLASSIFICATION OF MACRO AND MICROSCOPIC FEATURES

Gastric cancer is divided into early gastric and advanced gastric cancers. Early gastric cancer (EGC) is defined as a carcinoma that is confined to the mucosa (intra-mucosal cancer) or to the mucosa and submucosa (submucosal cancer) regardless of metastasis (Japanese Research Society for Gastric Cancer: JRSGC 1993).

1.1. Macroscopic classification

The macroscopic classification of EGC includes type I (protruded type), type II (superficial type), and type III (excavated type), as shown in Figs 4.1 and 4.2. Type II cancers are further subdivided into three types: type IIa is the elevated type, which is slightly raised above the surrounding mucosa (Fig. 4.3); type IIb is the flat type, which shows no obvious changes macroscopically; and type IIc is the depressed type, which is slightly depressed or associated with superficial erosion (Fig. 4.4). Combined types of EGC often occur in a single cancer. For example, in the case of EGC which has the co-existence of IIa and IIc, the type occupying the larger area is written first (e.g. IIa + IIc or IIc + IIa). In Japanese national statistics, type IIc is the most frequent EGC (34%), followed by type IIc + III (23%), type I (10%), and type IIa + IIc (7%) (Hirota *et al.* 1993).

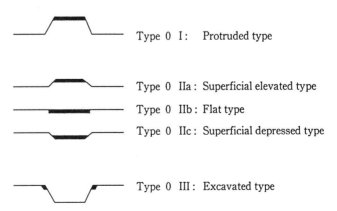

Type 0 I : Protruded type

Type 0 IIa : Superficial elevated type

Type 0 IIb : Flat type

Type 0 IIc : Superficial depressed type

Type 0 III : Excavated type

Fig. 4.1.   Schematic representation of the Japanese classification of early gastric cancer. (EGC).

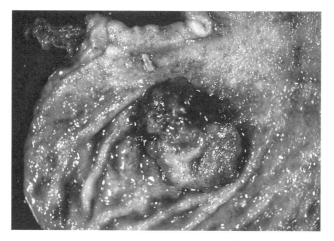

Fig. 4.2. Type I (protruded type) of EGC.

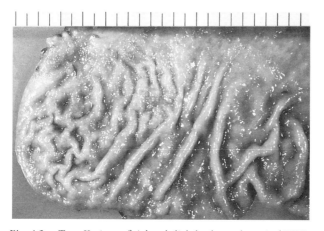

Fig. 4.3. Type IIa (superficial and slightly elevated type) of EGC.

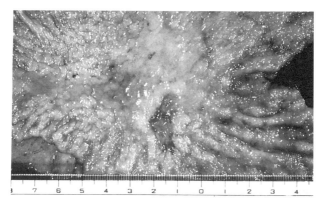

Fig. 4.4. Type IIc (superficial and slightly depressed type) of EGC.

According to the JRSGC (1993) macroscopic classification, EGC is classified as type O^3 (e.g. in the case of IIc, it is described as O IIc).

Macroscopic classification for advanced gastric cancer (AGC) is mainly based on Borrmann's classification (Borrmann 1926). These are four types: type 1, polypoid cancer; type 2, circumscribed excavating cancer; type 3, ulcerated and infiltrating cancer; and type 4, diffusely infiltrating cancer. Type 1 of AGC frequently occurs in the antrum or angulus, its incidence being in about 2.0% of the surgically resected cases. Type 2 is also most frequently found in the antrum. Type 3 is intermediate between types 2 and 4; its incidence being close to that of type 2 (30–40%) (Hirota *et al.* 1993). Type 4 is a scirrhous-type cancer and occurs that occur in the antrum or fundus, which type 4 has been termed linitis plastica', characterized by diffuse thickening and hardening of almost the entire gastric wall. This scirrhous-type cancer is often in younger age groups and the male/female sex ratio is almost 1.0. The incidence of type 4 is about 10–20% (Hirota *et al.* 1993).

1.2.   Histological classification

There are a variety of histological classifications of gastric cancer. Lauren (1965) divided gastric cancer into two types: intestinal-type and diffuse-type and the JRSGC (1993) classified these into five common types, as listed in detail below. This classification is similar to that of the World Health Organization (Watanabe *et al.* 1989).

Papillary adenocarcinoma   This type shows papillary or villous structures which mainly consist of cuboidal to cylindrical tumor cells, and is often associated with tubular structures (papillotubular adenocarcinoma) (Fig. 4.5). The majority of this type are EGC type I or IIa.

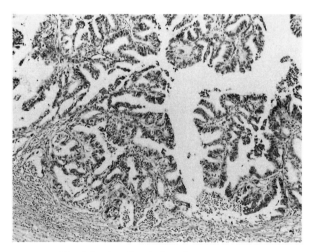

Fig. 4.5.   Papillotubular adenocarcinoma.

Tubular adenocarcinoma This is divided into well-differentiated and moderately differentiated subtypes. The former have a distinct tubular formation of cylindrical tumor cells that are often arranged in a single layer (Fig. 4.6). Fibrous stroma is not abundant. The moderately differentiated subtypes consist of incomplete and irregular gland structures of cuboidal tumor cells (Fig. 4.7).

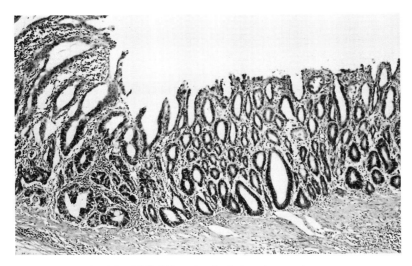

Fig. 4.6. Well-differentiated tubular adenocarcinoma.

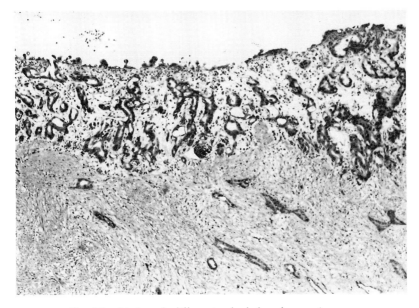

Fig. 4.7. Moderately differentiated tubular adenocarcinoma.

Poorly differentiated adenocarcinoma   This shows few distinct glandular structures but there is either acinar or microgland formation in a part of the tumor.
Depending on the growth pattern of tumor cells and the amount of stroma, this
type is subclassified into solid and non-solid type. The former corresponds to
medullary carcinoma and the latter has diffusely infiltrative or disperse growth of
individual cells (Fig. 4.8). Both these subtypes often occur in EGC types IIc or III.
Most of type 4 advanced cancer or scirrhous cancer demonstrates the non-solid
type with abundant fibrous stroma (Fig. 4.9).

Signet-ring cell carcinoma   Most of these tumor cells resemble a finger-ring with a
signet or seal because of a large amount of mucin within the cells (Fig. 4.10): this
type is frequently observed in EGC type IIc. When signetring cells infiltrate the submucosa and deeper tissue, they often induce diffusely productive fibrosis resulting
in scirrhous cancer.

Mucinous carcinoma   This type is characterized by mucous lakes or pools, within
which tumor cells float (Fig. 4.11). Over 50% of the total tumor volume can be
replaced by mucin.

Special types   These are as follows: (1) adenosquamous carcinoma; (2) squamous
cell carcinoma; (3) carcinoid tumor; and (4) miscellaneous carcinoma, including
undifferentiated carcinoma, endocrine cell carcinoma (ECC) (Ito and Tahara
1993), and choriocarcinoma.

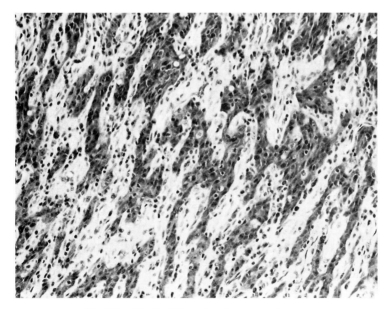

Fig. 4.8.   Poorly differentiated adenocarcinoma.

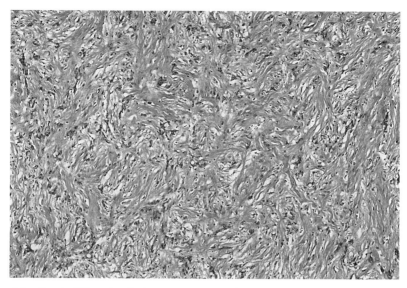

Fig. 4.9.   Poorly differentiated adenocarcinoma (scirrhous type). See also colour plate section.

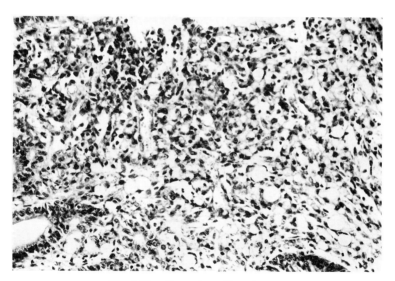

Fig. 4.10.   Signet-ring cell carcinoma.

Gastric ECC, which histologically shows poorly differentiated adenocarcinoma or undifferentiated carcinoma, should be distinguished from carcinoid tumor because of different biological behavior and prognosis (Ito and Tahara 1993).

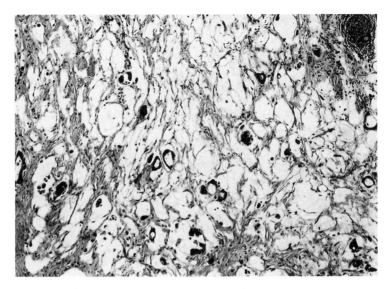

Fig. 4.11.   Mucinous carcinoma.

2. HANDLING OF RESECTION SPECIMENS

The resected specimen should be carefully opened along the greater curvature and fixed in buffered formalin. When a tumor exists in a greater curvature, it should be opened along the lesser. The location, size, and gross pattern of the tumor should be assessed. Factors of most importance are the extent of tumor invasion, metastasis, and involvement of resection margins, as these affect patient prognosis. The JRSGC (1993) provide general techniques for cutting away specimens, for example, in case of EGC, the full length of the tumor and non-neoplastic mucosa adjacent to it should be removed, as shown in Fig. 4.12. All specimens of lesser curvature including from the oral resection margin (ow) to the anal resection margin (aw) should always be cut away. In the case of AGC, the deepest portion of tumor invasion should be carefully investigated and removed. Other associated lesions, including gastritis, intestinal metaplasia, and polyp are also described (JRSGC 1993).

The sections should be histologically examined and meticulous attention should be paid to confirming the tumor stage (i.e. depth of tumor invasion, vascular invasion, lymphatic invasion, and lymph node metastases).

3. TUMOR STAGING

The TNM classification system for gastric cancer staging is generally used (Kennedy 1970). This is defined by three principal factors: (1) the depth of invasion of the primary tumor (T); (2) metastasis of the regional lymph nodes (N); and

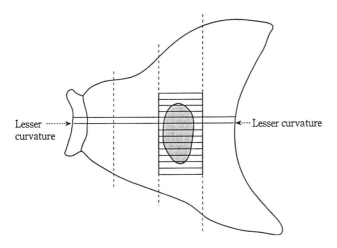

a . Sectioning of superficial flat tumor (Type 0)

Fig. 4.12.   The General Rule (JRSGC 1993) of techniques for cutting away specimens of EGC.

(3) distant metastasis (M). For clinical classification, T, N, or M are designated by the letters cT, cN, or cM; and for pathological classification, by the letters pT, pN, or pM.

3.1.   Primary sites

The stomach comprises the esophagogastric junction, the cardia, the fundus, and the antrum. The JRSGC (1993) divides the primary sites of stomach cancer into three regions, as shown in Fig. 4.13. If a tumor occupies two regions of the stomach, the major sites should be classified first, followed by invading sites (e.g. MC). When tumor invasion involves three regions, the most infiltrated part should be classified first (e.g. MCA or CEM).

3.2.   Classification of the primary tumor (T)

The classification of a primary tumor (T) depends on the degree of stomach wall invasion by carcinoma:

T_X: primary tumor cannot be assessed.
T_0: no evidence of primary tumor.
T_{is}: carcinoma *in situ* (i.e. intraepithelial tumor without invasion of the lamina propria).
T_1: tumor invades lamina propria or submucosa.
T_2: tumor invades the muscularis propria or the subserosa.
T_3: tumor penerates the serosa (viseral peritoneum) without invasion of adjacent structures.
T_4: tumor invades adjacent structures.

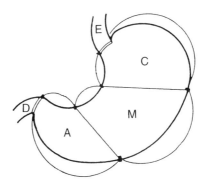

Fig. 4.13. The primary sites of gastric cancer: E, esophagus; C, one-third of the cardia; M, central region of the stomach; A, one-third of the antrum.

When a tumor penerates the muscularis propria with extension into the gastro-colic greater or lesser omentum without perforation of the visceral peritoneum, it is classified as T_2. If a tumor shows perforation of the visceral peritoneum covering the gastric ligaments or omenta, the tumor is classified as T_3. However, in the JRSGC (1993) classification, this does not apply to the stage grouping.

3.3. Classification of regional lymph nodes (N)

The principal factor is the distance of metastatic nodes from the primary tumor. Classification of N is as follows:

N_X: regional lymph node(s) cannot be assessed.
N_0: no regional lymph node metastasis.
N_1: metastasis in perigastric lymph node(s) within 3 cm of the edge of the primary tumor.
N_2: metastasis in perigastric lymph node(s) more than 3 cm from the edge of the primary tumor, or in lymph nodes along the left gastric, common hepatic, splenic, or celiac arteries.

The JRSGC (1993) has its own classification as follows:

N_0: no metastasis of the first group node to the fourth group node.
N_1: metastasis in the first group node but no metastasis in the second group, the third group, and the fourth group nodes.
N_2: metastasis in the second group node but no metastasis in the third and fourth group nodes.
N_3: metastasis in the third group node but no metastasis in the fourth group node.
N_4: metastasis in the fourth group node.

The group classification of lymph nodes slightly differs, depending on primary sites.

3.4. Classification of distant metastasis (M)

The classification of M is as follows:

M_X: presence of distant metastasis cannot be assessed.
M_0: no distant metastasis.
M_1: distant metastasis.

The Japanese Research Society for Gastric Cancer, in addition to the above, has its own classification of peritoneal dissemination (P) and liver metastasis (H). Metastasis in distant lymph nodes further away than the fourth group is classified M1.

Following the TNM classification, stage grouping is surgically or conclusively defined (see Table 4.1). The JRSGC stage grouping is almost the same as that of the TNM system. However, stage IV is classified into two types, stage IVa and stage IVb, in terms of P and H factors, which are indicators of the worst prognosis.

4. PRECANCEROUS LESIONS

These lesions involve chronic gastritis, regenerative hyperplasia, intestinal metaplasia, and adenoma (Correa and Tahara 1993). Among them, intestinal metaplasia and adenoma are most frequently implicated in the development of intestinal-type stomach cancer.

Intestinal metaplasia can be classified into complete or type 1, and incomplete metaplasia or type II, in terms of histological findings. Complete intestinal metaplasia comprises non-mucin-secreting absorptive cells expressing small intestinal

Table 4.1. Stage grouping of gastric cancers

	N_0	N_1	N_2	N_3	P_0H_1 under N_2
T_1 (M, SM)	Ia	Ib	II	IIIa	
T_2 (MP, SS)	Ib	II	IIIa	IIIb	IVa
T_3 (SE)	II	IIIa	IIIb	IVa	
T_4 (SI)	IIIa	IIIb	IVa		
P_1H_0 under T_3	IVa				IVb*

* IVb Involves two or more than two factors among T_4 (one organ), N_3, P_1, and H_1, or T_4 (multiple organs), N_4, $P_{2,3}$, $H_{2,3}$, M_1.

brush border enzymes, Paneth cells, and sialomucin-secreting goblet cells. Incomplete intestinal metaplasia includes mucin-secreting cells and absence of Paneth cells. Incomplete intestinal metaplasia can be further reclassified into two types on the basis of the mucin histochemistry (Jass 1983). When this is mainly a neutral mucin, it is classified as type II. In the case of sulphomucin, it is called type IIB or type III. Types IIB or III of incomplete intestinal metaplasia is frequently associated with both intestinal-type stomach cancer and adenoma. Therefore, incomplete intestinal metaplasia, as well as adenoma, may play an important role in the development of intestinal-type stomach cancer (Jass 1983).

Gastric adenoma is a circumscribed benign tumor comprising tubular and/or villous structures lined by dysplastic epithelium. Most tubular adenomas show slightly raised, sessile polypoid lesions. They are lined by columnar cells with dysplasia, including goblet cells, Paneth cells, and intestinal-type endocrine cells, often associated with cystic dilatation of non-neoplastic glands in deep regions of the mucosa. With increasing dysplasia, the number of goblet cells, Paneth cells, and endocrine cells decreases. The majority of gastric adenomas are under 2 cm in size. The frequency of malignant transformation depends on size: up to 2% in adenomas under 2 cm, and 40–50% in adenomas larger than 2 cm.

In this chapter, the term 'dysplasia' is not used as being synonymous with 'precancerous lesion'. Adenomatous dysplasia described by Correa (1993) or 'atypical epithelium' described by Sugano and co-workers (1971) is involved in adenoma.

5. BIOPSY DIAGNOSIS

In Japan, the group classification proposed by the JRSGC (1993) is widely used for biopsy diagnosis of gastric tumors. This is divided in to five groups according to structural and cellular atypia in the epithelium, and to standardize the interpretation of biopsy specimens:

Group I: normal epithelium and metaplastic or hyperplastic epithelium without atypia.
Group II: atypical changes interpreted as regenerated or metaplastic epithelium (Fig. 4.14).
Group III: atypical changes corresponding to adenoma and borderline lesions where it is difficult to distinguish between benign lesions and carcinoma (Fig. 4.15).
Group IV: changes strongly suggestive of carcinoma.
Group V: overt carcinoma.

Groups III and IV belong to categories where it is necessary for a follow-up study or re-examination of biopsy specimens to make a definite diagnosis and provide the most appropriate treatment. Among group III lesions, the most frequent is adenoma, which is usually of the flat, elevated type. Group III lesions showing ulcerative or depressed appearance may have a high probability of well-differentiated tubular adenocarcinoma.

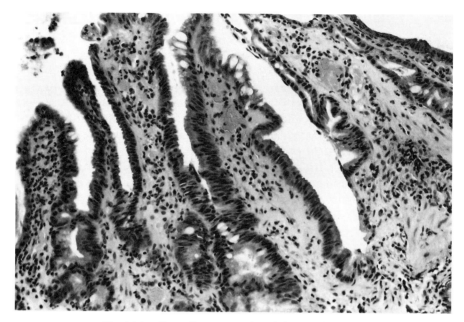

Fig. 4.14. Group II: regenerated epithelium with atypia.

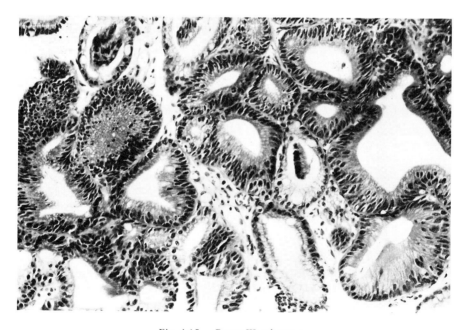

Fig. 4.15. Group III: adenoma.

Concerning causes of errors in biopsy diagnosis, there are a number of reasons for false-negative results. The major reason is inadequate sampling of the tumor, as the tumor may be small and crushed or necrotic. In such instances deeper cutting of biopsy specimens is recommended. Kato's group (1993) compared original and deeper cut sections from the same block and found that 12% of the specimens revealed distinct variations between the two. The next reason for a false-negative result is failure to recognize cancer. Particularly in the case of signet-ring cell carcinoma or poorly differentiated adenocarcinoma, cancer diagnose is sometimes difficult. The routine use of periodic acid–Shiff (PAS) staining is most helpful in recognizing infiltrating cancer cells. Conversely, false-positive results may occur. For example, regenerating mucosa at the margins of an ulcer, or atypical epithelial changes after radiation therapy, or embolization for liver cancer may sometimes be confused with adenocarcinoma.

6. MOLECULAR DIAGNOSIS

Striking advances in immunocytochemical and molecular analysis of gastrointestinal cancers have been made from clinical studies, including surgery and endoscopy. For example, recent evidence indicates that the development and progression of gastric cancer, as well as colon cancer, require multiple alterations affecting DNA mismatch repair genes, oncogenes, and tumor-suppressor genes (Tahara 1993; Tahara *et al.* 1993, 1996). Moreover, common and uncommon genetic changes are detected in esophageal, gastric, and colorectal carcinomas (Table 4.2). In addition to these genetic changes, the majority of gastrointestinal cancer express telomerase activity, which is necessary for cell immortality (H. Tahara *et al.* 1995), suggesting that telomerase activity may serve as a powerful additional tool for cancer diagnosis.

By transferring the principles of cancer biology to the clinic, we are now able to make accurate cancer diagnosies, thus determing the grade of malignancy and patient prognosis. Also, we can identify patients at high risk for developing cancer, and possibly new discover types of therapeutic approach.

Later in this chapter, a new routine strategy for molecular diagnosis of gastrointestinal cancers is described, which began at the Hiroshima City Medical Association Clinical Laboratory in August 1993 (Tahara 1995).

3.6.1. Molecular techniques

A variety of techniques including DNA extraction from formalin- fixed, paraffin-embedded tissue specimens, amplification of DNA by polymerase chain reaction (PCR), sequencing and expression of PCR products, single-strand conformation polymorphism (SSCP) analysis, and *in situ* hybridization can be used routinely in diagnostic laboratories, particularly as non-radioactive methods for nucleic acid detection have become less complicated and more sensitive.

Table 4.2. Genetic changes in gastrointestinal cancers

Genetic change	Esophageal cancer (%)	Gastric cancer (%)		Colorectal cancer (%)
		Well-differentiated type	Poorly differentiated type	
Mutation				
ras	–	9	–	47
APC	NE	41	–	60
p53	35	43	66	90
Deletion				
5q (APC)	77	60	–	35
p53	45	68	76	75
18q (DCC)	NE	50	–	73
E-cadherin	–		50	
Abnormal transcript				
CD44	NE	100	100	100
Amplification				
erbB	10	1	1	–
c-erbB2	–	20	–	2
K-sam	–	–	33	–
c-met	–	19	39[a]	3
cyclin D_1/hst-1/int-2	50	–	–	–
Replication errors	29	33	18	18[b] (92)
Telomerase activity	NE	100	90	100

NE, not examined; [a] scirrhous cancer; [b] sporadic (92), non-polyposis colorectal cancer.

The protocol for the extraction of genomic DNA from archival paraffin sections is described below (Yasui *et al.* 1992):

Day 1

1. De-wax a 4 μm-wide paraffin section with xylene and rehydrate with 70% ethanol.
2. Scrape out the lesion of interest with a razor blade or the tip of a fine needle. Transfer the tissue fragment into a 1.5 ml microcentrifuge tube containing 12.5 μl proteinase K (10 mg/ml), 25 μl, 10% SDS, and 212.5 μl TE (pH 9.0). Mix thoroughly by voltexing and incubate the tube at 45 °C for 3–4 hours.
3. Add 12.5 μl proteinase K (10 mg/ml) and 25 μl 10% SDS to the tube, voltex and incubate at 45 °C overnight.

Day 2

1. Extract with 200 μl phenol (saturated with TE, pH 9.0, and 200 μl chloroform/ isoamylalcohol (24:1) for 30 minutes.

2. Centrifuge for 10 minutes. Extract the upper aqueous phase with 200 μl phenol (saturated with TE, pH 9.0, and 200 μl chloroform/isoamylalcohol (24:1) for 30 minutes.

3. Centrifuge for 10 minutes. Extract the upper aqueous phase with 300 μl chloroform/isoamylalcohol (24:1) for 30 minutes.

4. Centrifuge for 10 minutes. Extract the upper aqueous phase with 300 μl chloroform/isoamylalcohol (24:1) for 30 minutes.

5. Centrifuge for 10 minutes. Carefully pipebte the aqueousphase into a new 1.5 ml microcentrifuge tube then add 30 μl sodium acetate (pH 5.2) and 660 μl chilled ethanol. Precipitate the DNA at −80 °C.

6. Centrifuge at 4 °C for 15 minutes. Wash the resulting pellet with 70% ethanol, centrifuge for 15 minutes. Air dry the pellet and dissolve with 10 μl TE (pH 7.4).

See Yasui *et al.* (1992) for references to other molecular techniques.

6.2. Immunocytochemical techniques

A large number of proteins including growth factor/receptors, cell adhesion molecules, and oncogene or tumor-suppressor gene proteins are specifically detected by immunocytochemical techniques using specific antibodies. For instance, an accumulation of the p53 protein in tumor cells is useful for screening the p53 gene mutation. Overexpression of growth factor receptor or cycline suggests gene amplification. A modification of the immunoglobulin enzyme bridge technique (ABC method) is used on formalin-fixed, paraffin-embedded sections.

6.3. Strategy

A new strategy for molecular diagnosis for gastrointestinal cancers is shown in Fig. 4.16. Initially, histological results are reported within a week after receiving biopsies or surgical specimens from the clinic. Then, if there is evidence of cancer, molecular analyses are performed in order to determine the grade of malignancy. This molecular diagnosis is then reported to the clinic within the week following the histological diagnosis report. Depending on the molecular diagnosis, clinical treatment, including surgery, chemotherapy, and radiation therapy will be decided. On the other hand, in instances of adenoma or borderline lesions, molecular analysis will also be carried out for a differential diagnosis. Depending on the molecular diagnosis, clinical treatment, such as polypectomy or surgery, will be performed.

6.4. Biomarkers

Practical biomarkers for molecular diagnosis are illustrated in Table 4.3. Among them, mutation and allele loss of the p53 gene and abnormal transcript of the CD44 gene are the common events of three gastrointestinal carcinomas (Tahara 1993a). Immunocytochemical staining of the p53 protein is useful for screening

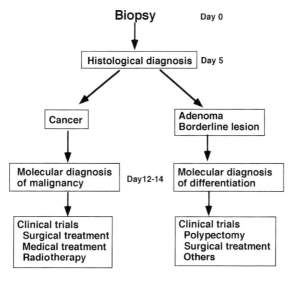

Fig. 4.16. A new strategy for molecular diagnosis of gastrointestinal cancers.

Table 4.3. Markers in the molecular diagnosis of gastrointestinal cancers

Tumor	Markers	Purpose
Esophagus	p53 EGF/TGFα/EGFR Cyclin D	Diagnosis Malignancy Metastasis
Stomach	p53, APC EGF/TGFα/EGFR/*cripto*/c-*erb*B2 c-*met*, K-*sam* nm23, CD44	Diagnosis Malignancy Scirrhous Metastasis
Colon	K-*ras*, p53, APC EGF/TGFα/EGFR/*cripto* nm23, CD44	Diagnosis Malignancy Metastasis

From the Hiroshima City Medical Association Laboratory (1994).

changes in the p53 gene to identify missence mutation. The detection of CD44 transcript variants, which is very easy and rapid, using non-radioactive techniques, will serve as a powerful tool in the diagnosis of gastrointestinal cancers (Yokozaki *et al.* 1995, Yoshida *et al.* 1995, Higashikawa *et al.* 1996). In instances of gastric cancer, overexpression of EGF-related growth factor/receptor and c-*erb*B2 is investigated immunocytochemically, in order to identify the grade of malignancy, as their overexpression is closely correlated with tumor staging and liver metastasis. In addition, reduction in adhesion molecules (cadherin, catenin), and nm23 protein are good markers for metastasis (Nakayama *et al.* 1993). Screening of DNA replication errors at microsatellite foci or mutation in MSH2 and MLH1 is a potentially useful way to identify patients at high risk for developing multiple primary cancers (Horii *et al.* in press 1995). In Chapter 7, the reason why these markers are selected for molecular diagnosis of gastric cancer is described. All biomarkers should be examine on end of cases simultaneously. For instance, in the case of esophageal tumor, p53 mutation, overexpression of EGF, TGFα, EGFR, and cyclin D1 as well as Ki-67 expression will be investigated on the same tumor.

6.5.   Evaluation

A total of 6094 cases were examined from August 1993 to October 1994, of which 93 were esophageal tumors, 2501 were gastric tumors, and 3497 were colorectal tumors, respectively. According to the results of molecular diagnosis on gastric lesions, 15 (2%) of 733 adenoma cases were regarded as adenocarcinoma. Out of 254 borderline cases, 38 (15%) and 30 (12%) were diagnosed as adenocarcinoma and suspected adenocarcinoma, respectively. Of 1495 cases of adenocarcinoma, 165 (11%) revealed a high grade of malignancy. This low rate of high grade malignancy on molecular diagnosis might be due to the fact that the majority of the cases were early stage or mucosal cancer.

We recently asked clinicians two questions regarding their opinions concerning molecular diagnosis. The first question was concerning the use of molecular diagnosis in practical medicine. More than 50% of the clinicians answered that molecular diagnosis was useful in deciding on whether to implement cancer therapy, and 38% answered that it is a good reference for following up. The second question was concerning the style of report, and 60% of clinicians replied that the report on molecular diagnosis is understandable. Although the evaluation of this strategy needs continuous assessment and follow-up studies, the evidence described above indicates that it can provide new opportunities for cancer diagnosis and more accurate evaluation of prognosis.

REFERENCES

Borrmann, R. (1926). Geschwülste des Magens und Duodenums. In *Handbuch der speziellen pathologischen Anatomie und Histologie*, (ed. Henke, F. and Lubarsh, O.), Vol. 4, p. 865. Springer, Berlin.
Correa, P. and Tahara, E. (1993). Stomach. In *Pathology of incipient neoplasia*, pp. 85–103. Saunders, London.
Higashikawa, K., Yokozaki, H., Ue, T., Taniyama, K., Ishikawa, T., Tarin, D., *et al.* (1996). Evaluation of CD44 transcription variants in human digestive tract carcinomas and normal tissues. *Int. J. Cancer*, **65**, 1–7
Hirota, T., Ming, S.C., and Itabashi, M. (1993). Pathology of early gastric cancer. In *Gastric cancer*, (ed. Nishi, M., Ichikawa, H., Nakajima, T., Maruyama, K., and Tahara, E.), pp. 66–87. Springer, Tokyo.

Horii, A., Han, H.-J., Shimada, M., Yanagisawa, A., Kato, Y., Ohta, H., *et al.* (1995). Frequent replication errors at microsatellite loci in tumors of patients with multiple primary cancers. *Cancer Res.* **54**, 3373–5.

Ito, H. and Tahara, E. (1993). Endocrine cell tumor of the stomach. In *Gastric cancer*, (ed. Nishi, M., Ichikawa, H., Nakajima, T., Maruyama, K., and Tahara, E.), pp. 151–67. Springer, Tokyo.

JRSGC (Japanese Research Society for Gastric Cancer) (1993). *Japanese classification of gastric carcinoma.* English edition, (ed. Mitsuma, N., Omori, Y., and Miwa, K.). Kanehara, Tokyo.

Jass, J.R. (1983). A classification of gastric dysplasia. *Histopathology*, **7**, 181–93.

Kato, Y., Yanagisawa, A., and Sugano, H. (1993). Biopsy interpretation in diagnosis of gastric carcinoma. In *Gastric cancer*, (ed. Nishi, M., Ichikawa, H., Nakajima, T., Maruyama, K., and Tahara, E.), pp. 133–50. Springer, Tokyo.

Kennedy, B.J. (1970). TNM classification for stomach cancer. *Cancer*, **26**, 971–83.

Lauren, P. (1965). The two histological main types of gastric carcinoma. Diffuse and so-called intestinal type carcinoma. An attempt at histochemical classification. *Acta. Path. Microbiol. Scand.*, **64**, 31–49.

Nakayama, H., Yasui, W., Yokozaki, H., and Tahara, E. (1993). Reduced expression of nm23 is associated with metastasis of human gastric carcinomas. *Jpn. J. Cancer Res.*, **84**, 184–90.

Sugano, H., Nakamura, K., and Takagi, K. (1971). An atypical epithelium of the stomach. A clinico-pathological entity. *Gann Monograph on Cancer Research*, **11**, 257–69.

Tahara, E. (1993). Molecular mechanism of stomach carcinogenesis. *J. Cancer Res. Clin. Oncol.*, **119**, 265–72.

Tahara, E. (1995). Genetic alterations in human gastrointestinal cancers. Cancer 75 (supplement), 1410–1417.

Tahara, E., Yokozaki, H., and Yasui, W. (1993). Growth factors in gastric cancer. In *Gastric cancer*, (ed. Nishi, M., Ichikawa, H., Nakajima, T., Maruyama, K., and Tahara, E.), pp. 209–17, Springer, Tokyo.

Tahara, E., Semba, S., and Tahara, H. (1996). Molecular biological observations in gastric cancer. *Seminars in Oncology*, **23**, 1–6.

Tahara, H., Kuniyasu, H., Yokozaki, H., Yasui, W., Shay, J.W., Ide, T., and Tahara, E. (1995). Telomerase activity in preneoplastic and neoplastic gastric and colorectal lesions. *Clinical Cancer Research*, **1**, 1245–51.

Watanabe, H., Jass, J.R., and Sobin, L.H. (1989). Histological typing of esophageal and gastric tumours. *World Health Organization international histological classification of tumours*, pp. 20–6. Springer, Berlin.

Yasui, W., Ito, H., and Tahara, E. (1992). DNA analysis of archival material and its application to tumour pathology. In *Diagnostic molecular pathology*, (ed. Herrington, C.S. and McGee, J.O'D.), Vol. 2, pp. 193–206. Oxford University Press.

Yokozaki, H., Ito, R., Nakayama H., Kuniyasu, H., Taniyama, K., and Tahara, E. (1994). Expression of CD44 abnormal transcripts in human gastric carcinomas. *Cancer Letters*, **83**, 229–34.

Yoshida, K., Bolodeoku, J., Sugino, T., Goodison, S., Matsumura, Y., Warren, B.F., *et al.* (1995). Abnormal retention of intron 9 in CD44 gene transcripts in human gastrointestinal tumors. *Cancer Res.*, **55**, 4273–7.

Part III: Biology and molecular genetics

5

Experimental gastric cancer

Hiroko Ohgaki and Takashi Sugimura

1. INTRODUCTION

Stomach cancer is still the most common cancer in some countries including Japan, Chile, and Eastern Europe. However, there are clear indications that the incidence of gastric cancer has decreased greatly, even in these countries during recent decades. This suggests that improvement in lifestyle, especially changes in diet, decreases the risk of gastric carcinogenesis (Mettlin 1988). In the past, many attempts to induce gastric cancer in experimental animals were not successful. However, in 1967, Sugimura and Fujimura selectively induced gastric adenocarcinomas in rats by chronic administration of N-methyl-N'-nitro-N-nitrosoguanidine (MNNG) in their drinking water. Since then, experimental models for the induction of gastric adenocarcinomas in various species by using MNNG and its ethyl derivative, N-ethyl-N'-nitro-N-nitrosoguanidine (ENNG), have been established. More recently, N-methyl-N-nitrosourea (MNU) was also demonstrated to induce selectively a high incidence of gastric adenocarcinomas in rats and mice when given in their drinking water (Hirota *et al.* 1987; Tatematsu *et al.* 1993*b*). These experimental models provide much valuable information about the mechanisms of gastric carcinogenesis, lesions related to gastric carcinogenesis, and modulating factors.

2. MNNG-INDUCED GASTRIC CANCER: MECHANISM OF TARGET ORGAN SPECIFICITY

MNNG is a direct-acting mutagenic compound. It causes methylation of nucleic acids and proteins (Lawley and Shah 1970, 1972; Sugimura *et al.* 1968). However, non-enzymatic decomposition of MNNG, which is accelerated by SH compound (L-cysteine and reduced glutathion), is necessary for its macromolecular binding (Lawley and Shah 1970). Methylated bases caused by exposure to MNNG are mainly 7-methylguanine with smaller amounts of 3-methyladenine, 1-methyladenine, 3-methylcytosine, and O^6-methylguanine (Lawley and Shah 1970, 1972). Of these, O^6-methylguanine is considered to be the most critical adduct for mutation.

MNNG was first shown to be carcinogenic by Schoental (1966) and Sugimura *et al.* (1966) who succeeded in inducing subcutaneous fibrosarcoma in rats by subcutaneous injection. Rats administered MNNG in their drinking water developed adenocarcinomas selectively in the glandular stomach (usually in the pyloric region) without developing tumors in the upper digestive tract. The organ specificity of MNNG within the digestive tract correlates well with the level of DNA methylation. After a single oral dose in rats, the concentration of methylpurines in the glandular stomach was 9 times higher than in the forestomach, 20 times higher than in the esophagus, and 1.3 times higher than in the duodenum (Wiestler *et al.* 1983). Similarly, during chronic administration of MNNG (80 μg/ml in drinking water) to inbred Wistar rats, the amount of O^6-methylguanine in the pylorus was about three times higher than in the fundus and duodenum (Kobori *et al.* 1988). These regional differences in DNA methylation correlate with the concentrations of cellular thiols, which enhance the decomposition of MNNG and the extent of its macromolecular binding (Wiestler *et al.* 1983). This is considered to be the major reason for the selective induction of tumors in the glandular stomach without concurrent development of tumors in the esophagus and forestomach of rats given MNNG in their drinking water. The fact that under the acidic conditions of gastric juice, MNNG is rapidly converted to *N*-methyl-*N'*-nitroguanidine which is not mutagenic (McKay and Wright 1947), may explain the low tumor incidence within the small and large intestine despite the high thiol concentration in these tissues. The amount of O^6-methylguanine DNA methyltransferase, which repairs O^6-methylguanine, has been reported to be low in rat glandular stomach (0.9–1.3 units/mg protein) and this value was about 15% of the amount of O^6-methylguanine DNA methyltransferase in the forestomach, and 2% of that in the liver (Weisburger *et al.* 1988). The low repair capacity of O^6-methylguanine may also play an important role in selective induction of adenocarcinomas in the glandular stomach by MNNG.

3. ANIMAL MODELS

3.1 Rat

Experimental conditions for induction of stomach cancer with MNNG

Young adult male rats are given MNNG in their drinking water at concentrations of 50–167 μg/ml for 4–8 months. After an observation period lasting several months, 60–100% of rats developed gastric adenocarcinomas (Sugimura *et al.* 1970; Sugimura and Kawachi 1973, 1978; Ohgaki and Sugimura 1988*a*; Ohgaki *et al.* 1991*a*). In order to determine the minimum induction period, Kobori *et al.* (1980) treated inbred Wistar rats with MNNG (80 μg/ml) for 3–17 weeks and then observed for 20–25 weeks. The stomach epithelium of rats given MNNG for 3–9 weeks showed no significant histologic changes, but those given MNNG for 11 or 13 weeks showed hyperplasia and adenomatous changes. Adenocarcinomas were found in almost all rats treated with MNNG for 15–17 weeks. From these results, Kobori *et al.* (1980) suggested that the threshold period of MNNG administration for inducing gastric carcinomas is approximately 15 weeks in this dose condition. More recently, Zaidi *et al.* (1993) carried out the experiment with various doses of MNNG and suggested that an 8-week treatment of MNNG

(80–160 μg/ml) may induce a high incidence of gastric adenocarcinomas. A single intragastric dose of MNNG (50–250 mg/body weight) to ACI or Wistar rats produced a high incidence of forestomach tumors but only a few adenocarcinomas in the glandular stomach (Hirono and Shibuya 1972; Zaidi *et al.* 1993).

Location and histopathology of tumors induced by MNNG

Most tumors induced by MNNG in drinking water are located in the pyloric region of the glandular stomach but tumors are also induced in the fundic region, duodenum, and jejunum (Ohgaki and Sugimura 1988*a*; Zaidi *et al.* 1993). Histologically, most gastric tumors are adenomas or adenocarcinomas but sarcomas also develop. Most adenocarcinomas induced in rats are well-differentiated adenocarcinomas, and poorly differentiated or signet-ring cell carcinomas are rare. Gastric adenocarcinomas frequently invade the muscle layers or serosa, but metastasis of gastric adenocarcinomas are extremely rare.

Sex and age

Male rats are generally more susceptible to gastric cancer induced by MNNG than females (Ohgaki *et al.* 1983). Castrated male rats developed gastric adenocarcinomas at a lower frequency (Furukawa *et al.* 1982*a*). Injections of estradiol reduced the incidence of gastric adenocarcinomas induced by MNNG in male rats (Furukawa *et al.* 1982*b*). These results suggest that female hormones suppress, and male hormones enhance, gastric carcinogenesis. Younger animals are more susceptible than older rats (Kimura *et al.* 1979).

Strain difference

Although most strains of rats develop gastric adenocarcinomas when given MNNG in their drinking water, there are considerable strain difference in MNNG susceptibility. Bralow *et al.* (1973) reported that the incidence of gastric adenocarcinomas in random-bred Wistar, inbred Wistar–May–Furth, and inbred Buffalo strain of rats were 73%, 10%, and 0%, respectively, after administration of 83 μg/ml MNNG for 52 weeks. Similarly, Martin *et al.* (1974) reported that the incidence of gastric adenocarcinomas in BDIX, BN, Lewis, and Wistar rats treated with 83 μg/ml MNNG for 7 months were 75%, 92%, 38%, and 55%, respectively. Treatment with MNNG in susceptible ACI rats, resistant Buffalo rats, and their F_1 and F_2 offspring demonstrated that susceptibly to MNNG was genetically determined and the resistance to MNNG in the Buffalo strain was a dominant trait (Ohgaki *et al.* 1983). Hypertensive SHR rats developed more gastric adenocarcinomas than WKY rats, from which SHR rats are derived, after MNNG treatment. Increased sympathetic nervous system activity and increased cell proliferation in gastric mucosa was suggested to enhance gastric carcinogenesis in SHR rats (Tatsuta *et al.* 1989, 1992).

Location of cells chronically exposed to MNNG

When rats were given MNNG in their drinking water, the distribution of cells exposed to MNNG were identified in the surface epithelium of fundus and pylorus of the glandular stomach by immunohistochemistry using O^6-methylguanine antibody and histoautoradiography using [^{3}H]-methyl-MNNG (Kobori *et al.* 1988; Ohgaki *et al.* 1988). Since fixation of DNA damage by cell proliferation is necessary for the acquisition of a mutation, most superficial pyloric epithelial cells must be considered non-susceptible to the initiation of malignant transformation. The proliferating cell zone is located deeper in the pyloric glands where the level of exposure to MNNG is much lower. Due to this difference in the location of chronically exposed cells and proliferating cells within the mucosa, the mutation frequency is predicted to be low when normal gastric mucosa is exposed to MNNG.

Cell proliferation

During MNNG treatment, the number of proliferating cells increases and the range of the proliferative cell zone extends greatly, which leads to the increase in the number of epithelial cells in the pyloric pit column and thickening of the pyloric mucosa (Deschner *et al.* 1979; Ohgaki *et al.* 1986*b*, 1988). In these conditions, the gastric mucosa is considered to be much more susceptible to additional MNNG exposure. Interestingly, resistant strain Buffalo rats showed less proliferative response during MNNG treatment than susceptible ACI rats, which may constitute a key factor determining the susceptibility to MNNG-induced gastric carcinogenesis in these two strains of rat (Ohgaki *et al.* 1988).

Sequential histologic changes and related lesions during gastric carcinogenesis

Sequential histologic changes   These changes during MNNG-induced gastric carcinogenesis have been vigorously investigated. Saito *et al.* (1970) reported that erosion, regenerative hyperplasia at the margin of erosions (until 21 weeks), adenomatous hyperplasia (21–30 weeks), and adenocarcinoma (31–60 weeks) were sequentially observed in male Wistar rats which were given MNNG in their drinking water at 167 µg/ml for 40 weeks and then 84 µg/ml until the end of the experiment. Ohgaki *et al.* (1986*b*) compared the sequential histologic changes during MNNG induced gastric carcinogenesis in susceptible ACI rats and resistant Buffalo rats. In ACI rats, sequential histologic changes were similar to those observed in Wistar rats. In resistant Buffalo rats, the major histologic changes by MNNG treatment were consistent erosions and glandular hyperplasia of pyloric glands at the margin of erosions, but no atypical changes were observed. Following cessation of MNNG treatment, glandular hyperplasia of pyloric glands subsided and was followed by atrophy of these glands. Kunze *et al.* (1979) reported that adenocarcinomas developed predominantly from atypical foci in the mucosa in female Wistar rats given MNNG, and this process was observed independently from erosion, intestinal metaplasia, chronic atrophic gastritis, or benign proliferative lesions. The weak gastric carcinogen *N*-propyl-*N'*-nitro-*N*-nitrosoguanidine (PNNG) was found to induce gastric carcinomas in male Wistar rats without previous ulceration or regenerative changes (Matsukura *et al.* 1980). From these results it is suggested that: (1) the first histologically detectable changes that eventually lead to adenocarcinoma are atypical glands or adenomatous hyperplasia; and (2) erosions and regenerative hyperplasia are not directly related to gastric carcinogenesis.

Biochemical changes Pyloric glands exposed to MNNG show biochemical changes well before preneoplastic changes are histologically detected. Pg1, one of the three pepsinogen isozymes, is normally present in the pyloric mucosa, but decreases or disappears about one week after the start of MNNG treatment (Tatematsu *et al.* 1980; Furihata *et al.* 1975). Decrease or disappearance of Pg1 is also consistently observed in gastric adenocarcinomas (Tatematsu *et al.* 1977). Tatematsu *et al.* (1993*a*) analysed the methylation pattern in CCGG and GCGC sites of the Pg1 gene in gastric adenocarcinomas and adenomatous hyperplasias induced by MNNG. The Pg1 gene was more methylated in adenocarcinoma or adenomatous hyperplasia than untreated pyloric mucosa.

Intestinal metaplasia There is a close relationship between the presence of intestinal metaplasia and human gastric cancer, suggesting that intestinal metaplasia is a possible precancerous lesion. Intestinal metaplasia is rarely seen in untreated rat stomach but is frequently observed in the stomach of rats given MNNG or PNNG (Matsukura *et al.* 1978; Sasajima *et al.* 1979). This finding suggests that intestinal metaplasia and gastric adenocarcinomas can be induced by a common cause. However, there is no direct evidence that intestinal metaplasia is a precancerous lesion in rat stomach (Watanabe and Ito 1986; Tatematsu *et al.* 1983).

Factors modulating gastric carcinogenesis

Many experimental studies have shown that gastric carcinogenesis is significantly modulated by various environmental and host factors. Most enhancing factors have been shown to have significant effects on cell proliferation in gastric mucosa (Ohgaki *et al.* 1989).

Sodium chloride Intragastric administration of saturated sodium chloride (NaC1) solution with MNNG treatment increased the incidences of gastric carcinomas induced by MNNG (Tatematsu *et al.* 1975). Administration of NaCl in the diet (10%) during the treatment with MNNG increased both the incidence and the size of gastric carcinomas (Takahashi *et al.* 1983). Treatment with saturated NaCl solution before a single dose of MNNG increased the incidence of carcinomas in the glandular stomach (Shirai *et al.* 1982). These results indicate that NaCl enhances the initiation of gastric carcinogenesis induced by MNNG in rats. The enhancing effect of NaCl was also observed when it was given to rats after cessation of MNNG treatment, suggesting that it also acts as a tumor promoter in gastric carcinogenesis (Takahashi *et al.* 1984; Ohgaki *et al.* 1984).

Dietary calcium, protein, and other nutrients Epidemiologic studies have shown that populations who drink milk have a low risk of developing gastric cancer (Sugimura and Wakabayashi 1990). The effect of calcium was tested in rats treated with MNNG (100 ppm in the drinking water) and NaCl (5% in the diet) for 8 weeks, followed by calcium chloride (0.2%) in their drinking water (Nishikawa *et al.* 1992). The incidence of adenomatous hyperplasia was significantly lower in rats given calcium chloride in a dose-dependent manner. On the other hand, when rats were given a calcium-deficient diet following MNNG treatment, the incidence of gastric adenocarcinomas was significantly increased (Tatsuta *et al.* 1993).

Populations having a poor diet (i.e. low in protein and high in carbohydrate) have a high risk of gastric cancer. Tatsuta *et al.* (1991) reported that the incidence of gastric adenocarcinomas in Wistar rats given MNNG (50 µg/ml) for 25 weeks followed by a low protein diet (5% casein) was 63% whereas those given a higher protein diet (10% and 25% casein) were 15% and 18%, respectively,. The serum gastrin, norepinephrine level, and the labeling index in pyloric mucosa were significantly higher in rats fed the low protein diet. It was suggested that the enhanced sympathetic nervous system, a result of the low protein diet, increased cell proliferation and enhanced gastric carcinogenesis (Tatsuta *et al.* 1991).

Ascorbate in the diet (2%) suppressed infiltrative growth of gastric adenocarcinomas induced by MNNG in rats (Kawasaki *et al.* 1982). Selenium (4 ppm in the diet) also decreased the incidence of gastric adenocarcinomas induced by MNNG (Kobayashi *et al.* 1986).

Gastrectomy and bile acid   Gastrectomy of rats, before or after MNNG treatment, resulted in a higher incidence of gastric adenocarcinomas (Kobori *et al.* 1984; Salmon *et al.* 1985; Kondo *et al.* 1984; Sano *et al.* 1984). A correlation between bile reflux and the increase in the incidence of gastric carcinomas has been suggested (Kobori *et al.* 1984; Salmon *et al.* 1985; Kondo *et al.* 1984; Sano *et al.* 1984; Langhans *et al.* 1984). Kondo *et al.* (1984) reported that even without MNNG treatment, adenocarcinomas developed at an incidence of 23% in the remnant of the stomach of Wistar rats. All of these carcinomas were located in the vicinity of the gastrojejunal anastomosis, which is directly exposed to duodenal contents (Kondo *et al.* 1984). Among the duodenal contents, bile acids (sodium taurocholate and taurocholic acid) were shown to enhance gastric carcinogenesis induced by MNNG (Kobori *et al.* 1984; Salmon *et al.* 1984).

Phenolic compounds   Catechol is a major industrial chemical as well as a phenolic component of cigarette smoke. It is not mutagenic to *Salmonella* mutagenicity assay but it greatly enhances cell proliferation in the gastric mucosa when given in the diet (Ohgaki *et al.* 1989). Administration of catechol in the diet (0.8%), after a single intragastric dose of 150 mg/kg of MNNG, greatly enhanced both forestomach and glandular stomach carcinogenesis (Hirose *et al.* 1987). Moreover, catechol alone induced adenomatous hypersplasia and adenocarcinomas in the pyloric region (Hirose *et al.* 1987). The other derivatives, including *p*-tert-butylcatechol and *p*-methylcatechol also significantly enhanced gastric carcinogenesis induced by MNNG. *p*-Methylcatechol alone also induced 100% of adenomatous hyperplasias and 6.7% of the adenocarcinomas (Hirose *et al.* 1989).

MNU-*induced gastric carcinogenesis*

N-methyl-*N*-nitrosourea (MNU) is a multipotent carcinogen and induces tumors in various tissues depending on the route of administration. Recently, it has been reported that MNU induced a high incidences of gastric adenocarcinomas in F344 male rats when given in their drinking water. Maekawa *et al.* (1985) reported that gastric adenocarcinomas developed in about 40% of F344 rats exposed to MNU (100 ppm) for 42 weeks. Hirota *et al.* (1987) reported that gastric adenocarcinomas were selectively induced in 100% of rats given MNU (400 ppm) for 25 weeks and then maintained without carcinogens for a further 20 weeks. Administration of MNU at 100 ppm for 15 weeks was found to be an optimal condition for the selective induction of gastric adenocarcinomas in F344 rats without toxicity (Fujita *et al.* 1989). Most gastric tumors developed in the pyloric region and they were histologically well-differentiated to poorly differentiated adnocarcinomas (Hirota *et al.* 1987; Fujita *et al.* 1989).

The amount of O^6-methylguanosine was measured in various organs in F344 rats given MNU (400 ppm) in the drinking water for two weeks (Ohgaki *et al.* 1991*b*). In contrast to MNNG treatment, chronic administration of MNU produced the highest levels of O^6-methylguanosine in the brain and significant levels in all the digestive tract tissues measured (i.e. esophagus, forestomach, pylorus, and fundus of the glandular stomach, duodenum, and colon). There was no clear correlation between target organ specificity and the extent of methylation. It was also found that the distribution of cells exposed to MNU was not restricted to the surface epithelium and most gastric mucosal cells were equally affected (Ohgaki *et al.* 1991*b*). In contrast to MNNG, MNU is stable in the acidic conditions of the intragastric environment and its decomposition to a methylating intermediate (i.e. methyldiazonium hydroxide) is not affected by intracellular thiols. Thus, it is likely that gastric mucosa is exposed to MNU both from the gastric lumen and the bloodstream when rats are given this carcinogen in drinking water. MNU-induced gastric adenocarcinomas in rats will provide useful information, particularly as the model of gastric cancer induced by chemicals may affect the mucosa both from the lumen and the circulation.

3.2. Dog

A high incidence of gastric adenocarcinomas were induced in mongrels and Beagles given MNNG (50–83 µg/ml) in their drinking water (Sugimura *et al.* 1971). The most common types of gastric carcinoma were well-differentiated adenocarcinomas of the fundic region (Shimosato *et al.* 1971). However, because MNNG also induces sarcomas in the small intestine, which causes early death (Koyama *et al.* 1976), MNNG is not recommended in dogs.

Administration of ENNG, mixed with either a pellet diet or in the drinking water (100–150 µg/ml for 3–9 months), produces a high incidence of gastric carcinomas in mongrels and beagles but no development of small intestinal tumors (Kurihara *et al.* 1974; Matsukura *et al.* 1981; Ohgaki and Sugimura 1988). The preferential sites for the induction of carcinomas in dogs are angulus and antrum but carcinomas also develop in the corpus. At concentrations of ENNG higher than 150 µg/ml, esophageal squamous cell carcinomas also developed frequently (Sasajima *et al.* 1977). Histologically, these gastric carcinomas are well-or poorly differentiated adenocarcinomas, and signet-ring cell carcinomas. Different histologic types of carcinomas often develop in the same stomach (Matsukura *et al.* 1981). The conditions of ENNG treatment appear to affect the incidence, histological types, and location of gastric carcinomas (Matsukura *et al.* 1981; Sunagawa *et al.* 1985). Only signet-ring cell carcinomas and poorly differentiated adenocarcinomas developed in the antrum in 50% of the dogs treated with ENNG for three months (total dose per dog: 6 g). After treatment for six and nine months (total dose per dog: 12–18 g), well-differentiated adenocarcinomas also developed in addition to poorly differentiated adenocarcinomas and/or signet-ring cell carcinomas in 90% of dogs (Sunagawa *et al.* 1985). Metastases of gastric adenocarcinomas to regional lymph nodes, liver, and other organs are frequent (Kurihara *et al.* 1977, 1979; Fujita *et al.* 1975; Sasajima *et al.* 1977). The advantages of the dog as an experimental model is the development of gastric carcinogenesis and the effect of treatment are easily followed-up by X-ray examination and endoscopy (Kurihara *et al.* 1979).

3.3.   Monkey

Macaque monkeys (rhesus and cynomolugus) given ENNG at a concentration of 200 or 300 µg/ml in their drinking water for 11–26 months developed gastric adenocarcinomas after 11–38 months (Ohgaki *et al.* 1986a). All the tumors were located in the pyloric region and they were poorly differentiated adenocarcinomas and signet-ring cell carcinomas, with a few moderate to well-differentiated adenocarcinomas. The histological appearance of these carcinomas was similar to those with the respective human cancer. However, metastasis was not found in any of the monkeys. One cynomolugus monkey given ENNG for 26 months was examined sequentially by endoscopy and biopsy. A tumor was first detected in the angulus of the stomach on the 31st month and was diagnosed as a signet-ring cell carcinoma. At the autopsy, in the 109th experimental month, this tumor was found to still be in the early (intramucosal) stages (Szentirmay *et al.* 1990). Two cynomolugus monkeys given ENNG (100 µg/ml) for 10 months and two rhesus monkeys given MNNG (83 µg/ml) for 10 months did not develop gastric carcinomas after 54–104 months of observation (Ohgaki *et al.* 1986a). Although the number of monkeys tested is limited, these animals appear to be more resistant to ENNG and MNNG than rats or dogs.

3.4.   Other animals

Mouse

Several attempts to induce gastric adenocarcinomas by MNNG or ENNG in various strains of the mouse, have been unsuccessful (Sugimura and Kawachi 1973), suggesting that mice are generally resistant to gastric carcinogenesis. Recently, Tatematsu *et al.* (1992) reported that BALB/c mice given 10-weekly MNU by intragastric intubations (0.5 mg/mouse) developed high incidences of carcinomas in both the forestomach and glandular stomach. More recently, Tatematsu *et al.* (1993b) succeeded in selectively inducing adenocarcinomas in the glandular stomach in C3H mice. C3H mice given MNU (30–120 ppm) in drinking water for 30 weeks developed adenocarcinomas in a dose-dependent manner. Adenocarcinomas were histologically well-differentiated, poorly differentiated, and signet-ring cell carcinomas.

Hamster

Golden hamsters administered ENNG (91 µg/ml) in drinking water for 12 months developed adenocarcinomas at an incidence of 50% after 36 months (Kawachi *et al.* 1974). When golden hamsters were given MNNG, most tumors developed were fibrosarcomas in the pyloric region (Fujimura *et al.* 1970*a,b*; Kogure *et al.* 1974).

Ferret

Ferrets given a single dose of MNNG (50–100 mg/kg) developed adenocarcinomas 29–55 months after treatment. Since these animals have *Helicobacter mustelae*, which naturally colonizes the ferret stomach and causes chronic gastritis, this species would be a good model for the study of the role of H. *mustelae* during the development of gastric cancer (Fox *et al.* 1993).

4. FUTURE PROSPECTS

Since the first success in induction of gastric adenocarcinomas in rats by MNNG by Sugimura and Fujimura (1967) experimental gastric cancer in various species has been successfully established. In animals, there is accumulating evidence that gastric carcinogenesis is modified considerably by both host and environmental factors. Although possible gastric carcinogens in man have not been clearly identified, results from animal experiment suggest that avoidance of enhancing factors, especially those affections cell proliferation could greatly prevent gastric carcinogenesis in humans.

During the past decade, the understanding of molecular genetics of human gastric cancer has rapidly increased, as summarized in Chapter 7 of this volume. However, knowledge of molecular mechanisms in experimental gastric cancer is still limited and should be expanded. Generations of transgenic mice with similar genetic alterations to human gastric cancer would also be an interesting future approach for studying the mechanisms of gastric carcinogenesis.

REFERENCES

Bralow, S.P., Gruenstein, M., and Meranze, D.R. (1973). Host resistance to gastric adeno-carcinomatosis in three strains of rats ingesting N-methyl-N'-nitro-N-nitrosoguanidine. *Oncology*, **27**, 168–80.

Deschner, E.E., Tamura, K., and Bralow, S.P. (1979). Sequential histopathology and cell kinetic changes in rat pyloric mucosa during gastric carcinogenesis induced by N-methyl-N'-nitro-N-nitrosoguanidine. *J. Natl. Cancer Inst.*, **63**, 171–9.

Fox, J.G., Wishnok, J.S., Murphy, J.C., Tannenbaum, S.R., and Correa, P. (1993). MNNG-induced gastric carcinoma in ferrets infected with *Helicobacter mustelae*. *Carcinogenesis*, **14**, 1957–61.

Fujimura, S., Kogure, K., Oboshi, S., and Sugimura, T. (1970*a*). Production of tumors in the glandular stomach of hamsters by *N*-methyl-*N'*-nitro-*N*-nitrosoguanidine. *Cancer Res.*, **30**, 1444–8.

Fujimura, S., Kogure, K., Sugimura, T., and Takayama, S. (1970*b*). The effects of limited administration of *N*-methyl-*N'*-nitro-*N*-nitrosoguanidine on the induction of stomach cancer in rats. *Cancer Res.*, **30**, 842–8.

Fujita, M., Taguchi, T., Takami, M., Usugane, M., and Takahashi, A. (1975). Lung metastasis of canine gastric adenocarcinoma induced by *N*-methyl-*N'*-nitro-*N*-nitrosoguanidine. *Gann*, **66**, 107–8.

Fujita, M., Ishi, T., Tsukahara, Y., Scimozuma, K., Nakano, Y., Taguchi, T., *et al.* (1989). Establishment of optimum conditions for induction of stomach carcinoma in rats by continuous oral administration of *N*-methyl-*N*-nitrosourea. *J. Toxicol. Pathol.*, **2**, 27–32.

Furihata, C., Sasajima, K., Kogure, T., Kawachi, T., Sugimura, T., Tatematsu, M. *et al.* (1975). Changes in pepsinogen isozymes in stomach carcinogenesis in rats by *N*-methyl-*N'*-nitro-*N*-nitrosoguanidine. *J. Natl. Cancer Inst.*, **55**, 925–30.

Furukawa, H., Iwanaga, T., Koyama, H., and Taniguchi, H. (1982*a*). Effect of sex hormones on carcinogenesis in the stomachs of rats. *Cancer Res.*, **42**, 5181–2.

Furukawa, H., Iwanaga, T., Koyama, H., and Taniguchi, H. (1982*b*). Effect of sex hormones on the experimental induction of cancer in rat stomach: a preliminary study. *Digestion*, **23**, 151–5.

Hirono, I. and Shibuya, C. (1972). Induction of stomach cancer by a single dose of *N*-methyl-*N'*-nitro-*N*-nitrosoguanidine through a stomach tube. In Topics in chemical carcinogenesis, (ed. W. Nakahara, S. Takayama, T. Sugimura and S. Odashima, pp. 121–31. University of Tokyo, Tokyo and University Park, Baltimore.

Hirose, M., Kurata, Y., Tsuda, H., Fukushima, S., and Ito, N. (1987). Catechol strongly enhances rat stomach carcinogenesis: a possible new environmental stomach carcinogen. *Jpn. J. Cancer Res. (Gann)*, **8**, 1144–9.

Hirose, M., Yamaguchi, S., Fukushima, S., Hasegawa, R., Takahashi, S., and Ito, N. (1989). Promotion by dihydroxybenzene derivatives of *N*-methyl-*N'*-nitro-*N*-nitrosoguanidine-induced F344 rat forestomach and glandular stomach carcinogenesis. *Cancer Res.*, **49**, 5143–7.

Hirota, N., Aonuma, T., Yamada, S., Kawai, T., Saito, K., and Yokoyama, T. (1987). Selective induction of glandular stomach carcinoma in F344 rats by *N*-methyl-*N*-nitrosourea. *Jpn. J. Cancer Res. (Gann)*, **78**, 634–8.

Kawachi, T., Kogure, K., Tanaka, N., Tokunaga, A., Fujimura, S., and Sugimura, T. (1974). Induction of tumors in the stomach and duodenum of hamsters by *N*-methyl-*N'*-nitro-*N*-nitrosoguanidine. *Z. Krebsforsch*, **81**, 29–36.

Kawasaki, H., Morishige, F., Tanaka, H., *et al.* (1982). Influence of oral supplimation of ascorbate upon the induction of *N*-methyl-*N'*-nitro-*N*-nitrosoguanidine. *Cancer Lett.*, **16**, 57–63.

Kimura, M., Fukuda, T., and Sato, K. (1979). Effect of aging on the development of gastric cancer in rats induced by *N*-methyl-*N'*-nitro-*N*-nitrosoguanidine. *Gann*, **70**, 521–5.

Kobayashi, M., Kogata, M., Yamamura, M., *et al.* (1986). Inhibitory effect of dietary selenium on carcinogenesis in rat glandular stomach induced by *N*-methyl-*N'*-nitro-*N*-nitrosoguanidine. *Cancer Res.*, **46**, 2266–70.

Kobori, O. (1980). Analytical study of precancerous lesions in rat stomach mucosa induced by N-methyl-N′-nitro-N-nitrosoguanidine. *Gann Monogr.*, **25**, 141–50.

Kobori, O., Simizu, T., Maeda, M., Atomi, Y., Watanabe, J., Shoji, M., *et al.* (1984). Enhancing effect of bile and bile acid on stomach tumorigenesis induced by N-methyl-N′-nitro-N-nitrosoguanidine in Wistar rats. *J. Natl. Cancer Inst.*, **73**, 853–61.

Kobori, O., Schmerold, I., Ludeke, B., Ohgaki, H., and Kleihues, P. (1988) DNA methylation in rat stomach and duodenum following chronic exposure to N-methyl-N′-nitro-N-nitrosoguanidine and the effect of dietary taurocholate. *Carcinogenesis*, **9**, 2271–4.

Kogure, K., Sasadaira, H., Kawachi, T., Shimosato, Y., Tokunaga, A., Fujimura, S., *et al.* (1974). Further studies on induction of stomach cancer in hamsters by N-methyl-N′-nitro-N-nitrosoguanidine. *Br. J. Cancer*, **29**, 132–42.

Kondo, K., Suzuki, H., and Nagayo, T. (1984). The influence of gastro-jejunal anastomosis on gastric carcinogenesis in rats. *Gann*, **75**, 362–9.

Koyama, Y., Omori, K., Hirota, T., Sano, R., and Ishihara, K. (1976). Leiomyosarcomas of the small intestine induced in dogs by N-methyl-N′-nitro-N-nitrosoguanidine. *Gann*, **67**, 241–51.

Kunze, E., Schauer, A., Eder, M., *et al.* (1979). Early sequential lesions during development of experimental gastric cancer with special reference to dysplasias. *J. Cancer Res. Clin. Oncol.*, **95**, 247.

Kurihara, M., Shirakabe, H., Murakami, T., Yasui, A., Izumi, T., Sumida, M., *et al.* (1974). A new method for producing adenocarcinomas in the stomach of dogs with N-methyl-N′-nitro-N-nitrosoguanidine. *Gann*, **65**, 163–77.

Kurihara, M., Shirakabe, H., Izumi, T., Miyasaka, K., Yamaya, F., Maruyama, T., *et al.* (1977). Adenocarcinomas of the stomach induced in beagle dogs by oral administration of N-methyl-N′-nitro-N-nitrosoguanidine. *Z. Krebsforsch.*, **90**, 241–52.

Kurihara, M., Izumi, T., Miyakawa, K., *et al.* (1979). Radiological and endoscopic analyses of growth of experimental dog gastric cancer and morphological alteration of human gastric cancer treated with anticancer agents. *Prog. Dig. Endosc.*, **15**, 16.

Langhans, P., Heger, R.A., and Stegamann, B. (1984). The cancer risk in the stomach subjected to nonresecting procedures. An experimental long-term study. *Scand. J. Gastroenterol.*, **92** (suppl. 19), 138–41.

Lawley, P.D. and Shah, S.A. (1970). Methylation of deoxyribonucleic acid in cultured mammalian cells by N-methyl-N′-nitro-N-nitrosoguanidine. The influence of cellular thiol concentrations on the extent of methylation and the 6-oxygen of guanine as a site of methylation. *Biochem. J.*, **116**, 693.

Lawley, P.D. and Shah, S.A. (1972). Methylation of ribonucleic acid by the carcinogens dimethylsulphate, N-methyl-N-nitrosourea and N-methyl-N′-nitro-N-nitrosoguanidine. Comparisons of chemical analyses at the nucleoside and base levels. *Biochem. J.*, **128**, 117–32.

Maekawa, A., Matsuoka, C., Onodera, H., Tanigawa, H., Furuta, K., Ogiu, T., *et al.* (1985). Organ-specific carcinogenicity of N-methyl-N-nitrosourea in F344 and ACI/N rats. *J. Cancer Res. Clin. Oncol.*, **109**, 178–82.

Martin, M.S., Martin, F., Justrabo, E., Michiels, R., Bastien, H., and Knobel, S. (1974). Susceptibility of inbred rats to gastric and duodenal carcinomas induced by N-methyl-N′-nitro-N-nitrosoguanidine. *J. Natl. Cancer Inst.*, **53**, 837–40.

Matsukura, N., Kawachi, T., Sasajima, K., Sano, T., Sugimura, T., and Hirota, T. (1978). Induction of intestinal metaplasia in the stomachs of rats by N-methyl-N′-nitro-N-nitrosoguanidine. *J. Natl. Cancer Inst.*, **61**, 141–4.

Matsukura, N., Itabashi, M., Kawachi, T., *et al.* (1980). Sequential studies on the histopathogenesis of gastric carcinoma in rats by a weak gastric carcinogen, N-propyl-N'-nitro-N-nitrosoguanidine. *J. Cancer Res. Clin. Oncol.*, **98**, 153–63.

Matsukura, N., Morino, K., Ohgaki, H., and Kawachi, T. (1981). Canine gastric carcinoma as an animal model of human gastric carcinoma. *Stom. Intes.*, **16**, 715–22.

McKay, A.F. and Wright, G.F. (1947). Preparation and properties of N-methyl-N'-nitro-N-nitrosoguanidine. *J. Am. Chem. Soc.*, **69**, 3028–30.

Mettlin, C. (1988). Epidemiologic studies in gastric adenocarcinoma. In *Gastric cancer*, (ed. H.O. Douglas, Jr.). Churchill Livingstone, New York.

Nishikawa, A., Furukawa, F., Mitsui, M., Enami, T., Kawanishi, T., Hasegawa, T., *et al.* (1992). Inhibitory effect of calcium chloride on gastric carcinogenesis in rats after treatment with N-methyl-N'-nitro-N-nitrosoguanidine and sodium chloride. *Carcinogenesis*, **13**, 1155–8.

Ohgaki, H. and Sugimura, T. (1988). Experimental stomach cancer. In *Gastric cancer* (ed. H.O. Douglass, Jr.), pp. 27–54. Churchill Livingstone, New York.

Ohgaki, H., Kawachi, T., Matsukura, N., Morino, K., Mlyamoto, M., and Sugimura, T. (1983). Genetic control of susceptibility of rats to gastric carcinoma. *Cancer Res.*, **43**, 3663–7.

Ohgaki, H., Kato, T., Morino, K., Matsukura, N., Sato, S., Takayama, S., *et al.* (1984). Study of the promoting effect of sodium chloride on gastric carcinogenesis by N-methyl-N'-nitro-N-nitrosoguanidine in inbred Wistar rats. *Gann*, **75**, 1053–7.

Ohgaki, H., Hasegawa, H., Kusama, K., Morino, K., Matsukura, N., Sato, S., *et al.* (1986*a*). Induction of gastric carcinomas in nonhuman primates by N-methyl-N'-nitro-N-nitrosoguanidine. *J. Natl. Cancer Inst.*, **77**, 179–86.

Ohgaki, H., Kusama, K., Hasegawa, H., Sato, S., Takayama, S., and Sugimura, T. (1986*b*). Sequential histologic changes during gastric carcinogenesis induced by N-methyl-N'-nitro-N-nitrosoguanidine in susceptible ACI and resistant Buffalo strain rats. *J. Natl. Cancer Inst.*, **77**, 747–55.

Ohgaki, H., Tomihari, M., Sato, S., Kleihues, P., and Sugimura, T. (1988). Differential proliferative response of gastric mucosa during carcinogenesis induced by N-methyl-N'-nitro-N-nitrosoguanidine in susceptible ACI rats, resistant Buffalo rats, and their F1 hybrid cross. *Cancer Res.*, **48**, 5275–9.

Ohgaki, H., Szentirmay, Z., Take, M., and Sugimura, T. (1989). Effects of 4-week treatment with gastric carcinogens and enhancing agents on proliferation of gastric mucosa cells in rats. *Cancer Lett.*, **46**, 117–22.

Ohgaki, H., Kleihues, P., and Sugimura, T. (1991*a*). Experimental gastric cancer. *Ital. J. Gastroenterol.*, **23**, 371–7.

Ohgaki, H., Lüdeke, B.I., Meier, I., Kleihues, P., and Lutz, W.K. (1991*b*). DNA methylation in the digestive tract of F344 rats during chronic exposure to N-methyl-N-nitrosourea. *J. Cancer Res. Clin. Oncol.*, **117**, 13–18.

Saito, T., Inokuchi, K., Takayama, S., and Sugimura, T. (1970). Sequential morphological changes in N-methyl-N'-nitro-N-nitrosoguandine carcinogenesis in the glandular stomach of rats. *J. Natl. Cancer Inst.*, **44**, 769–83.

Salmon, R.J., Laurrent, M., and Thierry, J.P. (1984). Effect of taurocholic acid feeding on N-methyl-N'-nitro-N-nitrosoguanidine induced gastric tumors. *Cancer Lett.*, **22**, 315–20.

Salmon, R.J. Merle, S., Zafrani, B., Decosse, J.J., Sherlock, P., and Deschner, E.E. (1985). Gastric carcinogenesis induce by N-methyl-N'-nitro-N-nitrosoguanidine: Role of gastrectomy and duodenal reflux. *Gann*, **76**, 167–72.

Sano, C., Kumashiro, R., Saito, T., and Inokuchi, K. (1984). Promoting effect of partial gastrectomy on carcinogenesis in the remnant stomach of rats after oral administration of N-methyl-N'-nitro-N-nitrosoguanidine. *Oncology*, **41**, 124–8.

Sasajima, K., Kawachi, T., Sano, T., Sugimura, T., Shimosato, Y., and Shirota, A. (1977). Esophageal and gastric cancers with metastases induced in dogs by N-methyl-N'-nitro-N-nitrosoguanidine. *J. Natl. Cancer Inst.*, **58**, 1789–94.

Sasajima, K., Kawachi, T., Matsukura, N., *et al.* (1979). Intestinal metaplasia and adenocarcinoma induced in the stomach of rats by N-propyl-N'-nitro-N-nitrosoguanidine. *J. Cancer Res. Clin. Oncol.*, **94**, 201–6.

Schoental, R. (1966). Carcinogenic activity of N-methyl-N'-nitro-N-nitrosoguanidine. *Nature*, **209**, 726–7.

Shimosato, Y., Tanaka, N., Kogure, K., Fujimura, S., Kawachi, T., and Sugimura, T. (1971). Histopathology of tumors of canine alimentary tract produced by N-methyl-N'-nitro-N-nitrosoguanidine, with particular reference to gastric carcinomas. *J. Natl. Cancer Inst.*, **47**, 1053–70.

Shirai, T., Imaida, K., Fukushima, S., Hasegawa, R., Tatematsu, M., and Ito, N. (1982). Effects of NaCl, tween 60 and a low dose of N-methyl-N'-nitro-N-nitrosoguandine on gastric carcinogenesis of rat given a single dose of N-methyl-N'-nitro-N-nitrosoguanidine. *Carcinogenesis*, **3**, 1419–22.

Sugimura, T. and Fujimura, S. (1967). Tumor production in glandular stomach of rats by N-methyl-N'-nitro-N-nitrosoguanidine. *Nature*, **216**, 943–4.

Sugimura, T. and Kawachi, T. (1973). Experimental stomach cancer. In *Methods in cancer research*, (ed. H. Busch), Vol. 7, pp. 245–308. Academic Press, Orlando, FL.

Sugimura, T. and Kawachi, T. (1978). Experimental stomach carcinogenesis. *In Gastrointestinal tract cancer*, (ed. M. Lipkin, R.A. Good, pp. 327–41. Plenum, New York.

Sugimura, T. and Wakabayashi, K. (1990). Gastric carcinogenesis: Diet as a causative factor. *Med. Oncol. Tumor Pharmacother.*, **7**, 87–92.

Sugimura, T., Nagao, M., and Okada, Y. (1966). Carcinogenic action of N-methyl-N'-nitro-N-nitrosoguanidine. *Nature*, **210**, 962–3.

Sugimura, T., Fujimura, S., Nagao, M., Yokoshima, T., and Hasegawa, S. (1968). Reaction of N-methyl-N'-nitro-N-nitrosoguanidine with protein. *Biochem. Biophys. Acta.*, **170**, 427–29.

Sugimura, T., Fujimura, S., and Baba T. (1970). Tumor production in the glandular stomach and alimentary tract of the rat by N-methyl-N'-nitro-N-nitrosoguanidine. *Cancer Res.*, **30**, 455–65.

Sugimura, T., Tanaka, N., Kawachi, T., Kogure, K., Fujimura, S., and Shimosato, Y. (1971). Production of stomach cancer in dogs by N-methyl-N'-nitro-N-nitrosoguanidine. *Gann*, **62**, 67.

Sunagawa, M., Takeshita, K., Nakajima, A., Ochi, K., Habu, H., and Endo, M. (1985). Duration of ENNG administration and its effect on histological differentiation of experimental gastric cancer. *Br. J. Cancer*, **52**, 771–9.

Szentirmay, Z., Ohgaki, H., Maruyama, K., Esumi, H., Takayama, S., and Sugimura, T. (1990). Early gastric cancer induced by N-methyl-N'-nitro-N-nitrosoguanidine in a cynomolugus monkey six years after initial diagnosis of the lesion. *Jpn. J. Cancer Res.*, **81**, 6–9.

Takahashi, M., Kokubo, T., Furukawa, F., Kurokawa, Y., Tatematsu, M., and Hayashi, Y. (1983). Effect of high salt diet on rat gastric carcinogenesis induced by N-methyl-N'-nitro-N-nitrosoguanidine. *Gann*, **74**, 28–34.

Takahashi, M., Kokubo, T., Furukawa, F., Kurokawa, Y., and Hayashi, Y. (1984). Effects of sodium chloride, saccharin, phenobarbital and aspirin on gastric carcinogenesis in rats after initiation with N-methyl-N'-nitro-N-nitrosoguanidine. *Gann*, 75, 494–501.

Tatematsu, M., Takahashi, M., Fukushima, S., Ito, N., Kokubo, T., Furukawa, F., *et al.* (1975). Effects in rats of sodium chloride on experimental gastric cancers induced by N-methyl-N'-nitro-N-nitrosoguanidine or 4-nitroquinoline-1-oxide. *J. Natl. Cancer Inst.*, 55, 101–6.

Tatematsu, M., Furihata, C., Hirose, M., Shirai, T., Ito, N., Nakajima, Y., *et al.* (1977). Changes in pepsinogen isozymes in stomach cancer induced in Wistar rats by N-methyl-N'-nitro-N-nitrosoguanidine and transplantable gastric carcinoma (SG2B). *J. Natl. Cancer Inst.*, 58, 1709–16.

Tatematsu, M., Saito, D., Furihata, C., *et al.* (1980). Initial DNA damage and heritable permanent change in pepsinogen isozyme pattern in the pyloric mucosa of rats after short-term administration of N-methyl-N'-nitro-N-nitrosoguanidine. *J. Natl. Cancer Inst.*, 64, 775–81.

Tatematsu, M., Furihata, C., Katsuyama, T., *et al.* (1983). Independent induction of intestinal metaplasia and gastric cancer in rats treated with N-methyl-N'-nitro-N-nitrosoguanidine. *Cancer Res.*, 43, 1335–41.

Tatematsu, M., Ogawa, K., Hoshiya, T., Schichino, Y., Kato, T., Imaida, K., *et al.* (1992). Induction of adenocarcinomas in the glandular stomach of BALB/c mice treated with N-methyl-N-nitrosourea. *Jpn. J. Cancer Res.*, 83, 915–18.

Tatematsu, M., Ichinose, M., Tsukada, S., Kakei, N., Takahashi, S., Ogawa, K., *et al.* (1993*a*). DNA methylation of the pepsinogen 1 gene during rat glandular stomach carcinogenesis induced by N-methyl-N'-nitro-N-nitrosoguanidine or catechol. *Carcinogenesis*, 14, 1415–19.

Tatematsu, M., Yamamoto, M., Iwata, H., Fukami, H., *et al.* (1993*b*). Induction of glandular stomach cancers in C3H mice treated with N-methyl-N-nitrosourea in the drinking water. *Jpn. J. Cancer Res.*, 84, 1258–64.

Tatsuta, M., Iishi, H., Baba, M., and Taniguchi, H. (1989). Enhancement of experimental gastric carcinogenesis induced in spontaneously hypertensive rats by N-methyl-N'-nitro-N-nitrosoguanidine. *Cancer Res.*, 49, 794–8.

Tatsuta, M., Iishi, H., Baba, M., Uehara, H., Nakaizumi, A., and Taniguchi, H. (1991). Enhanced induction of gastric carcinogenesis by N-methyl-N'-nitro-N-nitrosoguanidine in Wistar rats fed a low-protein diet. *Cancer Res.*, 51, 3493–6.

Tatsuta, M., Iishi, H., Baba, M., Uehara, H., Nakaizumi, A., and Taniguchi, H. (1992). Protection by muscimol against gastric carcinogenesis induced by N-methyl-N'-nitro-N-nitrosoguanidine in spontaneously hypertensive rats. *Int. J. Cancer*, 52, 924–7.

Tatsuta, M., Ishii, H., Baba, M., Uehara, H., Nakaizumi, A., and Taniguchi, H. (1993). Enhancing effects of calcium-deficient diet on gastric carcinogenesis by N-methyl-N'-nitro-N-nitrosoguanidine in Wistar rats. *Jpn. J. Cancer Res.*, 84, 945–50.

Watanabe, H. and Ito A. (1986). Relationship between gastric tumorigenesis and intestinal metaplasia in rats given X-radiation and/or N-methyl-N'-nitro-N-nitrosoguanidine. *J. Natl. Cancer Inst.*, 76, 865–70.

Weisburger, J.H., Jones, R.C., Barnes, W.S., and Pegg, A.E. (1988). Mechanisms of differential strain sensitivity in gastric carcinogenesis. *Jpn. J. Cancer Res. (Gann)*, 79, 1304–10.

Wiestler, O., Deimling, A., Kobori, O., and Kleihues, P. (1983). Location of N-methyl-N'-nitro-N-nitrosoguanidine induced gastrointestinal tumors correlates with thiol distribution. *Carcinogenesis*, 4, 879–83.

Zaidi, N.H., O'Connor, P.J., and Butler, W.H. (1993). N-methyl-N'-nitro-N-nitrosoguanidine-induced carcinogenesis: differential pattern of upper gastrointestinal tract tumors in Wistar rats after single or chronic oral doses. Carcinogenesis, 14, 1561–7.

6

Multiple genetic alterations in gastric cancer

Atsushi Ochiai and Setsuo Hirohashi

1. INTRODUCTION

Recent molecular genetic studies have established that most human tumors display multiple genetic alterations (Marx 1989). These alterations are considered to underlie the multistage process of carcinogenesis and tumor progression, although in most cases the precise sequence of the genetic events remains unclear. The genetic changes associated with the development of colorectal carcinomas have been well characterized by Vogelstein and his co-workers (Fearon and Vogelstein 1990; Fearon *et al.* 1990; Vogelstein *et al.* 1988; Baker *et al.* 1989. These changes include loss of heterozygosity (LOH) of chromosome 5q, on which tumor-suppressor genes *APC* and *MCC* (mutated in colon cancer) are located, mutation of c-Ki-*ras*, and LOH of chromosomes 17p and 18q, which carry the tumor-suppressor genes p53 and *DCC* (deleted in colon cancer), respectively.

In early studies, the incidence of genetic alterations detected in gastric cancers was low probably because of heavy contamination of non-cancerous cells in tissue samples for DNA extraction (Hirohashi and Sugimura 1991). However, with the application of more refined molecular genetic techniques, it has recently become clear that gastric carcinoma also displays multiple genetic alterations. These alterations include oncogenes, tumor-suppressor genes, and chromosomal LOH. As a novel mechanism for carcinogenesis, a genome-wide tendency to replication errors was recently found in a subset of colorectal carcinomas especially in those of hereditary non-polyposis colorectal carcinoma (HNPCC) patients (Aaltonen *et al.* 1993; Peltomaeki *et al.* 1993). A heritable susceptibility also may be involved in gastric carcinogenesis, and the presence of DNA replication error (RER) as representing genetic instability was recently reported in gastric cancer using microsatellite probes. Microsatellite alterations containing RER and LOH have been detected in some adenomas and adenocarcinomas of the stomach (Tamura *et al.* 1995).

2. ONCOGENES

2.1. The *ras* family

The members of *ras* oncogene family (c-Ha-*ras* located on chromosome 11p, c-Ki-*ras* on chromosome 12p, and N-*ras* on chromosome 1p) were first detected in human cancers as transforming genes in transfection assay using NIH/3T3 cells (Land *et al.* 1983). These genes, encoding closely related 21 kDa proteins, are highly conserved among species (Barbacid 1987). The *ras* protein binds guanine nucleotides with high affinity and serves as a transducer molecule for signals regulating cell proliferation and differentiation (Barbacid 1987). Amplification of c-Ki-*ras* has been reported in a few human cancers (Sukumar 1990). Mutations at codon 12, 13, and 61 amino acid positions confer transforming activity, and the point mutation of the c-Ki-*ras* oncogene has been detected at high frequency in adenocarcinoma of the colon, pancreas, and bile duct (Sukumar 1990). In contrast, point mutation of c-Ki-*ras* (or the other *ras* family members, c-Ha-*ras* and N-*ras*) has been found only infrequently in gastric carcinomas, even when the tumors were analysed by the highly sensitive polymerase chain reaction (PCR) (Bos *et al.* 1986; Deng 1988; Jiang *et al.* 1989; Nagata *et al.* 1990; Lee *et al.* 1995). For example, c-Ki-*ras* mutation at codon 12 was reported in 3 out of 35 cases (9%) of gastric carcinomas, and the three positive were all well-differentiated adenocarcinoma (Kihana *et al.* 1991). A few benign adenomas also have been reported to possess c-Ki-*ras* mutation (Kihana *et al.* 1991).

Studies on *ras* expression have generally shown increased p21 protein levels in carcinomas. Although the results correlating the *ras* expression with histological features or stages of progression varied in all studies, advanced carcinomas consistently showed higher frequency of *ras* immunopositivity than early stages of gastric cancers (Czerniak *et al.* 1989). The *ras* overexpression was also found in noncancerous epithelia such as dysplasia, intestinal metaplasia, and regenerating epithelium adjacent to peptic ulceration and neoplastic lesions (Czerniak *et al.* 1989).

2.2.   The c-*erb* B-2 gene

This gene is a v-*erb*B-related gene that encodes a growth factor receptor highly homologous to the epidermal growth factor receptor, and is localized on chromosome 17q21 (Semba *et al.* 1985; Fukushige *et al.* 1986). The protein encoded by c-*erb*B-2 is a transmembrane glycoprotein of the tyrosine kinase family with a molecular weight of 185 kDa. Amplification of the c-*erb*B-2 gene has been demonstrated in various adenocarcinomas including breast carcinomas (Tal *et al.* 1988) (Berger *et al.* 1988). A significant association between c-*erb*B-2 gene was amplification and poor prognosis, as well as lymph node metastasis has been reported. In gastric cancer, the amplification of c-*erb*B-2 gene was detected in 5 out of 13 cases of well-differentiated adenocarcinomas (intestinal-type) but undetectable in 30 cases of undifferentiated ones (diffuse-type) (Yokota *et al.* 1988). Amplification of oncogenes is usually associated with overexpression of the gene product, and overexpression of the c-*erb*B-2 gene product in some intestinal-type adenocarcinomas has been confirmed by immunohistochemical analysis (Park *et al.* 1989). The amplification/overexpression of c-*erb*B-2 gene product in the intestinal-type gastric carcinomas appears to be a marker for poor prognosis as observed in breast carcinoma (Yonemura *et al.* 1991; Uchino *et al.* 1993*a*; McCulloch *et al.* 1995; Lin *et al.* 1995).

2.3. The K-*sam* gene

This gene was originally isolated as an amplified sequence from KATO-III cell line which was derived from a diffuse-type carcinoma of the stomach (Nakatani *et al.* 1986; 1990; Hattori *et al.* 1996). The K-*sam* has been proven to be identical to human *bek* or keratinocyte growth factor (KGFR) or fibroblast growth factor receptor-2 (FGFR-2) gene and is located on chromosome 10q25 (Jaye *et al.* 1992). The KGF-binding motif and carboxyl-terminal portion has been proven to import-ant for carcinogenesis (Ishii *et al.* 1995). In gastric cancer, amplification of K-*sam* gene has been reported in 10 of 48 diffuse-type carcinoma cases compared with none of 35 intestinal-type carcinoma cases (Hattori *et al.* 1990). The amplification/ overexpression of this gene is thought to play an important role in the development of diffuse-type gastric carcinomas. Recent studies revealed that K-*sam* gene gener-ates multiple transcripts by the mechanism of alternative splicing, K-*sam* I/*bek*, and K-*sam* II/KGFR (keratinocyte growth factor receptor). Different biological activi-ties of these K-*sam* gene products (K-*sam* I/*bek* and K-*sam* II/KGFR) with different ligand-binding specificities (fibroblast growth factors and keratinocyte growth factor, respectively) were reported in gastric cancer cells (Ishii *et al.* 1994).

2.4. The *hst*/*int*-2 gene

The transfection assays with NIH-3T3 cells have been performed in several labora-tories in order to identify potential transforming genes in human gastric carcinoma. The *hst*-1 originally identified as a transforming gene from DNA samples of a gastric carcinoma and of an adjacent non-neoplastic gastric mucosa, is homologous to fibroblast growth factors, and is located on chromosome 11q13 (Sakamoto *et al.* 1986). Co-amplification of *hst*-1 gene and *int*-2 has been reported in various carci-nomas including urinary bladder carcinoma, melanoma, esophageal carcinoma, and gastric carcinoma (Yoshida *et al.* 1988). The *int*-2 is a gene implicated in mouse mammary carcinogenesis, activated by viral insertion, and located adjacent to *hst*-1 on chromosome 11. However, a recent co-amplification study showed no ampli-fication of either gene in 42 gastric adenocarcinomas while demonstrating co-amplification of both genes in 50% of esophageal carcinoma (Tsuda *et al.* 1989). In esophageal carcinomas, cyclin D, one of the G1 cyclins, is also included in the amplicon and overexpressed in cases with amplification.

2.5. The c-*met* gene

This gene was originally identified as a transforming gene of a human osteogenic sarcoma cell line (HOS) transformed with N-methyl-N'-nitro-N-nitrosoguanidine (MNNG) (Cooper *et al.* 1984). It encodes a heterodimeric transmembrane protein p190 consisting of an α and β-subunit with structural features of a tyrosine kinase receptor. The gene is located on chromosome 7q (Giordano *et al.* 1989). Hepatocyte growth factor (HGF) has been identified as a ligand for c-*met*, and it stimulates the tyrosine kinase activity of the c-*met* gene product (Bottaro *et al.* 1990). Various biological responses to HGF have been demonstrated to be all transduced by the c-*met* receptor in cell proliferation, cell movement, and cell differentiation (Montesano *et al.* 1991). HGF is expressed on both fibroblasts and epithelial cells and acts by in autocrine and pracrine mechanism (Rahimi *et al.* 1996). In gastric cancer, overexpression and amplification of c-*met* has been reported in a human gastric carcinoma cell line GTL-16 derived from poorly differentiated adenocarcinoma (Giordano *et al.* 1989). Amplification of c-*met* gene has been reported frequently in gastric carcinomas especially in diffuse-type scirrhous carcinomas, and it is closely correlated with advanced tumor stage and poor prognosis (Kuniyasu *et al.* 1992). In addition, abnormal transcript of 6.0 kb c-*met* gene has been reported to be closely associated with tumor stages (Kuniyasu *et al.* 1993).

The *tpr-met* oncogenic rearrangement was also first observed in MNNG-transformed HOS cells. The rearrangement involved the fusion of *tpr* (translocated promoter region) locus present on chromosome 1 to the 5' region of *met* gene sequences located on chromosome 7. The *tpr-met* protein, p65 *tpr-met*, induces meiotic maturation in *Xenopus* oocytes and activates maturation producing factor through a *mos*-dependent pathway (Daar *et al.* 1991). Expression of *tpr-met* was detected not only in gastric carcinomas but also in non-neoplastic mucosa of chronic gastritis (Soman *et al.* 1991).

2.6.   The c-*myc* gene

Human c-*myc* oncogene located on chromosome 8q is a cellular gene homologous to the transforming gene of avian myelocytosis virus MC29. The *myc* gene encodes a nuclear protein p62 that may have a role in transcription and cell cycle control. Overexpression of c-*myc* detected by immunohistochemistry has been reported in advanced gastric carcinomas (Yamamoto *et al.* 1987). Amplification of c-*myc* gene has been detected in some gastric carcinomas (Nakasato *et al.* 1984). In addition to c-*myc*, there have been sporadic reports on amplification of *yes, akt1, erb*B-1 in gastric carcinomas (Seki *et al.* 1985; Staal 1987; Nomura *et al.* 1986).

3 . TUMOR-SUPPRESSOR GENES

3.1.   The *APC* gene

The *APC* gene isolated as a tumor-suppressor gene for the familial adenomatous polyposis (FAP) is located at chromosome 5q21 (Joslyn *et al.* 1991; Kinzler *et al.* 1991). The *APC* gene is predicted to encode a protein of 312 kDa and the mechanism of tumor-suppressor function of this molecule has not yet been elucidated (Smith *et al.* 1993). Somatic mutations of this gene have been detected in patients with colorectal carcinoma as an early event because mutations have been detected in adenomas as small as 5 mm in diameter and the frequency of mutations has remained constant as tumors progressed from the benign to the malignant stage. The mutations of *APC* gene were detected not only in colorectal carcinomas in

FAP and sporadic patients, but also in pancreas carcinomas (Horii *et al.* 1992*a*). The vast majority of the mutations lead to truncation of the *APC* gene product. In gastric carcinomas, mutations of *APC* gene have been detected in both intestinal-type carcinomas (9/32) especially in very well-differentiated adenocarcinoma (7/17), and signet-ring cell carcinoma (3/44), which is classified as diffuse-type (Horii *et al.* 1992*b*; Nakatsuru *et al.* 1992; Tamura *et al.* 1994). The mutations of the *APC* gene have also been reported in 20% (6/30) of adenomas of the stomach (Tamura *et al.* 1994).

3.2. The *p53* gene

The p53 protein was originally identified as a protein forming a stable complex with the SV40 large T antigen. Subsequent studies made it clear that the human *p53* gene, located on chromosome 17p13, is a tumor-suppressor gene whose inactivation is suggested to be involved in carcinogenesis of various organs. Mutations of the *p53* gene are clustered at four hot spots in highly conserved regions (domains II–V) and the locations of the mutations and the types of base changes they show have been demonstrated to differ in cancers of different organs. In gastric cancers, high incidence of *p53* mutations has been reported in both early and advanced cancers (Tamura *et al.* 1991; Yokozaki *et al.* 1992; Uchino *et al.* 1993*a*; Cho *et al.* 1994). The G:C to A:T transitions at CpG sites, which were reported as frequent mutation patterns in colorectal cancer, are also frequent in gastric carcinomas. The mutation of *p53* is accompanied by simultaneous loss of heterozygosity of chromosome 17p in many cancers.

Accumulation of the p53 protein in the cell nucleus can be taken as evidence for the presence of a mutated *p53* allele, since the mutant protein has a longer half-life than the wild-type protein. Nuclear accumulation of p53 protein was more frequently observed in intestinal-type carcinoma 44/101 (43%) than in diffuse-type adenocarcinoma 2/48 (4%) (Uchino *et al.* 1992). This result suggests that *p53* mutations play a significant role in the development of gastric carcinomas of intestinal type. The *p53* mutations were also detected at the earliest stages of gastric carcinogenesis such as gastric dysplasia and chronic atrophic gastritis with intestinal metaplasia (Shiao *et al.* 1994; Ochiai *et al.* 1996).

4. LOSS OF HETEROZYGOSITY IN CHROMOSOMES

There is growing evidence from restriction fragment length polymorphism (RFLP) analysis that most human tumors display loss of heterozygosity (LOH) of one or more chromosomes. Indeed, the incidence of this type of genetic alteration is much higher than that of oncogene activation. For example, the LOH of chromosomes 3p, 13q, and 17p has been detected in nearly 100% of small-cell lung carcinomas (Yokota *et al.* 1987). Hepatocellular carcinomas frequently exhibit LOH of chromosomes 4,16q, and 17p. LOH of 16q in these tumors is a late event, marking their progression to a less differentiated and more malignant state (Tsuda *et al.*

1990). Chromosomal LOH has also been reported in gastric cancer, as listed in Table 6.1 (Motomura *et al.* 1988; Wada *et al.* 1987, 1988). However, several RFLP analysis of gastric carcinomas have failed to detect LOH at high incidence. The exceptionally low incidence of LOH in gastric carcinoma is inconsistent with the observation that these tumors often display DNA aneuploidy and other karyotypic abnormalities. It is highly probable that previous RFLP studies underestimated the incidence of LOH in gastric carcinomas, since this method of genetic analysis is particularly sensitive to the presence of contaminating DNA from normal cells.

Chromosomal LOH in tumors is often associated with inactivation of a tumor-suppressor gene on the remaining allele. Using the combination of flow cytometric cell sorting and molecular genetic analysis, frequent LOH (87%) on chromosome 5q where tumor-suppressor genes *APC* and *MCC* (mutated in colon cancer) are located, has been reported (Tamura *et al.* 1993; McKie *et al.* 1993). LOH on both loci is considered to be one of the most prevalent alteration of gastric carcinoma. LOH on *DCC* (deleted in colon cancer) locus located on chromosome 18q was detected in 61% of gastric cancer of intestinal type (Uchino *et al.* 1992). In addition, LOH on chromosome 17p, on which p53 gene is located has also been frequently observed (42%). LOH on chromosome 18q was reported to occur at an earlier stage than LOH on chromosome 17p in gastric carcinogenesis and progression (Uchino *et al.* 1992).

5. GENETIC INSTABILITY

Genetic alterations in simple repeated sequences constitute a newly recognized class of human mutations causing disease. These regions are genetically unstable and susceptible to replication error (RER) as judged by their unusually high mutation rates *in vivo* and *in vitro*, and by their highly polymorphic nature in the human population. The genetic instability, due to error during replication/repair by strand misalignment, correlates with tumorigenesis in colorectal and other carcinomas that developed in affected members of HNPCC families (Peltomaeki *et al.* 1993; Lothe *et al.* 1993). Gastric carcinoma frequently occur in cancer family syndrome and in HNPCC. RER abnormality examined by microsatellite probes reported in gastric cancer were 18% in Finland and 39% in Japan. In addition, RER positive cases were more frequent in diffuse-type carcinomas than that in intestinal-type (Peltomaeki *et al.* 1993; Tamura *et al.* 1995; Han *et al.* 1993; Horii *et al.* 1994; Mironov *et al.* 1994; Sano *et al.* 1991).

6. CONCLUSION

Evidence obtained by molecular genetic analyses of gastric carcinomas suggests that these, like other tumors, develop through multiple steps accumulating multiple genetic alterations. First, some genetic changes occur in the gastric mucosa showing

Table 6.1. Alterations of oncogenes, tumor-suppressor genes, and chromosomes in gastric cancers

Oncogenes
1. *ras* family
   Ki-*ras* mutation at codon 12 and 13   Kihana *et al.* (1991)
   Ha-*ras* mutation at codon 12   Deng (1988)
   Overexpression of *ras* p21   Czerniak *et al.* (1989)
2. c-*erb*B-2
   Amplification   Yokota *et al.* (1988);
                                                                    Park *et al.* (1989)

   Rearrangement   Yokota *et al.* (1988)
   Overexpression   Park *et al.* (1989);
                                                                    Uchino *et al.* (1993*b*)

3. K-*sam*
   Amplification   Nakatani *et al.* (1986);
                                                                    Nakatani *et al.* (1990);
                                                                    Hattori *et al.* (1990)

4. *hst/int*-2
   Transforming activity   Sakamoto *et al.* (1986);
                                                                    Tsuda *et al.* (1989)

5. c-*met*
   Amplification   Kuniyasu *et al.* (1992)
   Aberrant expression of 6.0 kb c-*met* mRNA   Kuniyasu *et al.* (1993)
   Rearrangement *tpr-met*   Soman *et al.* (1991)
6. c-*myc*
   Amplification   Montesano *et al.* (1991);
                                                                    Bottaro *et al.* (1990)

Tumor-suppressor genes
1. *APC*
   Mutation (somatic mutation)   Horii *et al.* (1992*a,b*);
                                                                    Nakatsuru *et al.* (1992)

2. p53
   Mutation   Yokozaki *et al.* (1992);
                                                                    Uchino *et al.* (1993*a*)

   Nuclear accumulation of p53 gene product   Uchino *et al.* (1992).

Loss of heterozygosity of chromosomes
   1p   Sano *et al.* (1991)
   5q   Tamura *et al.* (1993)
   7q   Sano *et al.* (1991)
   12q   Sano *et al.* (1991)
   13q   Wada *et al.* (1988)
   17p   Sano *et al.* (1991)
   18q   McKie *et al.* (1993)
   Y   Wada *et al.* (1987)

Genomic instability
   Replication error (RER) examined by microsatellite probes   Han *et al.* (1993);
                                                                    Horii *et al.* (1994);
                                                                    Mironov *et al.* (1994)

chronic atrophic gastritis or intestinal metaplasia as the earliest change. Those epithelial cells with genetic alterations, if acquiring advantages in growth and/or genetic instability, will expand clonally and accumulate additional mutations, leading to early carcinoma, a locally aggressive tumor, and finally, to an advanced tumor with metastatic ability.

The data accumulated on genetic alterations in gastric cancer also indicate that these multiple steps of gastric carcinogenesis differ in two histological subtypes of gastric cancer: intestinal and diffuse. Intestinal-type gastric cancer, which associated intestinal metaplasia in the vicinity of the tumor, may have a similar carcinogenic pathway as that of colorectal cancer, since these two cancers share mutations of *ras*, p53 gene, *APC* gene, and LOH of chromosomes 5q, 17p, and 18q. On the other hand, genetic changes in the early stage of diffuse-type gastric cancer has not yet been elucidated, and amplification of the K-*sam* gene and c-*met* gene has only been detected in advanced gastric cancer of this type.

The genetic alterations discussed here undoubtedly play important roles in the multistage progression of gastric carcinomas. Studies are needed to clarify the genetic alterations in the early stages of gastric carcinogenesis in order to discover the risk factors and the mechanism of genetic susceptibility. Elucidation of these multiple genetic alterations in gastric carcinogenesis will clarify differences of the natural history of gastric cancers of both intestinal- and diffuse-type, and should provide important information for gastric cancer prevention.

References

Aaltonen, L.A., Peltomaeki, P., Leach, F.S., Sistonen, P., Pylkkaenen, L., Mecklin, J.-P., *et al.* (1993). Clues to the pathogenesis of familial colorectal cancer. *Science*, 260, 812–16.

Baker, S., Fearon, E., Nigro, J., Hamilton, S., Preisinger, A., Jessup, J., *et al.* (1989). Chromosome 17 deletions and p53 gene mutations in colorectal carcinomas. *Science*, 244, 217–21.

Barbacid, M. (1987). *ras* genes. *Ann. Rev. Biochem.*, 561, 779–827.

Berger, M.S., Locher, G.W., Saurer, S., Gullick, W.J., Waterfield, M.D., Groner, B., *et al.* (1988). Correlation of c-*erb* B-2 gene amplification and protein expression in human breast carcinoma with nodal status and nuclear grading. *Cancer Res.*, 48, 1238–43.

Bos, J.L., Varis, M.V.-d., Marshall, C.J., Veeneman, G.H., Boom, J.H. v., and Eb, A.J. v. d. (1986). A human gastric carcinoma contains a single mutated and an amplified normal allele of the Ki-*ras* oncogene. *Nucleic Acids Res.*, 14, 1209–17.

Bottaro, D.P., Rubin, J.S., Faletto, D.L., Chan, A.M.-L., Kmiecik, T.E., Woude, G.F.V., *et al.* (1990). Identification of the hepatocyte growth factor receptor as the c-*met* proto-oncogene product. *Science*, 251, 802–4.

Cho, J.-H., Noguchi, M., Ochiai, A., Uchino, S., and Hirohashi, S. (1994). Analysis of regional differences of p53 mutation in advanced gastric carcinoma: relation to heterogeneous differentiation and invasiveness. *Modern Pathol.*, 7, 205–11.

Cooper, C.S., Park, M., Blair, D.G., Tainsky, M.A., Huebner, K., Croce, C.M., *et al.* (1984). Molecular cloning of a new transforming gene from a chemically transformed human cell line. *Nature*, 311, 29–34.

Czerniak, B., Herz, F., Gorczyca, W., and Koss, L.G. (1989). Expression of *ras* oncogene p21 protein in early gastric carcinoma and adjacent gastric epithelia. *Cancer*, **64**, 1467–73.

Daar, I.O., White, G.A., Schuh, S.M., Ferris, D.K., and Van de Woude, G.F. (1991). *tpr-met* oncogene product induces maturation-producing factor activation in *Xenopus* oocytes. *Mol. Cell Biol.*, **11**, 5985–91.

Deng, G. (1988). A sensitive non-radioactive PCR-RFLP analysis for detecting point mutations at 12th codon of oncogene c-Ha-*ras* in DNAs of gastric cancer. *Nucleic Acid Res.*, **16**, 6231.

Fearon, E.R. and Vogelstein, B. (1990). A genetic model for colorectal tumorigenesis. *Cell*, **61**, 759–67.

Fearon, E.R., Cho, K.R., Nigro, J.M., Kern, S.E., Simons, J.W., Ruppert, J., *et al.* (1990). Identification of a chromosome 18q gene that is altered in colorectal cancers. *Science*, **247**, 49–56.

Fukushige, S., Matsubara, K., Yoshida, M., Sasaki, M., Suzuki, T., Semba, K., *et al.* (1986). Localization of a novel v-*erb*B-related gene, c-*erb*B-2, on human chromosome 17 and its amplification in a gastric cancer cell line. *Mol. Cell. Biol.*, **6**, 955–8.

Giordano, S., Ponzetto, C., Renzo, M.F.D., Cooper, C.S., and Comoglio, P.M. (1989). Tyrosine kinase receptor indistinguishable from the c-*met* protein. *Nature*, **339**, 155–6.

Han, H.-J., Yanagisawa, A., Kato, Y., Park, J.-G., and Nakamura, Y. (1993). Genetic instability in pancreatic cancer and poorly differentiated type of gastric cancer. *Cancer Res.*, **53**, 5087–9.

Hattori, Y., Odagiri, H., Nakatani, H., Miyagawa, K., Naito, K., Sakamoto, H., *et al.* (1990). K-*sam*, an amplified gene in stomach cancer, is a member of the heparin-binding growth factor receptor genes. *Proc. Natl. Acad. Sci. USA*, **87**, 5983–7.

Hattori, Y., Itoh, H., Uchino, S., Ino, Y., Ochiai, A., Ishii, H., *et al.* (1996). K-sam expression in undifferentiated type of stomach cancer correlates with poor prognosis. *Clinical Cancer Res.*, **2**, 1373–81.

Hirohashi, S. and Sugimura, T. (1991). Genetic alterations in human gastric cancer. *Cancer Cells*, **3**, 49–52.

Horii, A., Nakatsuru, S., Miyoahi, Y., Ichii, S., Nagase, H., Ando, H., *et al.* (1992*a*). Frequent somatic mutations of the *APC* gene in human pancreatic cancer. *Cancer Res.*, **52**, 6696–8.

Horii, A., Nakatsuru, S., Miyoshi, Y., Ichii, S., Nagase, H., Kato, Y., *et al.* (1992*b*). The *APC* gene, responsible for familial adenomatous polyposis, is mutated in human gastric cancer. *Cancer Res.*, **52**, 3231–3.

Horii, A., Han, H.-J., Shimada, M., Yanagisawa, A., Kato, Y., Ohta, H., *et al.* (1994). Frequent replication errors at microsatellite loci in tumors of patients with multiple primary cancers. *Cancer Res.*, **54**, 3373–5.

Ishii, H., Hattori, Y., Itoh, H., Kishi, T., Yoshida, T., Sakamoto, H., *et al.* (1994). Preferential expression of the third immunoglobulin-like domain of K-*sam* product provides keratinocyte growth factor-dependent growth in carcinoma cell lines. *Cancer Res.*, **54**, 518–22.

Ishii, H., Yoshida, T., Oh, H., Yoshida, S., and Terada, M. (1995). A truncated K-sam product lacking the distal carboxyl-terminal portion provides a reduced level of autophosphorylation and greater resistance against induction of differentiation. *Mol. Cell Biol.*, **15**, 3664–71.

Jaye, M., Schlessinger, J., and Dionne, C.A. (1992). Fibroblast growth factor receptor tyrosne kinase: molecular analysis and signal transduction. *Biochim. Biophys. Acta*, **1135**, 185–99.

Jiang, W., Kahn, S.M., Guillem, J.G., Lu, S.-H., and Weinstein, I.B. (1989). Rapid detection of *ras* oncogenes in human tumors: applications to colon, esophageal, and gastric cancer. *Oncogene*, **4**, 923–928.

Joslyn, G., Carlson, M., Thliverris, A., Albertsen, H., Gelbert, L., Samowits, W., *et al.* (1991). Identification of deletion mutations and three new genes at the familial polyposis locus. *Cell*, **66**, 601–13.

Kihana, T., Tsuda, H., Hirota, T., Shimosato, Y., Sakamoto, H., Terada, M., *et al.* (1991). Point mutation of c-Ki-*ras* oncogene in gastric adenoma and adenocarcinoma with tubular differentiation. *Jpn. J. Cancer Res.*, **82**, 308–14.

Kinzler, K.W., Nilbert, M.C., Su, L.-K., Vogelstein, B., Bryan, T.M., Levy, D.B., *et al.* (1991). Identification of FAP locus genes from chromosome 5q21. *Science*, **253**, 661–5.

Kuniyasu, H., Yasui, W., Kitadai, Y., Yokozaki, H., Ito, H., and Tahara, E. (1992). Frequent amplification of the c-*met* gene in scirrhous type stomach cancer. *Biochem. Biophys. Res. Commun.*, **189**, 227–32.

Kuniyasu, H., Yasui, W., Yokozaki, H., Kitadai, Y., and Tahara, E. (1993). Aberrant expression of c-*met* mRNA in human gastric carcinomas. *Int. J. Cancer*, **55**, 72–5.

Land, H., Parada, L.F., and Weinberg, R.A. (1983). Cellular oncogenes and multistep carcinogenesis. *Science*, **222**, 771–8.

Lee, K.H., Lee, J.S., Suh, C., Kim, S.W., Kim, S.B., Lee, H.H., *et al.* (1995). Clinicopathologic significance of the K-ras gene codon 12 point mutation in stomach cancer. An analysis of 140 cases. *Cancer*, **75**, 2794–801.

Lin, J.T., Wu, M.S., Shun, C.T., Lee, W.J., Sheu, J.C., and Wang, T.H. (1995). Occurrence of microsatellite instability in gastric carcinoma is associated with enhanced exression of erbB-2 oncoprotein. *Cancer Res.*, **55**, 1428–30.

Lothe, R.A., Peltomaeki, P., Meling, G.I., Aaltonen, L.A., Nystroem-Lahti, M., *et al.* (1993). Genomic instability in colorectal cancer: relationship to clinicopathological variables and family history. *Cancer Res.*, **53**, 5849–52.

Marx, J. (1989). Many gene changes found in cancer. *Science*, **246**, 1386–88.

McCulloch, P.G., Ochiai, A., O'Dowd, G.M., Nash, H.R.G., Sasako, M., and Hirohashi S. (1995). Comparison of the molecular genetics of stomach cancers in Britain and Japan: cerbB-2 and p53. *Cancer*, **75**, 920–5.

McKie, A.B., Filipe, I.M., and Lenoine, N.R. (1993). Abnormalities affecting the *APC* and *MCC* tumor suppressor gene loci on chromosome 5q occur frequently in gastric cancer but not in pancreatic cancer. *Int. J. Cancer*, **55**, 598–603.

Mironov, N.M., Aguelon, M.A.-M., Potapova, G.I., Omori, Y., Gorbunov, O.V., Klimenkov, A.A., *et al.* (1994). Alterations of (CA)n DNA repeats and tumor suppressor genes in human gastric cancer. *Cancer Res.*, **54**, 41–4.

Montesano, R., Matsumoto, K., Nakamura, T., and Orci, L. (1991). Idenification of a fibroblast-deribed epithelial morphogen as hepatocyte growth factor. *Cell*, **67**, 901–8.

Motomura, K., Nishisho, I., Takai, S., Tateishi, H., Okazaki, M., Yamamoto, M., *et al.* (1988). Loss of alleles at loci on chromosome 13 in human primary gastric cancers. *Genomics*, **2**, 180–4.

Nagata, Y., Abe, M., Kobayashi, K., Yoshida, K., Ishibashi, T., and Naoe, T. (1990). Glycine to aspartic acid mutaions at codon 13 of the c-Ki-*ras* gene in human gastro-intestinal cancers. *Cancer Res.*, **50**, 480–2.

Nakasato, F., Sakamoto, H., Mori, M., Hayashi, K., Shimosato, Y., Nishi, M., *et al.* (1984). Amplification of the c-*myc* oncogene in human stomach cancers. *Gann*, **74**, 732–42.

Nakatani, H., Tahara, E., Yoshida, T., Sakamoto, H., Suzuki, T., Watanabe, H. *et al.* (1986). Detection of amplified DNA sequences in gastric cancers by a DNA renaturation method in gel. *Jpn. J. Cancer Res.*, **81**, 849–53.

Nakatani, H., Sakamoto, H., Yoshida, T., Yokota, J., Tahara, E., Sugimura, T., *et al.* (1990). Isolation of an amplified DNA sequence in stomach cancer. *Jpn. J. Cancer Res.*, **81**, 707–10.

Nakatsuru, S., Yanagisawa, A., Ichii, S., Tahara, E., Kato, Y., Nakamura, Y., *et al.* (1992). Somatic mutations of the *APC* gene in gastric cancer: frequent mutations in very well differentiated adenocarcinoma and signet-ring cell carcinoma. *Human Mol. Genet.*, **1**, 559–63.

Nomura, N., Yamamoto, T., Toyoshima, K., Ohami, H., Akimura, K., Sasaki, S., *et al.* (1986). DNA amplification of the c-*myc* and c-*erb*B-1 gene in a human stomach cancer. *Jpn. J. Cancer Res.*, **77**, 1188–92.

Ochiai, A., Yamauchi, U., and Hirohashi, S. (1996). p53 mutations in the non-neoplastic mucosa of the human stomach showing intestinal metaplasia. *Int. J. Cancer*, **69**, 28–33.

Park, J.-B., Rhim, J.S., Park, S.-C., Kimm, S.-W., and Kraus, M.H. (1989). Amplification, overexpression, and rearrangement of the *erb*B-2 protooncogene in primary human stomach carcinomas. *Cancer Res.*, **49**, 6605–9.

Peltomaeki, P., Lothe, R.A., Aaltonen, L.A., Pylkkaenen, L., Nystroem-Lahti, M., Seruca, R. *et al.* (1993). Microsatellite instability is associated with tumors that characterize the hereditary non-polyposis colorectal carcinoma syndrome. *Cancer Res.*, **53**, 5853–55.

Rahimi, N., Tremblay, E., McAdam, L., Park, M., Schwall, R., and Elliott, B. (1996). Identification of a hepatocyte growth factor autocrine loop in a murine mannary carcinoma. *Cell Growth and Differentiation*, **7**, 263–70.

Sakamoto, H., Mori, M., Taira, M., Yoshida, T., Matsukawa, S., Shimizu, K., *et al.* (1986). Transforming gene from human stomach cancers and a noncancerous protein of stomach mucosa. *Proc. Natl. Acad. Sci. USA*, **83**, 3997–4001.

Sano, T., Tsujino, T., Yoshida, K., Nakayama, H., Haruma, K., Ito, H., *et al.* (1991). Frequent loss of heterozygosity on chromosomes 1q, 5q, and 17p in human gastric carcinomas. *Cancer Res.*, **51**, 2926–31.

Seki, T., Fujii, G., Mori, S., Tamaoki, N., and Shibuya, M. (1985). Amplification of c-*yes*-1 proto-oncogene in a primary human gastric cancer. *Jpn. J. Cancer Res. (Gann)*, **76**, 907–10.

Semba, K., Kamata, N., Toyoshima, K., and Yamamoto, T. (1985). v-*erb*-related protooncogene, c-*erb*B-2, is distinct from the c-*erb*B-1/epidermal growth factor receptor gene and is amplified in a human salivary gland adenocarcinoma. *Proc. Natl. Acad. Sci. USA*, **82**, 6497–501.

Shiao, Y.-H., Rugge, M., Correa, P., Lehmann, P.H., and Scheer, D.W. (1994). p53 alteration in gastric precancerous lesions. *Am. J. Pathol.*, **144**, 511–17.

Smith, K.J., Johnson, K.A., Bryan, T.M., Hill, D.E., Markowits, S., Willson, J.K.V., *et al.* (1993). The *APC* gene product in normal and tumor cells. *Proc. Natl. Acad. Sci. USA*, **90**, 2846–50.

Soman, N.R., Correa, P., Ruiz, B.A., and Wogan, G.N. (1991). The *TPR-MET* oncogenic rearrangement is present and expressed in human gastric carcinoma and precursor lesions. *Proc. Natl. Acad. Sci. USA*, **88**, 4892–6.

Staal, S.P. (1987). Molecular cloning of the *akt* oncogene and its human homologues *AKT*1 and *AKT*2: amplification of *AKT*1 in a primary human gastric adenocaarcinoma. *Proc. Natl. Acad. Sci. USA*, **84**, 5034–7.

Sukumar, S. (1990). An experimental analysis of cancer: role of as oncogenes in multistep carcinogenesis. *Cancer Cells*, **2**, 199–244.

Tal, M., Wetzer, M., Josephberg, Z., Deutch, A., Gutman, M., Assaf, D., *et al.* (1988). Sporadic amplification of the *HER/neu* protooncogene in adenocarcinomas of various tissues. *Cancer Res.*, **48**, 1517–20.

Tamura, G., Kihana, T., Nomura, K., Terada, M., Sugimura, T., and Hirohashi, S. (1991). Detection of frequent p53 gene mutations in primary gastric cancer by cell sorting and polymerase chain reaction single-strand conformation polymorphism analysis. *Cancer Res.*, **51**, 3056–8.

Tamura, G., Maesawa, C., Suzuki, Y., Ogasawara, S., Terashima, M., Saito, K., *et al.* (1993). Primary gastric carcinoma cells frequently lose heterozygosity at the *APC* and *MCC* genetic loci. *Jpn. J. Cancer Res.*, **84**, 1015–18.

Tamura, G., Maesawa, C., Suzuki, Y., Tamada, H., Satoh, M., Ogasawara, S., *et al.* (1994). Mutations of the *APC* gene occur during early stages of gastric adenoma development. *Cancer Res.*, **54**, 1149–51.

Tamura, G., Sakat, K., Maesawa, C., Suzuki, Y., Terashima, M., Satoh, K., *et al.* (1995). Microsatellite alterations in adenoma and differentiated adenocarcinoma of the stomach. *Cancer Res.*, **55**, 1933–6.

Tsuda, T., Tahara, E., Kajiyama, G., Sakamoto, H., Terada, M., and Sugimura, T. (1989). High incidence of coamplification of *hst*-1 and *int*-2 genes in human esophageal carcinomas. *Cancer Res.*, **49**, 5505–8.

Tsuda, H., Zhang, W., Shimosato, Y., Yokota, J., Terada, M., Sugimura, T., *et al.* (1990). Allele loss on chromosome 16 associated with progression of human hepatocellular carcinoma. *Proc. Natl. Acad. Sci. USA*, **87**, 6791–4.

Uchino, S., Noguchi, M., Hirota, T., Itabashi, M., Saito, T., Kobayashi, M., *et al.* (1992). High incidence of nuclear accumulation of p53 protein in gastric cancer. *Jpn. J. Clin. Oncol.*, **22**, 225–31.

Uchino, S., Tsuda, H., Noguchi, M., Yokota, J., Terada, N., Saito, T., *et al.* (1992). Frequent loss of heterozygosity at the *DCC* locus in gastric cancer. *Cancer Res.*, **52**, 3099–102.

Uchino, S., Noguchi, M., Ochiai, A., Saito, T., Kobayashi, M., and Hirohashi, S. (1993*a*). p53 mutation in gastric cancer: a genetic model for carcinogenesis is common to gastric and colorectal cancer. *Int. J. Cancer*, **54**, 759–64.

Uchino, S., Tsuda, H., Maruyama, K., Kinoshita, T., Sasako, M., Saito, T., *et al.* (1993*b*). Overexpression of c-*erb*B-2 protein in gastric cancer: its correlation with long-term survival of patients. *Cancer*, **72**, 3179–84.

Vogelstein, B., Fearon, E.R., Hamilton, S.R., Kern, S.E., Preisinger, A.C., Leppert, M., *et al.* (1988). Genetic alterations during colorectal-tumor development. *New Engl. J. Med.*, **319**, 525–32.

Wada, M., Yokota, J., Mizoguchi, M., Terada, M., and Sugimura, T. (1987). Y chromosome abnormality in human stomach and lung cancer. *Jpn. J. Cancer Res.*, **78**, 780–3.

Wada, M., Yokota, J., Mizoguchi, H., Terada, M., and Sugimura, T. (1988). Infrequent loss of chromosomal heterozygosity in human stomach cancer. *Cancer Res.*, **48**, 2988–92.

Yamamoto, T., Yasui, W., Ochiai, A., Ito, H., Abe, K., Yanaihara, N., *et al.* (1987). Immunohistochemical detection of c-*myc* oncogene product in human gastric carcinomas: expression in tumor cells and stromal cells. *Jpn. J. Cancer Res. (Gann)*, **78**, 1169–74.

Yokota, J., Wada, M., Shimosato, Y., Terada, M., and Sugimura, T. (1987). Loss of heterozygosity on chromosomes 3,13, and 17 in small-cell carcinoma and on chromosome 3 in adenocarcinoma of the lung. *Proc. Natl. Acad. Sci. USA*, **84**, 9252–6.

Yokota, J., Yamamoto, T., Miyajima, N., Toyoshima, K., Nomura, N., Sakamoto, H., *et al.* (1988). Genetic alterations of the c-*erb*B-2 oncogene occur frequently in tubular adenocarcinoma of the stomach and often accompained by amplification of the v-*erb*A homoloque. *Oncogene*, **2**, 283–7.

Yokozaki, H., Kuniyasu, K., Kitadai, Y., Nishimura, K., Todo, H., Ayhan, A., *et al.* (1992). P53 point mutations in primary human gastric carcinomas. *Cancer Res. Clin. Oncol.*, **119**, 67–70.

Yonemura, Y., Ninomiya, I., Yamaguchi, A., Fushida, S., Kimura, H., Ohoyama, S., *et al.* (1991). Evaluation of immunoreactivity for *erb*B-2 protein as a marker of poor short term prognosis in gastric cancer. *Cancer Res.*, **52**, 1034–8.

Yoshida, M., Wada, C., Satoh, H., Yoshida, T., Sakamoto, H., Miyagawa, K., *et al.* (1988). Human *HST*1 (*HSTF*1) gene maps to chromosome band 11q13 and coamplifies with the *INT*2 gene in human cancer. *Proc. Natl. Acad. Sci. USA*, **85**, 4861–4.

7

Cell growth regulation and cancer: stromal interaction

Eiichi Tahara

1. INTRODUCTION

Gastric cancer exhibits aberrant expression or genetic alterations of multiple growth factor/receptors, gut hormones, and cytokines which confer growth autonomy or cell death on tumor cells themselves by autocrine, paracrine, and juxtacrine mechanisms (Tahara 1990). Some proto-oncogenes encode directly for growth factor/receptors and protein kinases in signal transduction system. Interestingly, genetic changes in proto-oncogenes encoding tyrosine kinase receptors, such as K-*sam* and c-*erb*B-2, differ depending on the histological types of gastric cancers (Tahara *et al.* 1993). The development of tumor progression and invasion requires the accumulation and interaction of multiple growth factor expression. Moreover, growth factors and cytokines produced by tumor cells of gastric cancer induce the complex interaction between tumor cells and stromal cells (Tahara 1993).

This chapter focuses on the concept of autocrine and paracrine mechanisms of neoplastic cell growth and the cancer–stromal interaction through growth factors and cytokines in gastric cancer.

2. GROWTH FACTORS AND THEIR RECEPTORS

2.1. The EGF family

The EGF family of growth factors includes epidermal growth factor (EGF), transforming growth factor alpha (TGFα), amphiregulin, heparin-binding EGF (HB-EGF), *cripto*, and heregulin (Prigent and Lemoine 1992). Among them, EGF, TGFα, amphiregulin, and HB-EGF each bind to the EGF receptor, whereas heregulin binds to c-*erb*B-2 but not the EGF receptor. However, the interaction of *cripto* with the EGF receptor, c-*erb*B-2 or c-*erb*B-3 receptors has not been clarified.

TGFα and EGF receptor genes are commonly co-expressed by gastric cancer, indicating that TGFα produced by tumor cells act as a positive autocrine growth factor for gastric cancer (Tahara 1990). Overexpression of EGF is frequently associated with advanced cases of the well-differentiated adenocarcinoma. Moreover, synchronous overexpression of EGF or TGFα and EGF receptor is closely correlated with depth of tumor invasion, tumor stage, and patient prognosis (Tahara 1990).

Amphiregulin, a selected heparin-binding growth factor, of which C-terminal 10-amino acid residue has 38% and 32% homology with EGF and TGFα (Shayob *et al.* 1989), respectively, can either stimulate or inhibit cell growth through tyrosine phosphorylation of the EGF receptor depending on the concentration of amphiregulin, expression of both TGFα and EGF, and the nature of the target cells (Prigent and Lemoine 1992). Overexpression of amphiregulin is observed in most gastric carcinoma tissues and cells (Kitadai *et al.* 1993). Interestingly, amphiregulin stimulates the growth of the gastric carcinoma cell lines TMK-1 and MKN-28 cells in a dose-dependent manner, whereas amphiregulin antisense *S*-oligo induces significant growth inhibition of MKN-28 cells. Moreover, amphiregulin induces expression of mRNAs for amphiregulin itself and TGFα in both cell lines (Akagi *et al.* 1995). It is very likely that amphiregulin may act as an autocrine growth stimulator for gastric cancer as well as colon carcinoma (Johnson *et al.* 1992).

In addition to EGF/TGFα and amphiregulin, the *cripto* gene, a new member of the EGF family gene that consists of 2020 base pairs (bp) with a 564 bp open reading frame encoding a protein of 188 amino acids (Ciccoicola *et al.* 1989), is overexpressed by most well-differentiated gastric carcinomas as well as colorectal adenocarcinoma (Kuniyasu *et al.* 1991). The *cripto* protein is overexpressed in intestinal metaplasia and 38% of gastric adenomas (Kuniyasu *et al.* 1994). Moreover, a good correlation is found between overexpression of *cripto* protein in tumor cells and tumor stage or patient prognosis, suggesting that overexpression of *cripto* has implication for both the development and progression of well-differentiated gastric adenocarcinoma (Kuniyasu *et al.* 1994).

Amplification and overexpression of c-*erb*B-2 are frequently associated with well-differentiated gastric adenocarcinoma (Kameda *et al.* 1990). Overexpression of c-*erb*B-2 is associated with poor prognosis and distant metastasis. However, c-*erb*B-3 is not amplified in gastric cancer.

2.2. The TGFβ/receptor system

There are now five isoforms of TGFβ (TGFβ1–5) expressed by mammalian tissues and cells (Massague 1990). TGFβ acts as a growth inhibitor for many cells including not only normal epithelial, endothelial, neuronal, lymphoid, and hematopoietic cells but also carcinoma cells such as the colon, breast, and gastric carcinomas (Moses *et al.* 1990). Furthermore, TGFβ induces apoptotic cell death of gastric carcinoma cell line HSC-39 (Yanagihara and Tsumuraya 1992). On the other hand, overexpression of TGFβ 1 is frequently observed in gastric carcinoma tissues, particularly in poorly differentiated adenocarcinoma or scirrhous carcinoma (Yoshida *et al.* 1989).

Recent evidence indicates that TGFβ signalings may occur through heteromeric serine/threonine kinase complex of TGFβ type I and type II receptors (Massague 1992). Interestingly, over 80% of gastric carcinoma tissues show a reduction in TGFβ type I receptor that is closely correlated with the depth of tumor invasion (M. Ito *et al.* 1992*a,b*). Recently, genetic changes in the type II receptor have been found in gastric cancer cell lines that were resistant to growth inhibition of TGFβ

(Park *et al.* 1994). Moreover, the level of the TGFβ inhibitory element (TIE) binding protein also displays reduction in tumor tissues as the tumor progressed (M. Ito *et al.* 1992*b*). It is highly probable that most advanced gastric cancers escape from growth inhibition by TGFβ through reduction in the type I receptor for TGFβ.

2.3.   The FGF family of growth factors and receptors

Fibroblast growth factor (FGF) has a family of at least seven related polypeptides involving FGF1/aFGF, FGF2/bFGF, FGF3/INT2, FGF4/HST/kFGF, FGF5, FGF6, and FGF7/KGF, respectively (Partanen *et al.* 1992). FGF 7/KGF acts specifically on epithelial cells and FGF6 has implication for muscle development. Scirrhous gastric carcinoma characterized by their fibrous stroma and rapid growth is frequently associated with overexpression of bFGF, suggesting that bFGF produced by tumor cells may cause productive fibrosis and angiogenesis as a paracrine growth factor on stromal fibroblast and endothelial cells (Tanimoto *et al.* 1991). HST-1, a trans-forming gene first isolated from gastric carcinoma, is not expressed in gastric cancer even if amplified (Yoshida *et al.* 1987). Moreover, co-amplification of HST-1 and INT-2 is rare in gastric cancer, although it does occur in 50% of esophageal carcinoma (Tsuda *et al.* 1989*a*).

Three types of receptors for FGF have been identified; the tyrosine kinase type, the proteoglycan type and the cystein-rich type (CFR) almost entirely made of external cysteine-rich repeats (Partanen *et al.* 1992). The K-*sam* gene, which encodes the tyrosine kinase receptor (Hattori *et al.* 1990), is amplified preferentially in poorly differentiated gastric adenocarcinoma (Tahara 1993), especially in scirrhous gastric carcinoma. In some instances, amplification of the K-*sam* gene is found only in metastatic tumors and not in primary tumors. Overexpression of the K-*sam* protein is correlated with metastatic potential and poor prognosis. Recently, three additional K-*sam* cDNAs have been cloned, of which the types III and IV cDNAs encoded secreted receptors with or without the tyrosine kinase domain (Katoh *et al.* 1992). Although the biological significance of the secreted receptors remains to be determined, the secreted receptors may modulate the response of target cells to ligands of families, by acting as a trap for those factors or by competing with the transmembrane receptors.

2.4.   PDGF and insulin-like growth factor

Platelet-derived growth factor (PDGF), a mitogen for fibroblasts and smooth muscle cells, is comprises disulfide-bonded dimers of A- and B-chains (PDGF-AA, -AB, -BB). The PDGF B-chain is encoded by the c-*sis* gene (Westermark and Heldin 1991). All gastric carcinoma cell lines and all gastric carcinoma tissues express mRNA for the PDGF A-chain (Tsuda *et al.* 1989*b*). TMK-1 and MKN-cells also express mRNA for PDGF receptor. Moreover, overexpression of PDGF receptor mRNA is frequently associated with scirrhous gastric carcinoma (Tsuda *et al.* 1989*b*). These results indicate that the PDGF produced by tumor cells acts as an autocrine or paracrine growth factor for the production of fibrous stroma.

Insulin-like growth factors (IGF) are polypeptides which are closely related in structure to insulin, and two types have been identified IGF-I and IGF-II (Nissley and Rechler 1986). There are distinct receptors for IGF-I and IGF-II. The mitogenic effects of both IGF-I and IGF-II are mediated by the IGF-I receptor. Gastric carcinoma also expresses mRNAs for IGF-I and IGF-II (Tahara 1990). In particular, most scirrhous gastric carcinomas overexpress IGF-I and IGF-II. In these cancers, IGF-II is produced by both the tumor cells and stromal fibroblasts, while IGF-I is produced only by stromal cells. Thus, the interaction between the tumor cells and stromal cells through the IGF–receptor system may play a role in the development of scirrhous gastric carcinoma.

Above all, these *in vitro* and *in vivo* results indicate that, the development of scirrhous gastric carcinoma, which corresponds to diffusely infiltrating carcinoma or Borrmann's type IV carcinoma of the stomach, may require synchronous overexpression of TGFβ, basic FGF, PDGF, and IGF-II in the same tumor, all of which may act mainly as paracrine growth factors, resulting in extensive progression and fibrosis. In addition, scirrhous gastric carcinoma is frequently associated with amplification of the K-*sam* and c-*met* genes which occurs independently (Tahara *et al.* 1993).

2.5. The HGF/c-*met* system

Hepatocyte growth factor (HGF), a heparin-binding polypeptide, is a heterodimetric molecule composed of a 69 kDa α-subunit and a 34 kDa β-subunit, and is derived from a single-chain precursor of 728 amino acids (Nakamura *et al.* 1989). Although HGF was initially identified as a mitogen for hepatocytes, HGF is produced by stromal cells and stimulates cell growth, cell motility, and tubular formation of epithelial cells expressing c-*met* protein. Interestingly, HGF may act as a paracrine mediator of cancer–stromal interaction in progression and morphogenesis of gastric cancer (Tahara *et al.* 1993, Tahara 1993). Stromal fibroblast stimulated by TGFα, TGFβ, or IL-1α, may secrete HGF in a paracrine manner which can bind to c-*met* protein on cancer cells. If this occurs, in the case of a clone maintaining expression of E-cadherin and catenins, HGF could stimulate the growth of cancer cells and promote tubular formation, leading to well-differentiated gastric adenocarcinoma. On the other hand, in the case of a clone having diminished expression or loss of E-cadherin and catenins, HGF could cause scattering and proliferation of cancer cells, resulting in poorly differentiated gastric adenocarcinoma or scirrhous carcinoma (Tahara *et al.* 1993, Tahara 1993).

The c-*met* gene encodes receptor for HGF composed of a 50 kDa α-subunit disutide-linked to a 145 kDa β-subunit to form a 190 kDa heterodimer (Cooper *et al.* 1984). The c-*met* gene amplification is found in 23% of advanced gastric cancer but not in early gastric cancer (Kuniyasu *et al.* 1992). In particular, the c-*met* gene is amplified in about 40% of scirrhous gastric carcinomas. Alleles of five scirrhous carcinoma cell lines, including HSC-39, KATO-III, NTAS, NKPS, and HSC-43 cells, share gene amplification. Overexpression of the 7.0 kb transcript is frequently associated with well-differentiated gastric adenocarcinoma. The

6.0 kb transcript, which is expressed preferentially in gastric cancer of both cell lines and cancer tissues, is closely correlated with tumor staging and lymph node metastasis (Kuniyasu *et al.* 1993).

2.6.   Cytokines

Gastric cancer can produce not only growth factors but also cytokines including IL-1, IL-6 and IL-8. Interleukin 1 (IL-1) is expressed by most gastric carcinoma cell lines, of which TMK-1 and MKN-7 cells secrete IL-1α into the culture fluid (R. Ito *et al.* 1993). Interestingly, IL-1α functions as an autocrine growth factor to these cell lines and induces overexpression of mRNA for TGFα, EGF receptor, amphiregulin, and IL-1α itself, respectively. On the other hand, the expression of IL-1α mRNA by these cell lines is induced by either IL-1α, EGF, amphiregulin, or TGFα. IL-1α affects the expression of various cell adhesion molecules by activating lymphocyte and vascular endothelial cells, and stimulates fibroblasts, resulting in their proliferation, prostaglandin production, and collagenase secretion. Moreover, IL-1α acts as a strong trigger for HGF secretion from stromal fibroblasts (Tahara 1993). Therefore, cytokines, as well as growth factors produced by cancer cells, may not only affect autocrine or paracrine growth and motility of cancer cells themselves, but also bind to each of the receptors on stromal cells, leading to fibrosis, angiogenesis, activation of cytokine network, and suppression of T cell function. Conversely, fibroblast, endothelial cells, macrophages, and lymphocytes stimulated by tumor cells may cause the secretion of multiple growth factors and cytokines, resulting in proliferation, enhanced motility, and cell death, or necrosis of tumor cells

3.   CELL CYCLE REGULATORS

Growth factors and cytokines positively or negatively regulate cell proliferation, differentiation, and cell death, or apoptosis, by the cell cycle operated by the cyclin-dependent kinases (CDKs) and the cyclin-dependent kinase inhibitors (CDIs). Many growth factors, except for TGFβ, are linked with cyclin D which may act as a growth factor sensor promoting cell division. On the other hand, TGFβ may function as a major inhibitor of cell growth through a cyclin-CDK inhibitors, including p27, p28, and p15 (Polyak *et al.* 1994; Karp *et al.*, 1995).

   Gene abnormalities and aberrant expression of various cyclins could have a pivotal role in the pathogenesis of gastrointestinal cancers. The majority of gastric cancers display overexpression of cyclin E, which correlates well with tumor staging invasiveness and histological grade as well as with the proliferative activity measured by Ki-67 antigen and p53 expression. The cyclin E gene is amplified in 15% of primary gastric cancer, all of which reveal lymph node metastasis (Akama *et al.* 1995). One of eight gastric cancer cell lines shares gene amplification of the cyclin E and all the gastric cancer cell lines express high levels of cyclin E mRNA and abnormal proteins, even without gene amplification. However, no gene amplification of the cyclin D1 is found in any gastric and colorectal cancers. This is in contrast to observations in esophageal cancer that co-amplification of cyclin D1, together with the HST-1 and INT-2 genes, takes place in 50% of primary tumors and in 100% of metastatic tumors (Yoshida *et al.* 1994). Therefore, overexpression of cyclin E and subsequent deregulation of the cell cycle could confer the development and progression of gastric cancer.

Recently, five different CDK inhibitor genes, which are attractive candidates for new tumor suppressor genes, have been identified in mammalian cells (Karp *et al.* 1995). Among them, the MTS1 gene encoding 16 has been found to be structurally abnormal in many human malignancies (Kamb *et al.* 1994). The p16 protein binds to CDK4 and inhibits cyclin D1/CDK4 complex that phosphorylates pRb (Serrano *et al.* 1993). The MTS2 gene that is adjacent to the MTS1 gene encodes p15 which also binds directly to CDK4 and CDK6. Although loss of heterozygosity on chromosome 9p [α-interferon (IFN) locus] is found in 18% of gastric cancer, no somatic mutation of the 16 gene is detected in any of primary gastric cancer (Sakata *et al.* 1995). However, two cells (MKN-45 and HSC-39) of eight gastric cancer cell lines harbor homozygous deletion of the 16 and 15 genes, and an other three cell lines (MKN-28, MKN-74, and KATO-III), as well as MKN-45 and HSC-39 cells, have no expression of p16 protein. Rearrangement of the 15 gene is found in TMK-1 cells: p15 also resembles p27 in that the net expression of both CDK inhibitors are induced by TGFβ (Karp *et al.* 1995). Rearrangement of the 27 gene is noted in MKN-45 cells, although the expression of p27 protein is well preserved in all gastric cancer cell lines. IFNα dramatically induced expression of p27 mRNA and protein by TMK-1, indicating existence of TGFβ-independent expression of p27.

The other CDK inhibitor, p21, also known as: sdi1 (Noda *et al.* 1994)/WAF1 (El-Deitry *et al.* 1993)/Cip1 (Harper *et al.* 1993), inhibits cyclins/CDK2 kinase and is transcriptionally induced by wild-type p53 but not by mutant p53. However, induction of p21 by a p53 independent pathway has been demonstrated not only in normal tissues but also in tumor cells (Parker *et al.* 1995). In gastric cancer cell line TMK-1, TGFβ induces p21 expression and consequently suppresses CDK2 kinase activity, followed by reduction in cyclin A and phosphorylation of Rb protein (Akagi *et al.* 1996). The expression of p21 in tumor cells of gastric cancer may account for both p53-dependent and p53-independent pathways, as an inverse correlation is observed between the expression of p21 and p53 in half of gastric cancer tissues. Interestingly, the expression of p21 protein in gastric cancer correlates with tumor aggressiveness as determined by immunohistochemical analysis and invasiveness (Yasui *et al.* 1996). Although the p21 gene exhibits a codon 31 polymorphism, no mutation of the p21 gene has yet been uncovered.

4. CONCLUSION

Gastric cancer cells express a broad spectrum of growth factors and cytokines which not only serve autocrine or paracrine growth of tumor cells themselves but also organize networks between tumor and stromal cells. However, the scenario of cancer–stromal interaction differs by the two histological types, well-differentiated or intestinal-type and poorly differentiated or diffuse-type, as different genetic pathways exist for the two types of gastric cancer. The interaction between HGF from activated fibroblast and cell-adhesion molecules in the c-*met* overexpressed tumor cells may be involved in the morphogenesis of gastric cancer. Gene amplification and aberrant expression of cyclin E are frequently associated with gastric cancer and also correlated with tumor progression. Although gene alteration in the p16 and p15 genes is found in cultured gastric cancer cells, it is a rare event in primary tumors. Both p53-dependent and p53-independent expression of the p21 gene exists in gastric cancer, but no remarkable changes in the p21 gene as well as in the p27 gene have been uncovered yet. Interestingly, the expression of p21 protein correlates with tumor aggressiveness.

References

Akagi, M., Yokozaki, H., Kitadai, Y., Ito, R., Yasui, W., Haruma, K., *et al.* (1995). Expression of amphiregulin in human gastric cancer cell lines. *Cancer*, **75** (suppl.), 1460–6.

Akagi, M., Yasui, W., Akama, Y., Yokozaki, H., Tahara, H., Haruma, K., *et al.* (1996). Inhibition of cell growth by transforming growth factor β1 is associated with p53-independent induction of p21 in gastric carcinoma cells. *Jpn. J. Cancer Res.*, **87**, 377–84.

Akama, Y., Yasui, W., Yokozaki, H., Kuniyasu, H., Kitahara, K., Ishikawa, T., *et al.* (1995). Frequent amplification of the cyclin E gene in human gastric carcinomas. *Jpn. J. Cancer Res.*, **86**, 617–21.

Ciccodicola, A., Dono, R., Obici, S., Simeone, A., Zollo, M., and Persico, M.G. (1989). Molecular characterization of a gene of the EGF family expressed in undifferentiated human NTERA2 teratocarcinoma cell. *EMBO*, **8**, 1987–91.

Cooper, C.S., Blair, D.G., Oskersson, M.K., Tainsky, M.A., Eader, L.A. and Van de Woude, G.F. (1984). Characterization of human transforming genes from chemically transformed, teratocarcinoma, and pancreatic carcinoma cell lines. *Cancer Res.*, **44**, 1–10.

El-Deiry, W.S., Tokino, T., Velculescu, V.E., Levy, D.B., Parsons, R., Trent, J.M., *et al.* (1993). WAF1, a potential mediator of p53 tumor suppression. *Cell*, **75**, 817–25.

Harper, J.W., Adami, G.R., Wei, N., Keyomarsi, K., and Elledge, S.J. (1993). The p21 cdk-interacting protein cip1 is a potent inhibitor of G1 cyclin-dependent kinases. *Cell*, **75**, 805–16.

Hattori, Y., Odagiri, H., Nakatani, H., Miyagawa, K., Naito, K., Sakamoto, H., *et al.* (1990). K-*sam*, an amplified gene in stomach cancer, and is a member of the heparin-binding growth factor receptor genes. *Proc. Natl. Acad. Sci. USA*, **87**, 5983–7.

Ito, M., Yasui, W., Kyo, E., Yokozaki, H., Nakayama, H., Ito, H., *et al.* (1992*a*). Growth inhibition of transforming growth factor β on human gastric carcinoma cells: receptor and postreceptor signaling. *Cancer Res.*, **52**, 295–300.

Ito, M., Yasui, W., Nakayama, H., Yokozaki, H., Ito, H., and Tahara, E. (1992*b*). Reduced levels of transforming growth factor-beta type I receptor in human gastric carcinomas. *Jpn. J. Cancer Res.*, **83**, 86–92.

Ito, R., Kitadai, Y., Kyo, E., Yokozaki, H., Yasui, W., Yamashita, U., *et al.* (1993). Interleukin 1α acts as an autocrine growth stimulator for human gastric carcinoma cells. *Cancer Res.*, **53**, 4102–6.

Johnson, G.R., Saeki, T., Gordon, A.W., Shoyab, M., Salomon, D.S., and Stromberg, K. (1992). Autocrine action of amphiregulin in a colon carcinoma cell line and immuno-cytochemical localization of amphiregulin in human colon. *J. Cell Biol.*, **118**, 741–51.

Kamb, A., Gruis, N.A., Weaver-Feldhaus, J., Liu, Q., Harshman, K., Tavtigian, S.V., *et al.* (1994). A cell cycle regulator potentially involved in genesis of many tumor types. *Science*, **264**, 436–40.

Kameda, T., Yasui, W., Yoshida, K., Tsujino, T., Nakayama, H., Ito, M., *et al.* (1990). Expression of *ERBB2* in human gastric carcinomas: relationship between p185*ERBB2* expression and the gene amplification. *Cancer Res.*, **50**, 8002–9.

Karp, J.E. and Broder, S. (1995). Molecular foundations of cancer: new targets for intervention. *Nature Medicine*, **1**, 309–20.

Katoh, M., Hattori, Y., Sasaki, H., Tanaka, M., Sugano, K., Yazaki, Y., *et al.* (1992). K-*sam* gene encodes secreted as well as transmembrane receptor tyrosine kinase. *Proc. Natl. Acad. Sci. USA*, **89**, 2960–4.

Kitadai, Y., Yasui, W., Yokozaki, H., Kuniyasu, H., Ayhan, A., Haruma, K., *et al.* (1993). Expression of amphiregulin, a novel gene of the epidermal growth factor family, in human gastric carcinomas. *Jpn. J. Cancer Res.*, **84**, 879–84.

Kuniyasu, H., Yoshida, K., Yokozaki, H., Yasui, W., Ito, H., Toge, T., *et al.* (1991). Expression of *cripto*, a novel gene of the epidermal growth factor family, in human gastrointestinal carcinomas. *Jpn. J. Cancer Res.*, **82**, 969–73.

Kuniyasu, H., Yasui, W., Kitadai, Y., Yokozaki, H, Ito, H., and Tahara, E. (1992). Frequent amplification of the c-*met* gene in scirrhous type stomach cancer. *Biochem. Biophys. Res. Comm.*, **189**, 227–32.

Kuniyasu, H., Yasui, W., Yokozaki, H., Kitadai, Y., and Tahara, E. (1993). Aberrant expression of c-*met* mRNA in human gastric carcinomas. *Int. J. Cancer*, **55**, 72–5.

Kuniyasu, H., Yasui, W., Akama, Y., Akagi, M., Tohdo, H., Ji, Z.Q., *et al.* (1994). Expression of cripto in human gastric carcinomas: an association with tumor stage and prognosis. *J. Exp. Clin. Cancer Res.*, **13**, 151–7.

Massague, J. (1990). The transforming growth factor-β family. *Ann. Rev. Cell Biol.*, **6**, 597–641.

Massague, J. (1992). Receptors for the TGF-β family. *Cell*, **69**, 1067–70.

Moses, M.L., Yang, E.Y., and Pietenpol, J.A. (1990). TGF-β stimulation and inhibition of cell proliferation: new mechanistic insights. *Cell*, **63**, 245–7.

Nakamura, T., Nishizawa, T., Hagiya, M., Seki, T., Shimonishi, M., Sugimura, A., *et al.* (1989). Molecular cloning and expression of human hepatocyte growth factor. *Nature*, **342**, 440–3.

Nissley, S.P. and Rechler, M.M. (1986). Insulin-like growth factors: biosynthesis, receptors, and carrier protein. *Hormon. Prot. Pept.*, **12**, 127–203.

Noda, A., Ning, Y., Venable, S.F., Smith, O.M., and Smith, J.R. (1994). Cloning of senescent cell derived inhibitors of DNA synthesis using an expression screen. *Exp. Cell Res.*, **11**, 90–8.

Park, K., Kim, S.-J., *et al.* (1994). Genetic changes in TGFβ type II receptor gene in human gastric cancer cells: Correlation with sensitivity to growth inhibition by TGFβ. *Proc. Natl. Acad. Sci. USA*, **91**, 8772–6.

Parker, S.B., Eichele, G., Zhang, P., *et al.* (1995). p53-independent expression of p21[cip1] in muscle and other terminally differentiated cells. *Science*, **267**, 1024–7.

Partanen, J., Vainikka, S., Korhonen, J., Armstrong, E., and Alitalo, K. (1992). Diverse receptors for fibroblast growth factors. *Prog. Growth Factor Res.*, **4**, 69–83.

Polyak, K., Kato, J.-Y., Solomon, M.J., Sherr, C.J., Massague, J., Roberts, J.M., *et al.* (1994). p27^{kip1}, a cyclin-cdk inhibitor, links transforming growth factor-β and contact inhibition to cell cycle arrest. *Genes Develop.*, **8**, 9–22.

Prigent, S.A. and Lemoine, N.R. (1992). The type 1 (EGFR-related) family of growth factor receptors and their ligands. *Prog. Growth Factor Res.*, **4**, 1–24.

Sakata, K., Tamura, G., Maesawa, C., *et al.* (1995). Loss of heterozygosity on the short arm of chromosome 9 without p16 gene mutation in gastric carcinomas. *Jpn. J. Cancer Res.*, **86**, 333–5.

Serrano, M., Hannon, G.J., and Beach, D. (1993). A new regulatory motif in cell-cycle control causing specific inhibition of cyclin D/CDK4. *Nature (London)*, **366**, 704–7.

Shoyab, M., Plowman, G.D., McDonald, V.L., Bradley, J.G., and Todaro, G.J. (1989). Structure and function of human amphiregulin: a member of the epidermal growth factor family. *Science*, **243**, 1074–6.

Tahara, E. (1990). Growth factors and oncogenes in human gastrointestinal carcinomas. *J. Cancer Res. Clin. Oncol.*, **116**, 121–31.

Tahara, E. (1993). Molecular mechanism of stomach carcinogenesis. *J. Cancer Res. Clin. Oncol.*, **119**, 265–72.

Tahara, E., Yokozaki, H., and Yasui, W. (1993). Growth factors in Gastric Cancer. In *Gastric cancer*, (ed. M. Nishi, H. Ichikawa, T. Nakajima, K. Maruyama, and E. Tahara), pp. 209–17. Springer, Tokyo.

Tanimoto, H., Yoshida, K., Yokozaki, H., Yasui, W., Nakayama, H., Ito, H., *et al.* (1991). Expression of basic fibroblast growth factor in human gastric carcinoma. *Virchows Archiv B Cell Pathol.*, **61**, 263–7.

Tsuda, T., Tahara, E., Kajiyama, G., Sakamoto, H., Terada, M., and Sugimura, T. (1989*a*). High incidence of coamplification of *hst*-1 and *int*-2 genes in human esophageal carcinomas. *Cancer Res.*, **49**, 5505–8.

Tsuda, T., Yoshida, K., Tsujino, T., Nakayama, H., Kajiyama, G., and Tahara, E. (1989*b*). Coexpression of platelet-derived growth factor (PDGF) A-chain and PDGF receptor genes in human gastric carcinomas. *Jpn J. Cancer Res.*, **80**, 813–17.

Westermark, B. and Heldin, C.-H. (1991). Platelet-derived growth factor in autocrine transformation. *Cancer Res.*, **51**, 5087–92.

Yanagihara, K. and Tsumuraya, M. (1992). Transforming growth factor β1 induces apoptotic cell death in cultured human gastric carcinoma cells. *Cancer Res.*, **52**, 4042–5.

Yasui, W., Akama, Y., Kuniyasu, H., Yokozaki, H., Semba, S., Shimamoto, F., *et al.* (1996). Expression of cyclin-dependent kinase inhibitor p21$^{WAFI/CIPI}$ in non-neoplastic mucosa and neoplasia of the stomach: Relationship with p53 status and proliferative activity. *J. Pathology*, **180**, 120–8.

Yoshida, K., Kawami, H., Kuniyasu, H., Nishiyama, M., Yasui, W., Hirai, T., *et al.* (1994). Coamplification of cyclin D, hst-1 and int-2 genes is a good biological marker of high malignancy for human esophageal carcinomas. *Oncology Reports*, **1**, 493–6.

Yoshida, T., Miyagawa, K., Odagiri, H., Sakamoto, H., Little, P.F.R., Terada, M., *et al.* (1987). Genomic sequence of *hst*, a transforming gene encoding a protein homologous to fibroblast growth factors and the *int*-2-encoded protein. *Proc. Natl. Acad. Sci. USA*, **84**, 7305–9.

Yoshida, K., Yokozaki, H., Niimoto, M., Ito, H., Ito, M., and Tahara, E. (1989). Expression of TGF-β and procollagen type I and type III in human gastric carcinomas. *Int. J. Cancer*, **44**, 394–8.

8

Invasion and metastasis

Yae Kanai and Setsuo Hirohashi

1. INTRODUCTION

Invasion and metastasis, which are the most life-threatening potentials of malignant tumors, are considered as later but critically important steps of multistage carcinogenesis. The processes of invasion and metastasis, consist of sequential steps involving host–tumor interactions. For the formation of a metastatic nodule, cancer cells must leave the primary cancer nests, invade the surrounding host tissue, enter the circulation, lodge at the distant vascular bed, extravasate into the target organ, and proliferate, resulting in formation of the metastatic nodule (Liotta *et al.* 1991) (Fig. 8.1). Table 8.1 shows the results of investigations on molecular mechanisms for each step of invasion and metastasis. Some molecules are tentatively classified according to the predicted main steps in which they play roles (Table 8.1) and are introduced in this chapter, although each molecule may participate, in a complex fashion, in several steps of invasion and metastasis.

2. DISSOCIATION OF CANCER CELLS

2.1. E-cadherin and catenins

The first step in invasion and metastasis is the dissociation of cancer cells from cancer nests. Members of the cadherin family act as Ca^{2+}-dependent dependent adhesion molecules in the cell–cell adherens junction and participate in morphogenesis (Takeichi 1991). Firm cell–cell adhesion is established when cadherins are connected to cytoskeletal actin filaments through undercoat proteins called catenins. The suppression of E (epithelial)-cadherin activity might trigger the release of tumor cells from the primary cancer nests. In fact, *in vitro* experiments using cell lines have revealed that E-cadherin does have invasion suppressor properties: non-invasive epithelial cells acquired the ability to invade collagen gels on addition of antibodies against E-cadherin (Behrens *et al.* 1989) or plasmids encoding E-cadherin-specific antisense RNA (Vleminckx *et al.* 1991). Invasiveness of human carcinoma cell lines has been reported to be reduced by transfection with E-cadherin cDNA (Vleminckx *et al.* 1991; Frixen *et al.* 1991). *In vivo*, scattered-type undifferentiated stomach adenocarcinomas, which lacked tight intercellular adhesion, frequently showed reduced or heterogeneous expression of E-cadherin and/or α-catenin, whereas these molecules were expressed uniformly at the cell

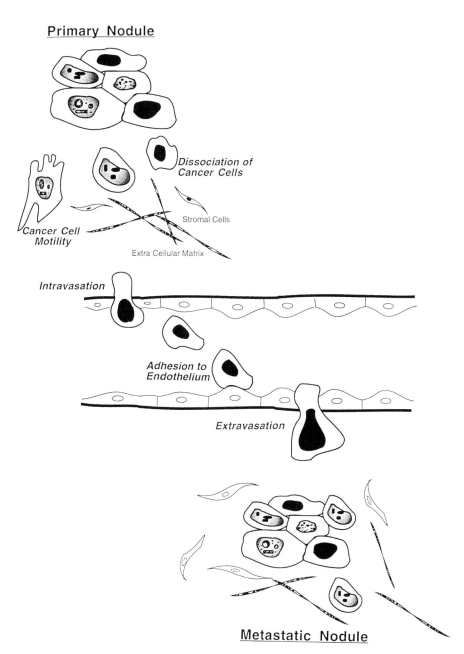

Fig. 8.1. Schematic view of stages in cancer invasion and metastasis.

Table 8.1. Molecular events in cancer invasion and metastasis

Process	Function	Molecule	Event	Study
Dissociation of cancer cells	Cell–cell adhesion	E-cadherin and catenins	Reduced expression; Gene mutation	Shimoyama & Hirohashi (1991); Ochiai et al. (1994b); Oda et al. (1994)
		DCC	Reduced expression; Deletion	Miyaki et al. (1990); Itoh et al. (1993); Uchino et al. (1992)
	Cell motility	Autocrine motility factor; Scatter factor; FGF	Overexpression	
Intravasation	Adhesion to extracellular matrix	Integrins	Reduced or overexpression	Koretz et al. (1991); Nakajima et al. (1990)
		ICAM-1	Overexpression	Staunton et al. (1988)
	Destruction of extracellular matrix	Matrix metalloproteinase; Tissue inhibitor of matrix metalloproteinase	Activation; Inactivation	Nakajima et al. (1990); Leonor et al. (1994)
		Matrix serine proteinase	Activation	Koshikawa et al. (1992)
	Neo-vascularization	FGF; VEGF	Overexpression	
Extravasation	Adhesion to endothelium and extracellular matrix	CD44	Expression of splicing variants	Wielenga et al. (1993); Heider et al. (1993); Mayer et al. (1993); Ma et al. (1993); Takahashi et al. (1994)
		Selectins and glycoproteins	Overexpression	
Proliferation in target organ	Growth factors	TGFβ; EGF		Horimoto et al. (1995); Iida et al. (1995)
	Growth factor receptors	EGFR; HGFR (*c-met*)	Aberrant expression	Kuniyasu et al. (1993); Seruca et al. (1995)
Unknown	NDP kinase	nm23	Reduced expression	Bevilacqua et al.(1989); Kodera et al. (1994)

membrane in most of the differentiated-and adherent-type stomach adenocarcinomas (Shimoyama and Hirohashi 1991; Ochiai *et al*. 1994*b*). CpG methylation of the promoter region inactivates the E-cadherin invasion-suppressor gene due to reduction of expression in human cancers (Yoshiura *et al*. 1995). In human stomach cancer cell lines, E-cadherin gene mutations resulting in mRNA splicing error caused dysfunction of E-cadherin molecules or markedly reduced expression of E-cadherin (Oda *et al*. 1994). In these cell lines, the wild-type allele of E-cadherin locus was lost, indicating that inactivation of an E-cadherin-mediated invasion suppressor system could be caused by a combination of a loss of one allele and a mutation in the remaining allele (Oda *et al*. 1994). Indeed, exon skipping-type mutation of the E-cadherin gene has been reported in surgically resected tissue from diffuse-type stomach cancer cases (Becker *et al*. 1994). Moreover, mutation of the E-cadherin gene has been detected in the intramucosal lesions of signet-ring cell carcinoma of the stomach, indicating that inactivation of the E-cadherin gene may participate in not only late events in multistage carcinogenesis, invasion and metastasis, but also in earlier developmental stages of stomach cancer (Muta *et al*. 1996). In other cell lines derived from signet-ring cell carcinoma of the stomach, homozygous deletion of a part of the β-catenin gene, resulting in the disruption of interaction between E-cadherin and α-catenin, caused the dysfunction of the cell adhesion system (Oyama *et al*. 1994). Recently, a tumor-suppressor gene product, APC protein (Rubinfeld *et al*. 1993; Su *et al*. 1993), and a oncogene product, c-*erb*B-2 protein (Ochiai *et al*. 1994*a*; Kanai *et al*. 1995), have been shown to interact with β-catenin. Further studies may elucidate the signal transduction pathways through which E-cadherin-mediated intercellular connections regulate cell growth and participate in the steps of multistage carcinogenesis.

2.2.   The DCC gene

The deleted in colorectal carcinomas (DCC) gene was identified at 18q21, where allelic deletions frequently occur in colorectal cancers, and were predicted to participate in normal cell–cell interactions because of the sequence similarity to NCAM (neural cell adhesion molecules) (Fearon *et al*. 1990). A loss of DCC gene product may also be involved in dissociation of cancer cells from cancer nests. In fact, exposure of cultured fibroblasts to DCC specific antisense RNA has been reported to inhibit cell adhesion to various extracellular matrices, providing the direct biological evidence for the possible role of DCC (Narayanan *et al*. 1992). Sixty-three per cent of examined sporadic colorectal carcinomas exhibited the loss of heterozygosity (LOH) on chromosome 18 and occurrence of LOH was closely correlated with the histopathological stage (Miyaki *et al*. 1990). Moreover, reduced expression of DCC mRNA in all examined colorectal carcinomas with liver metastasis has been reported, suggesting that the functional loss'of DCC in cancerous tissue might play a role in cancer invasion and metastasis (Itoh *et al*. 1993). As regards stomach cancer, Uchino *et al*. (1992) reported that 61% of examined intestinal-type stomach cancer cases showed LOH on chromosome 18, including the locus of the DCC gene, and proposed that the DCC gene is critically involved in the development of the majority of gastric cancers.

2.3. Cell motility factors

The potential of cancer cells to leave the primary tumor nodule might be augmented by increased cancer cell motility. AMF (autocrine motility factor), which stimulates motility of the producer cells, has been isolated and purified from the serum-free conditioned medium of human melanoma cells. Liotta *et al.* (1986) reported that AMF was produced in large amounts by three different clones of *ras* oncogene-transfected NIH3T3 cells with metastatic ability but not by the non-transfected parental cells, suggesting that AMF may play a major role in the local invasive behavior of tumor cells. AMF elicited increases in phosphoinositide metabolism via a pertussis toxin-sensitive G protein signal transduction pathway (Kohn *et al.* 1990). AMF has the possibility of acting as both a motility factor and a growth factor, thus evoking a similarity to SF (scattering factor)/HGF (hepatocyte growth factor), which exerts its function in a paracrine manner (Weidner *et al.* 1991). Aberrant expression of c-*met* mRNA-encoding HGF receptor has been reported to correlate with the clinical stage, serosal invasion, and nodal metastatic rates of stomach cancers (Kuniyasu *et al.* 1993). Other growth factors, such as acidic FGF (fibroblast growth factor), also induced human cancer cell lines to lose their cohesiveness and epithelial characteristics (Valles *et al.* 1990). Further clarification is needed for correlation between motility factors and growth factors in invasion and metastasis.

3. INTRAVASATION

3.1. Integrins

Interaction between cancer cells, which are dissociated from cancer nests, and extracellular matrices has been considered as a critical process that precedes the intravasation and metastasis to target organs (Liotta 1986). Immunoselection with antibodies that block cell adhesion and affinity chromatography with extracellular ligands have been used to isolate cell surface receptors for extracellular matrix glycoproteins such as fibronectin and vitronectin. Many of these receptors recognize sites that include the tripeptide, arginine-glycine-aspartic acid (RGD), a sequence which is common to many extracellular ligands and thought to play a key role in cell–matrix adhesion (Ruoslahti and Pierschbacher 1987). However, receptors isolated from different cell types and/or with different extracellular ligands are not identical. With a few exceptions, almost all of the receptors consist of two non-covalently linked α- and β-subunits; each subunit has a transmembrane domain, a large *N*-terminal extracellular domain and a small *C*-terminal cytoplasmic domain. Hynes (1987) named the family of cell surface glycoprotein receptors 'integrins'. Synthetic RGD peptides inhibited adhesion of malignant melanoma cells to fibronectin and metastasis to the lung in mice, indicating that integrins are involved in tumor invasion and metastasis (Humphries *et al.* 1986; Saiki *et al.* 1989). Subcutaneous injection of cancer cells with overproduction of integrins showed frequent metastasis to the liver (Takeda *et al.* 1991). On the other hand, immuno-histochemical examination showed reduced expression of α2/β1-, α6/β1-integrin (i.e. collagen and laminin receptors, respectively) in colon carcinomas with liver metastasis, when compared to normal colonic mucosa (Koretz *et al.* 1991). Therefore, either up- or down-regulation of integrins alone does not induce cancer metastasis, but the balance of integrin expression with other factors might determine the metastatic potential of cancer cells. Moreover, data on integrin-mediated signal transduction pathways are being accumulated (Juliano and Varner 1993; Sastry and Horwitz 1993). As regards stomach cancer, Fujita *et al.* (1992) reported that all of examined human gastric cancer cell lines expressed β1-subunit. Newly developed antihuman β1-subunit monoclonal antibody completely inhibited the adhesion of the cell lines to acetone-fixed lung, liver, and brain tissue and invasion of them through the artificial basement membrane in an *in vitro* invasion model. This suggests that β1-integrin plays an important role in tissue attachment, migration, and invasion of gastric cancer cells (Fujita *et al.* 1992). Involvement of β1-integrin expression in peritoneal metastasis of scirrhous gastric cancer has been suggested using a nude mice orthotopic implantation model (Yashiro *et al.* 1996). In addition, α3-integrin expression is considered to be correlated with cancer– stromal interaction in stomach cancer cases with abundant intestinal fibrosis (Boku *et al.* 1995).

3.2. Intercellular adhesion molecule-1

Intercellular adhesion molecule (ICAM-1) was isolated as a candidate of the ligand for LFA-1 (lymphocyte function-associated antigen-1), a member of the integrin family that promotes intercellular adhesion in immunological and inflammatory reactions (Marlin and Springer 1987). The amino acid sequence of ICAM-1 specified an integral membrane protein with an extracellular domain of 453 residues containing five immunoglobulin-like domains and showed the highest homology with NCAM, which also contains five immunoglobulin-like domains (Staunton *et al.* 1988). Unlike NCAM, the ICAM-1 and LFA-1 interaction is heterophilic and unusual, because it is between members of the immunoglobulin and integrin families. Since immunohistochemical examination revealed that expression of ICAM-1 was lacking in benign melanocytes and early melanomas, but detected in advanced human melanomas with increased risk of metastasis, it has been speculated that this cell adhesion molecule contributes to the development of metastasis of malignant cells (Johnson *et al.* 1989). The results of two-color flow-cytometric analysis on gastric cancer cells have been reported: all of the metastatic carcinoma cells from peritoneal effusions showed a high level expression of ICAM-1, although ICAM-1 was not detected in normal gastric mucosa but was detected in carcinoma cells from large volumes of tumor located in the stomach (Koyama *et al.* 1992).

3.3. Matrix metalloproteinase, tissue inhibitor of metalloproteinase, and matrix serine proteinase

Matrix proteinases, which can be divided into two groups, metalloproteinase and serine proteinase, are other key factors in cancer cell–host tissue interaction. MMP (matrix metalloproteinase)-2 (i.e. 72 kDa type IV collagenase), was purified as an enzyme, which was secreted by highly metastatic mouse sarcoma cells and degraded the main constituent of basement membrane type IV collagen (Salo *et al.* 1983; Collier *et al.* 1988). *In vivo*, MMP-2 was reported to be expressed mainly in stromal cells of lung carcinomas (Soini *et al.* 1993). The 92 kDa type IV collagenase, MMP-9, has also been isolated from SV40-transformed human lung fibroblasts (Wilhelm *et al.* 1989). MMP-9 activity correlated with metastatic potentials of cancer cells in metastatic models both *in vivo* and *in vitro* (Nakajima *et al.* 1990). In clinical cases of stomach cancers, expression of type IV collagenase has been examined immuno-histochemically. However, significant correlation between MMP expression and clin-icopathological factors has not yet been elucidated (Leonor *et al.* 1994). MMPs are secreted as inactive precursors and activated in invasive tumor tissue as a result of proteolysis. Recently, cDNA cloning of a new matrix metalloproteinase, which was expressed on the surface of invasive tumor cells and activated the precursor of MMP-2, has been performed (Sato *et al.* 1994). On the other hand, combination effects of TIMPs (tissue inhibitor of metalloproteinases) are also essential for control of MMP activity. To date, TIMP-1, -2, and -3 have been purified and cloned (Docherty *et al.* 1985; Stetler-Stevenson *et al.* 1989; Yang and Hawkes 1992). Mouse 3T3 cell lines transfected with TIMP-specific antisense RNA were invasive in a human amnion invasion assay and tumorigenic and metastatic in athymic mouse (Khokha *et al.* 1989). TIMP-1 cDNA transfection reduced the invasion of murine melanoma cells in a matrigel transwell invasion assay (Khokha *et al.* 1992). Although MMP and TIMP have been rather well studied with respect to cancer invasion and metastasis, some stomach cancer cell lines secrete not MMP but MSP (matrix serine proteinase), indi-cating the possible involvement of MSP in the destruction of extracellular matrices by stomach cancer cells (Koshikawa *et al.* 1992).

3.4. Angiogenetic factors

Newly developed tumor vessels are frequent sites for tumor cell entry into the cir-culation (Liotta *et al.* 1991). The well-known serine proteinase, urokinase, and its inhibitor PAI (plasminogen activator inhibitor)-1, have been considered to play a role in physiological and tumor- induced angiogenesis (Bacharach *et al.* 1992). Moreover, acidic (Gimenez-Gallego *et al.* 1985) and basic (Esch *et al.* 1985) FGF have been purified, and their powerful angiogenic effects have been demonstrated. VEGF (vascular endothelial growth factor, Leung *et al.* 1989)/VPF (vascular per-meability factor, Senger *et al.* 1983), another heparin-binding growth factor, is not only able to induce angiogenesis but also to increase vascular permeability resulting in an accumulation of ascites *in vivo*. However, further evaluation is necessary for the contribution of these molecules in the development of human cancers.

4. EXTRAVASATION

4.1. CD44

For the extravasation in the target organ, cancer cells must lodge on endothelial cells and adhere to extracellular matrices of host tissues. CD44 was first purified as receptor that was involved in the tissue-specific homing of lymphocytes (Jalkanen *et al.* 1987). Although CD44 showed molecular variation because of a different splicing and glycosylation pattern, a standard type was an 85 kDa protein and its cDNA cloning revealed that the core of CD44 was an 37 kDa membrane-spanning protein (Stamenkovic *et al.* 1989). CD44 was not only involved in heterophilic cell–cell adhesion but also acted as a principal cell receptor for collagen and hyaluronate (Carter and Wayner 1988; Aruffo *et al.* 1990; Miyake *et al.* 1990). This indicates the possibility that CD44 might participate in both the lodging of cancer cells on endothelial cells and adhesion to extracellular matrices. The cDNA cloning of a CD44 variant, which was strongly expressed in a metastasizing rat pancreatic cancer cell line, revealed that it possessed variant exon v6 (Günthert *et al.* 1991). Transfection of the cDNA with v6 exon in the non-metastasizing cultured cells was sufficient to establish full metastatic behavior (Günthert *et al.* 1991). Activated human lymphocytes and aggressive non-Hodgkin's lymphoma cells expressed a homologue of the v6 exon contained in a rat metastasis-associated variant of CD44 (Koopman *et al.* 1993). When injected intravenously into mice, human melanoma cells expressing low levels of CD44 gave significantly fewer lung nodules than the high-expressing clones, suggesting that CD44 molecules may play a vital role in determining the fate of hematogeneously disseminating melanoma cells (Birch *et al.* 1991). Expression of CD44 variants has also been examined in epithelial tumors. Some variants of the CD44 without exon v6 already appear in adenomas of the colon. Expression of variants containing exon v6 is largely restricted to the advanced stages of tumor development and, in addition, is more prevalent and intense in metastatic (Dukes C and D) than in non-metastatic (Dukes A and B) colonic cancer cases (Wielenga *et al.* 1993). Concerning stomach tissue, an immunohistochemical examination revealed that normal stomach mucosa was stained by an exon v5-specific monoclonal antibody within the foveolar proliferation zone and on mucoid surface epithelium, and areas of intestinal metaplasia reacted positively with monoclonal antibodies specific for exon v5 and v6 (Heider *et al.* 1993). Moreover, adenocarcinomas of the intestinal-type were strongly positive for epitopes encoded by variant exon v5 and v6, whereas diffuse-type adenocarcinomas predominantly expressed exon v5 only, supporting the theory of different origins for these two tumors (Heider *et al.* 1993). Another report indicated that v6 expression was associated with infiltrative tumor growth, depth of invasion, lymph node involvement, and a high incidence of distant metastasis in stomach cancers of the diffuse-type (Hong *et al.* 1995). Good correlation between the expression of total CD44 variant and exon v9-containing isoforms has been reported in human gastric cancers, and v9 expression in primary tumors was significantly and positively associated with recurrence of stomach cancers and mortality of the examined cases (Mayer *et al.* 1993).

4.2.   Selectins and their ligands

The selectin family is another factor participating in cancer cell adhesion to endothelium in hematogeneous metastasis. E-selectin (ELAM-1, endothelial leukocyte adhesion molecule-1) is expressed on activated endothelial cells and recognizes carbohydrate antigen sialyl Lewis X and A (Phillips *et al.* 1990; Takada *et al.* 1991). Adhesion of some cancer cell lines, including those derived from stomach carcinogenesis to human umbilical vein endothelial cells, has been demonstrated to be mediated by E-selectin molecules (Takada *et al.* 1993). Another member of the selectin family, P-selectin, is also expressed in endothelial cells and binds to sialyl Lewis X and A and sulfated glycans (Handa *et al.* 1991). P-selectin is expressed in activated platelets, suggesting that P-selectin might also participate in tumor thrombi formation which precedes cancer metastasis. Although expression of ligands for the selectin family is known to be elevated in the development of colonic adenocarcinomas, significant correlation between their expression and stomach carcinogenesis has not been clarified. Recently, a preoperative serum sialyl-Tn antigen level has been reported to be associated with a poor prognosis for gastric cancer patients (Ma *et al.* 1993; Takahashi *et al.* 1994). However, to date, the functions of the carbohydrate antigen have not been thoroughly investigated.

5. OTHER FACTORS

The functional significance of some factors that are considered to be involved in cancer metastasis, such as the nm23 gene and its product, has not been clarified to date. The nm23 gene was reported as being a tumor metastasis-associated gene first identified in a murine melanoma cell line with high metastatic potential (Steeg *et al.* 1988). The cDNA cloning of nm23 revealed that its product was identical to cytosolic nucleotide diphosphate kinase (Kimura *et al.* 1990). Transfection of nm23 cDNA into murine melanoma cells reduced the incidence of primary tumor formation and metastatic potential that was independent of tumor cell growth in mice, demonstrating the suppressive effects of nm23 on tumor metastasis (Leone *et al.* 1991). In human primary infiltrating ductal carcinoma of the breast, association of low nm23 expression levels correlated with lymph node involvement and other histopathological indicators of high metastatic potential (Bevilacqua *et al.* 1989). A significant down-regulation of the nm23 gene has been reported in stomach cancers with serosal invasion and nodal metastasis (Nakayama *et al.* 1993; Kodera *et al.* 1994; Livingstone *et al.* 1995).

6. CONCLUSION

Various molecules have been revealed to participate in cancer invasion and metastasis, some of which are introduced here. Many unknown factors may also play roles in this late and most life-threatening step of multistage carcinogenesis. Interaction and/or cumulative effects of these molecules could confer tumors' metastatic potentials. Further research is needed to elucidate which of the molecular events is most crucial for the successful formation of metastatic lesions. In the near future, the most crucial steps in invasion and metastasis will become the target of clinical therapy controlling the malignant potential of cancers and maintaining the quality of life of cancer patients.

REFERENCES

Aruffo, A., Stamenkovic, I., Melnick, M., Underhill, C.B., and Seed, B. (1990). CD44 is the principal cell surface receptor for hyaluronate. *Cell*, **61**, 1303–13.

Bacharach, E., Itin, A., and Keshet, E. (1992). *In vivo* patterns of expression of urokinase and its inhibitor PAI-1 suggest a concerted role in regulating physiological angiogenesis. *Proc. Natl. Acad. Sci. USA*, **89**, 10686–90.

Becker, K.-F., Atkinson, M.J., Reich, U., Becker, I., Nekarda, H., Siewert J. R., *et al.* (1994). E-cadherin gene mutation provide clues to diffuse type gastric carcinomas. *Cancer Res.*, **54**, 3845–52.

Behrens, J., Mareel, M.M., Van Roy, F.M., and Birchmeier, W. (1989). Dissecting tumor cell invasion: Epithelial cells acquire invasive properties after the loss of Uvomorulin-mediated cell–cell adhesion. *J. Cell Biol.*, **108**, 2435–47.

Bevilacqua, G., Sobel, M.E., Liotta, L.A., and Steeg, P.S. (1989). Association of low *nm*23 RNA levels in human primary infiltrating ductal breast carcinomas with lymph node involvement and other histopathological indicators of high metastatic potential. *Cancer Res.*, **49**, 5185–90.

Birch, M., Mitchell, S., and Hart, I.R. (1991). Isolation and characterization of human melanoma cell variants expressing high and low levels of CD44. *Cancer Res.*, **51**, 6660–7.

Boku, N., Yoshida, S., Ohtsu, A., Fujii, T., Koba, I., Oda, Y., *et al.* (1995). Expression of integrin α3 in gastric and colorectal cancers: Its relation to wall contraction and mode of invasion. *Jpn. J. Cancer Res.* **86**, 934–40.

Carter, W.G. and Wayner, E.A. (1988). Characterization of the class Ö° collagen receptor, a phosphorylated, transmembrane glycoprotein expressed in nucleated human cells. *J. Biol. Chem.*, **263**, 4193–201.

Collier, I.E., Wilhelm, S.M., Eisen, A.Z., Marmer, B.L., Grant, G.A., Seltzer, J.L., *et al.* (1988). H-ras oncogene-transformed human bronchial epithelial cells (TBE-1) secrete a single metalloproteinase capable of degrading basement membrane collagen. *J. Biol. Chem.*, **263**, 6579–87.

Docherty, A.J.P., Lyons, A., Smith, B.J., Wright, E.M., Stephens, P.E., and Harris, T.J.R. (1985). Sequence of human tissue inhibitor of metalloproteinases and its identity to erythroid-potentiating activity. *Nature*, **318**, 66–9.

Esch, F., Baird, A., Ling, N., Ueno, N., Hill, F., Denoroy, L., *et al.* (1985). Primary structure of bovine pituitary basic fibroblast growth factor (FGF) comparison with the amino-terminal sequence of bovine brain acidic FGF. *Proc. Natl. Acad. Sci. USA*, **82**, 6507–11.

Fearon, E.R., Cho, K.R., Nigro, J.M., Kern, S.E., Simons, J.W., Ruppert, J.M., *et al.* (1990). Identification of a chromosome 18q gene that is altered in colorectal cancers. *Science*, **247**, 49–56.

Frixen, U.H., Behrens, J., Sachs, M., Eberle, G., Voss, B., Warda, A., *et al.* (1991). E-cadherin-mediated cell–cell adhesion prevents invasiveness of human carcinoma cells. *J. Cell Biol.*, **113**, 173–85.

Fujita, S., Suzuki, H., Kinoshita, M., and Hirohashi, S. (1992). Inhibition of cell attachment, invasion and metastasis of human carcinoma cells by anti-integrin β_1 subunit antibody. *Jpn. J. Cancer Res.*, **83**, 1317–26.

Gimenez-Gallego, G., Rodkey, J., Bennett, C., Ricos-Candelore, M., DiSalvo, J., and Thomas, K. (1985). Brain-derived acidic fibroblast growth factor: Complete amino acid sequence and homologies. *Science*, **230**, 1385–8.

Günthert, U., Hofmann, M., Rudy, W., Reber, S., Zöler, M., Haussmann, I., *et al.* (1991). A new variant of glycoprotein CD44 confers metastatic potential to rat carcinoma cells. *Cell*, **65**, 13–24.

Handa, K., Nudelman, E.D., Stroud, M.R., Shiozawa, T., and Hakomori, S.-I. (1991). Selectin GMP-140 (CD62; PADGEM) binds to sialosyl-Le^a and sialosyl-Le^X, and sulfated glycans modulate this binding. *Biochem. Biophys. Res. Commun.*, **181**, 1223–30.

Heider, K.-H., Dämmrich, J., Skroch-Angel, P., Hans-Konrad, Müller-Hermelink, Vollmers, H.P., *et al.* (1993). Differential expression of CD44 splice variants in intestinal and diffuse-type human gastric carcinomas and normal gastric mucosa. *Cancer Res.*, **53**, 4197–203.

Hong, R.-L., Lee, W.-J., Shun, C.-T., Chu, J.-S., and Chen, Y.-C. (1995). Expression of CD44 and its clinical implication in diffuse-type and intestinal-type gastric adenocarcinomas. *Oncology*, **52**, 334–9.

Horimoto, M., Kato, R., Takimoto, R., Terui, T., Mogi, Y., and Niitsu, Y. (1995). Identification of a transforming growth factor beta-1 activator derived from a human gastric cancer cell line. *Br. J. Cancer Res.*, **72**, 676–80.

Humphries, M.J., Olden, K., and Yamada, K. (1986). A synthetic peptide from fibronectin inhibits experimental metastasis of murine melanoma cells. *Science*, **233**, 467–70.

Hynes, R.O. (1987). Integrins: A family of cell surface receptors. *Cell*, **48**, 549–54.

Iida, A., Hirose, K., Arai, M., Yamaguchi, A., and Nakagawara G. (1995). Relationships among the expression of epidermal growth factor receptor, proliferating cell nuclear antigen labeling index, and lymph node metastasis in gastric cancer. *Oncology*, **52**, 189–95.

Itoh, F., Hinoda, Y., Ohe, M., Ohe, Y., Ban, T., Endo, T., *et al.* (1993). Decreased expression of DCC mRNA in human colorectal cancers. *Int. J. Cancer*, **53**, 260–3.

Jalkanen, S., Bargatze, R.F., Toyos, J.D.L., and Butcher, E.C. (1987). Lymphocyte recognition of high endothelium: Antibodies to distinct epitopes of an 85–95-kD glycoprotein antigen differentially inhibit lymphocyte binding to lymph node, mucosal or synovial endothelial cells. *J. Cell Biol.*, **105**, 983–90.

Johnson, J.P., Stade, B.G., Holzmann, B., Schwäble, W., and Riethmüller, G. (1989). *De novo* expression of intercellular-adhesion molecule 1 in melanoma correlates with increased risk of metastasis. *Proc. Natl. Acad. Sci. USA*, **86**, 641–4.

Juliano, R. and Varner, J. (1993). Adhesion molecules in cancer: The role of integrins. *Curr. Opin. Cell Biol.*, **5**, 812–18.

Kanai, Y., Ochiai, A., Shibata, T., Oyama, T., Ushijima, S., Akimoto, S., *et al.* (1995). c-*erb*B-2 gene product directly associates with β-catenin and plakoglobin. *Biochem. Biophys. Res. Commun.*, **208**, 1067–72.

Khokha, R., Waterhouse, P., Yagel, S., Lala, P.K., Overall, C.M., Norton, G., *et al.* (1989). Antisense RNA-induced reduction in murine TIMP levels confers oncogenicity on Swiss 3T3 cells. *Science*, **243**, 947–50.

Khokha, R., Zimmer, M.J., Graham, C.H., Lala, P.K., and Waterhouse, P. (1992). Suppression of invasion by inducible expression of tissue inhibitor of metalloproteinase-1 (TIMP-1) in B16-F10 melanoma cells. *J. Natl. Cancer Inst.*, **84**, 1017–22.

Kimura, N., Shimada, N., Nomura, K., and Watanabe, K. (1990). Isolation and characterization of a cDNA clone encoding rat nucleoside diphosphate kinase. *J. Biol. Chem.*, **265**, 15744–9.

Kodera, Y., Isobe, K.-I., Yamauchi, M., Kondoh, K., Kimura, N., Akiyama, S., *et al.* (1994). Expression of nm23 H-1 RNA levels in human gastric cancer tissue. *Cancer*, **73**, 259–65.

Kohn, E.C., Liotta, L.A., and Schiffmann, E. (1990). Autocrine motility factor stimulates a three-fold increase in inositol trisphosphate in human melanoma cells. *Biochem. Biophys. Res. Commun.*, **166**, 757–64.

Koopman, G., Heider, K.-H., Horst, E., Adolf, G.R., Berg, F.V.D., Ponta, H., *et al.* (1993). Activated human lymphocytes and aggressive non-Hodgkin's lymphomas express a homologue of the rat metastasis-associated variant of CD44. *J. Exp. Med.*, **177**, 897–904.

Koretz, K., Schlag, P., Boumsell, L., and Möller, P. (1991). Expression of VLA-α2, VLA-α6, and VLA-β1 chains in normal mucosa and adenomas of the colon, and in colon carcinomas and their liver metastases. *Am. J. Pathol.*, **138**, 741–50.

Koshikawa, N., Yasumitsu, H., Umeda, M., and Miyazaki, K. (1992). Multiple secretion of matrix serine proteinases by human gastric carcinoma cell lines. *Cancer Res.*, **52**, 5046–53.

Koyama, S., Ebihara, T., and Fukao, K. (1992). Expression of intercellular adhesion molecule 1 (ICAM-1) during the development of invasion and/or metastasis of gastric carcinoma. *J. Cancer Res. Clin. Oncol.*, **118**, 609–14.

Kuniyasu, H., Yasui, W., Yokozaki, H., Kitadai, Y., and Tahara, E. (1993). Aberrant expression of c-*met* mRNA in human gastric carcinomas. *Int. J. Cancer*, **55**, 72–5.

Leone, A., Flatow, U., King, C.R., Sandeen, M.A., Margulies, I.M.K., Liotta, L.A., *et al.* (1991). Reduced tumor incidence, metastatic potential, and cytokine responsiveness of *nm*23-transfected melanoma cells. *Cell*, **65**, 25–35.

Leonor, D., Nesland, J.M., Holm, R., and Sobrinho-Simões, M. (1994). Expression of laminin, collagen IV, fibronectin, and type IV collagenase in gastric carcinoma. *Cancer*, **73**, 518–27.

Leung, D.W., Cachianes, G., Kuang, W.-J., Goeddel, D.V., and Ferrara, N. (1989). Vascular endothelial growth factor is a secreted angiogenic mitogen. *Science*, **246**, 1306–9.

Liotta, L.A. (1986). Tumor invasion and metastases—Role of the extracellular matrix. Rhoads memorial award lecture. *Cancer Res.*, **46**, 1–7.

Liotta, L.A., Mandler, R., Murano, G., Katz, D.A., Gordon, R.K., Chiang, P. K., *et al.* (1986). Tumor cell autocrine motility factor. *Proc. Natl. Acad. Sci. USA*, **83**, 3302–6.

Liotta, L.A., Steeg, P.S., and Stetler-Stevenson, W.G. (1991). Cancer metastasis and angiogenesis: An imbalance of positive and negative regulation. *Cell*, **64**, 327–36.

Livingstone, J.I., Yasui, W., Tahara, E., and Wastell, C. (1995). Are Japanese and European gastric cancer the same biological entity? An immunohistochemical study. *Br. J. Cancer Res.*, **72**, 976–80.

Ma, X.C., Terata, N., Kodama, M., Jancic, S., Hosokawa, Y., and Hattori, T. (1993). Expression of sialyl-Tn antigen is correlated with survival time of patients with gastric carcinomas. *Eur. J. Cancer*, **29**, 1820–3.

Marlin, S.D. and Springer, T.A. (1987). Purified intercellular adhesion molecule-1 (ICAM-1) is a ligand for lymphocyte function-associated antigen-1 (LFA-1). *Cell*, **51**, 813–19.

Mayer, B., Jauch, K. W., Gunthert, U., Figdor, C.G., Schilderg, F.W., Funke, I., *et al.* (1993). *De-novo* expression of CD44 and survival in gastric cancer. *Lancet*, **342**, 1019–22.

Miyake, K., Underhill, C.B., Lesley, J., and Kincade, P.W. (1990). Hyaluronate can function as a cell adhesion molecule and CD44 participates in hyaluronate recognition. *J. Exp. Med.*, **172**, 69–75.

Miyaki, M., Sek, M., Okamoto, M., Yamanaka, A., Maeda, Y., Tanaka, K., *et al.* (1990). Genetic changes and histopathological types in colorectal tumors from patients with familial adenomatous polyposis. *Cancer Res.*, **50**, 7166–71.

Muta, H., Noguchi, M., Kanai, Y., Ochiai, A., Nawata, H., and Hirohashi, S. (1996). E-cadherin gene mutations in signet ring cell carcinoma of the stomach. *Jpn. J. Cancer Res*, **87**, 843–8.

Nakajima, M., Morikawa, K., Fabra, A., Bucana, C.D., and Fidler, I.J. (1990). Influence of organ environment on extracellular matrix degradative activity and metastasis of human colon carcinoma cells. *J. Natl Cancer Inst.*, **82**, 1890–8.

Nakayama, H., Yasui, W., Yokozaki, H., and Tahara, E. (1993). Reduced expression of nm23 is associated with metastasis of human gastric carcinomas. *Jpn. J. Cancer Res.*, **84**, 184–90.

Narayanan, R., Lawlor, K.G., Schaapveld, R.Q.J., Cho, K.R., Vogelstein, B., Tran, P.B.-V., *et al.* (1992). Antisense RNA to the putative tumor-suppressor gene DCC transforms Rat-1 fibroblasts. *Oncogene*, **7**, 553–61.

Ochiai, A., Akimoto, S., Kanai, Y., Shibata, T., Oyama, T., and Hirohashi, S. (1994*a*). c-*erb*B-2 gene product associates with catenins in human cancer cells. *Biochem. Biophys. Res. Commun.*, **205**, 73–8.

Ochiai, A., Akimoto, S., Shimoyama, Y., Nagafuchi, A., Tsukita, S., and Hirohashi, S. (1994*b*). Frequent loss of α catenin expression in scirrhous carcinoma with scattered cell growth. *Jpn. J. Cancer Res.*, **85**, 266–73.

Oda, T., Kanai, Y., Oyama, T., Yoshiura, K., Shimoyama, Y., Birchmeier, W., *et al.* (1994). E-cadherin gene mutation in human gastric cancer cell lines. *Proc. Natl. Acad Sci. USA*, **91**, 1858–62.

Oyama, T., Kanai, Y., Ochiai, A., Akimoto, S., Oda, T., Yanagihara, K., *et al.* (1994). A truncated β-catenin disrupts the interaction between E-cadherin and α-catenin: A cause of loss of intercellular adhesiveness in human cancer cell lines. *Cancer Research*, **54**, 6282–7.

Phillips, M.L., Nudelman, E., Gaeta, F.C.A., Perez, M., Singhal, A.K., and Hakomori, S.-I. (1990). ELAM-1 mediates cell adhesion by recognition of a carbohydrate ligand, Sialyl-Le^X. *Science*, **250**, 1130–2.

Rubinfeld, B., Souza, B., Albert, I., Müller, O., Chamberlain, S.H., Masiarz, F.R., *et al.* (1993). Association of the APC gene product with β-catenin. *Science*, **262**, 1731–4.

Ruoslahti, E. and Pierschbacher, M.D. (1987). New perspectives in cell adhesion: RGD and integrins. *Science*, **238**, 491–7.

Saiki, I., Iida, J., Ogawa, R., Nishi, N., Sugimura, K., Tokura, S., *et al.* (1989). Inhibition of the metastasis of murine malignant melanoma by synthetic polymeric peptides containing core sequence of cell-adhesive molecules. *Cancer Res.*, **49**, 3815–22.

Salo, T., Liotta, L.A., and Tryggvason, K. (1983). Purification and characterization of a murine basement membrane collagen-degrading enzyme secreted by metastatic tumor cells. *J. Biol. Chem.*, **258**, 3058–63.

Sastry, S. and Horwitz, A. (1993). Integrin cytoplasmic domains: Mediators of cytoskeletal linkage and extra- and intracellular initiated transmembrane signaling. *Curr. Opin. Cell Biol.*, **5**, 819–31.

Sato, H., Takino, T., Okada, Y., Cao, J., Shinagawa, A., Yamamoto, E., *et al.* (1994). A matrix metalloproteinase expressed on the surface of invasive tumor cells. *Nature*, **370**, 61–5.

Senger, D.R., Galli, S.J., Dvorak, A.M., Perruzzi, C.A., Harvey, V.S., and Dvorak, H.F. (1983). Tumor cells secrete a vascular permeability factor that promotes accumulation of ascites fluid. *Science*, **219**, 983–5.

Seruca, R., Suijkerbuijk, R.F., Gärtner, F., Criado, B., Veiga, I., Olde-Weghuis, D., *et al.* (1995). Increasing levels of MYC and MET co-amplification during tumor progression of a case of gastric cancer. *Cancer Genet. Cytogenet.* **82**, 140–5.

Shimoyama, Y. and Hirohashi, S. (1991). E- and P-cadherin expression in gastric carcinomas. *Cancer Res.,* **51**, 2185–92.

Soini, Y., Pääkkö, P., and Autio-Harmainen, H. (1993). Genes of laminin B1 chain, α1 (IV) chain of type IV collagen, and 72-kd type IV collagenase are mainly expressed by the stromal cells of lung carcinomas. *Am. J. Pathol.,* **142**, 1622–30.

Stamenkovic, I., Amiot, M., Pesando, J. M., and Seed, B. (1989). A lymphocyte molecule implicated in lymph node homing is a member of the cartilage link protein family. *Cell,* **56**, 1027–62.

Staunton, D.E., Marlin, S.D., Stratowa, C., Dustin, M.L., and Springer, T.A. (1988). Primary structure of ICAM-1 demonstrates interaction between members of the immunoglobulin and integrin super gene families. *Cell,* **52**, 925–33.

Steeg, P.S., Bevilacqua, G., Kopper, L., Thorgeirsson, U.P., Talmadge, J. E., Liotta, L.A., *et al.* (1988). Evidence for a novel gene associated with low tumor metastasis potential. *J. Natl. Cancer Inst.,* **80**, 200–4.

Stetler-Stevenson, W.G., Krutzsch, H.C., and Liotta, L.A. (1989). Tissue inhibitor of metalloproteinase (TIMP-2): A new member of the metallopoteinase inhibitor family. *J. Biol. Chem.,* **264**, 17374–8.

Su, L.-K., Vogelstein, B., and Kinzler, K.W. (1993). Association of the APC tumor suppressor protein with catenins. *Science,* **262**, 1734–7.

Takada, A., Ohmori, K., Takahashi, N., Tsuyuoka, K., Yago, A., Zenita, K., *et al.* (1991). Adhesion of human cancer cells to vascular endothelium mediated by carbohydrate antigen, sialyl Lewis A. *Biochem. Biophys. Res. Commun.,* **179**, 713–19.

Takada, A., Ohmori, K., Yoneda, T., Tsuyuoka, K., Hasegawa, A., Kiso, M., *et al.* (1993). Contribution of carbohydrate antigens sialyl Lewis A and sialyl Lewis X to adhesion of human cancer cells to vascular endothelium. *Cancer Res.,* **53**, 354–61.

Takahashi, Y., Maehara, T., Kusumoto, T., Kohnoe, S., Kakeji, Y., Baba, H., *et al.* (1994). Combined evaluation of preoperative serum sialyl-Tn antigen and carcinoembryonic antigen levels is prognostic for gastric cancer patients. *Br. J. Cancer,* **69**, 163–6.

Takeda, K., Fujii, N., Nitta, Y., Sakihara, H., Nakayama, K., Rikiishi, H., *et al.* (1991). Murine tumor cells metastasizing selectively in the liver: Ability to produce hepatocyte-activating cytokines interleukin-1 and/or -6. *Jpn. J. Cancer Res.,* **82**, 1299–308.

Takeichi, M. (1991). Cadherin cell adhesion receptor as a morphogenetic regulator. *Science,* **251**, 1451–5.

Uchino, S., Tsuda, H., Noguchi, M., Yokota, J., Terada, M., Saito, T., *et al.* (1992). Frequent loss of heterozygosity at DCC locus in gastric cancer. *Cancer Res.,* **52**, 3099–102.

Valles, A.M., Boyer, B., Badet, J., Tucker, G.C., and Barritault, D. (1990). Acidic fibroblast growth factor is a modulator of epithelial plasticity in a rat bladder carcinoma cell line. *Proc. Natl. Acad. Sci. USA,* **87**, 1124–8.

Vleminckx, K., Vakaet, L. Jr., Mareel, M., Fiers, W., and Van Roy, F. (1991). Genetic manipulation of E-cadherin expression by epithelial tumor cells reveals an invasion suppressor role. *Cell,* **66**, 107–19.

Weidner, K.M., Arakaki, N., Hartmann, G., Vandekerckhove, J., Weingart, S., Rieder, H., *et al.* (1991). Evidence for the identity of human scatter factor and human hepatocyte growth factor. *Proc. Natl. Acad. Sci. USA,* **88**, 7001–5.

Wielenga, V.J.M., Heider, K.-H., Offerhaus, G.J.A., Adolf, G.R., Berg, F. M.V.D., Ponta, H., *et al.*. (1993). Expression of CD44 variant proteins in human colorectal cancer is related to tumor progression. *Cancer Res.*, **53**, 4754–6.

Wilhelm, S.M., Collier, I.E., Marmer, B.L., Eisen, A.Z., Grant, G.A., and Goldberg, G.I. (1989). SV40-transformed human lung fibroblasts secrete a 92-kDa type IV collagenase which is identical to that secreted by normal human macrophages. *J. Biol. Chem.*, **264**, 17213–21.

Yang, T.-T. and Hawkes, S.P. (1992). Role of the 21-kDa protein TIMP-3 in oncogenic transformation of cultured chicken embryo fibroblasts. *Proc. Natl. Acad. Sci. USA*, **89**, 10676–80.

Yashiro, M., Chung, Y.-S., Nishimura, S., Inoue, T., and Sowa, M. (1996). Peritoneal metastatic model for human scirrhous gastric carcinoma in nude mice. *Clin. Exp. Metastasis*, **14**, 43–54.

Yoshiura, K., Kanai, Y., Ochiai, A., Shimoyama, Y., Sugimura, T., and Hirohashi, S. (1995). Silencing of the E-cadherin invasion-suppressor gene by CpG methylation in human carcinomas. *Proc. Natl. Acad. Sci. USA*, **92**, 7416–19.

Part IV: Diagnosis

9

Diagnosis: general considerations

Hisanao Ohkura

1. TAKING A HISTORY

When taking a patient's history, the questionnaire should include not only details of abdominal symptoms, but also information on bowel movement, smoking and drinking habits, diet (e.g. meals comprising hot, salty, smoked, fermented, or spicy foods), change in body weight and any history of gastric and other cancers in the patient and his/her family.

As more than 90% of gastric cancers occur in the fifth or later decades and is associated with chronic atrophic gastritis or intestinal metaplasia, it is essential to screen those who have had this type of gastritis or symptoms of dyspepsia in the past (Landsdown *et al.* 1990). Any history of cancer in the stomach or other organs suggests a higher risk for gastric cancer (Lundegardh *et al.* 1991). Partial gastrectomy cannot eliminate the risk of a second primary cancer in the remaining stomach. A past history of peptic ulcer lowers but does not eliminate the possibility of getting gastric cancer (Lee *et al.* 1990).

As there are specific groups of people who have a higher risk for gastric cancer (e.g. Japanese, Korean, Finn, Icelandic, and Chilean), taking a history from these ethnic groups is important.

If patients have had screening tests for stomach cancer, the date, type of tests, and diagnosis should be recorded. Prior diagnosis of chronic atrophic gastritis, intestinal metaplasia, dysplasia, adenomas, atypical glands, pernicious anemia (Hsing *et al.* 1993), and helicobacter infection (Parsonnet *et al.* 1991) indicate a higher risk for gastric cancer.

2. EARLY GASTRIC CANCER: SIGNS AND SYMPTOMS

There are no specific clinical signs and symptoms of early gastric cancer. Most patients with early gastric cancer (EGC) are asymptomatic when they are diagnosed by a gastroscope or a double contrast barium meal X-ray examination. Some EGCs are diagnosed by *ad hoc* examination due to uncertain abdominal symptoms, such as dyspepsia, epigastric distress, epigastralgia, nausea, anorexia, and weight loss, where these are usually caused by associated benign diseases, such as chronic gastritis, esophagitis, irritable colon, etc. (Kagevi *et al.* 1989).

3. ADVANCED GASTRIC CANCER: SIGNS AND SYMPTOMS

The signs and symptoms listed below are accompanied not only by various benign and malignant diseases, but also by advanced gastric cancer. These are: dyspepsia, anorexia, epigastric distress, abdominal fullness, abdominal pain, nausea, vomiting, hiccups, back flow of sour or bitter gastric juice, increased oral odor, thick tongue moss, melena, dark stool, weight loss, and anemia (Snooks *et al.* 1989).

The vomitus contains undigested foods, blood streaks, or coagula, and has a foul odour in advanced cancer. Hematoemesis is a not common symptom of gastric cancer, but massive bleeding from a cancerous lesion can occur.

Abdominal pains are mostly epigastric, sticking, dull or colic, fasting, postprandial or spontaneous, radiating to the back and shoulder, which may be relieved by antacids or antispasmodics but may be increased by alcoholic drinks, and spicy and/or heavy meals. Borborygmi, hyperperistalsis, and irregular bowel movements associated with abdominal pain may signs of peritoneal involvement.

Progressive anemia, emaciation, palpable epigastric mass enlarged liver, and *peritonitis carcinomatosa* are symptoms of late-stage gastric cancer. The supraclavicular lymph node metastasis (Virchow's node), ascitic fluid, ovarian metastasis (Kruckenberg's tumor), or deep pelvic metastasis (Schnitzler's metastasis) diagnosed by an anal digital examination, indicate advanced disease and very poor prognosis.

4. DIAGNOSTIC METHODS

4.1. Barium meal

Details of barium meal studies are described in Chapter 10. There are two types: one is to screen those subjects with any prior abnormal findings for a subsequent screening—this test can be carried out by X-ray television and indirect films. The other type is to visualize precise findings: number, type, height or depth, margin, width, extension and rigidity of the lesions, and relation to the surrounding organs, by direct fluoroscopy or X-ray television. A double contrast barium meal test is recommended for both types of diagnosis (Ichikawa 1993).

The barium meal test can be repeated following surgery in order to determine the recurrence, dumping syndrome, or stenosis due to postoperative adhesions.

4.2. Endoscopy

Details of endoscopy are described in Chapter 11. There are three types of tests using the gastrofiberscope: one is to screen those patients with any signs or symptoms, or any risk factors, in order to detect abnormal findings for a subsequent screening. The second type is to visualize precise findings of the lesions and diagnose them (Kagevi *et al.* 1989, Hallissey *et al.* 1990). A double-angled panendoscope is recommended for both purposes. As there are several types of early gastric cancer, investigations regarding location, size, and classification of the lesion are critical for their prognosis. A dye-spraying test and an endoscope biopsy can be done at the same time (Yoshida *et al.* 1992). One must not forget the possibility of multicentric carcinomas or synchronous benign and malignant lesions.

The third test is presurgical endoscopy for those patients with resectable gastric cancer. Preoperative diagnosis of the location, depth, and width of the cancerous invasion, especially the distance from the cardiac ring are essential for resection procedure.

4.3. Laboratory tests

There is no specific laboratory test for diagnosing early gastric cancer. However, the following tests often reveal abnormal results in advanced cancer.

Patients with advanced gastric cancer may have anemia, mostly hypochromic, macrocytic or microcytic, due to continuous blood loss from the lesion. Platelet counts and coagulation tests usually remain within normal unless there is persistent bleeding, disseminated intravascular coagulopathy (DIC), or massive metastasis in the liver, pancreas, spleen, lung, or bone marrow.

Biochemical tests may show a slightly elevated level in lactic dehydrogenase (LDH) and alkaline phosphatase (ALP) and a decreased level in serum albumin and other proteins, irons, and ferritin.

4.4. Occult blood tests

A fecal occult blood test is negative in more than half of advanced gastric cancers by a Guiyack (Hemoccult) test, or by immunological hemoglobin tests, unless the patient has persistent and/or massive bleeding from the primary lesion in the stomach.

A positive occult blood test is non-specific as there are many sources of bleeding in the gastrointestinal (GI) tract: peptic ulcers, erosions, gingivitis, reflux esophagitis, hemorrhagic gastritis, hemobilia, colitis, colon polyps, colorectal malignancies, and hemorrhoids. A positive occult blood test indicates a colonoscopy or a barium enema study to find the source of bleeding in the lower GI tract. However, this test also indicates a barium meal study or an upper GI endoscopy. In order to avoid false-positive results, intake of iron-containing foods, such as meat and green vegetables, must be avoided prior to benzidine or Guiyack tests, but this precaution is not necessary for immunological hemoglobin tests.

4.5. Tumor markers

Serum tumor markers are not elevated in patients with early gastric cancer. If the patient does have an abnormal value, it suggests a possibility of production from occult metastasis.

The carbohydrate antigen of sialylated Lewis a (Le_a) group (CA19-9, CA50, and SPan1), core antigen of sialosyl Tn group (CA72-4, STn, or CA546), NCC-ST-439, or carcinoembryonic antigen (CEA) are produced by gastric cancer tissue in 70% of patients and appear in serum in 40–60% when the disease is advanced. The well- and moderately differentiated adenocarcinomas usually produce two or more markers, however, 60% of the undifferentiated type produce none of these markers (Table 9.1).

Human chorionic gonadotrophin (hCG), α1-fetoprotein (AFP), or heat-resistant alkaline phosphatase isoenzymes are produced in 2–3% cases of gastric cancer with special histological subtypes. The higher the level of a marker in serum, the larger the tumor mass; the more frequently the patient has metastasis, the higher the clinical stage, and the worse the prognosis. By multivariate analyses, some serum tumor markers are independent prognostic factors following the three major anatomical prognostic factors, such as depth of invasion (T), distant metastasis (M), and lymph node metastasis (N).

4.6. Gastric juice

Non-cytological laboratory tests for gastric juice are not diagnostic for gastric cancer but are useful for screening high-risk individuals. In the pioneer work of Haekkinen *et al.* (1979), a fetal sulphoglycoprotein (FSA) was determined immunologically in gastric juice as a screening test for gastric cancer in Finland.

Anacidity is a sign of atrophic gastritis, and is diagnosed by a gastric juice analysis, with or without gastrin, or histamine stimulation, or by Gastrotest using an acid-soluble dye tablet. The pepsinogen isoenzymes I and II, derived from gastric mucosa, can be determined in serum by immunoassays. Miki *et al.* (1989) reported that the level of type I enzyme and the ratio of types I/II enzymes are lower in those suffering from atrophic gastritis, chronic gastritis with intestinal metaplasia, and/or gastric cancer. For patients whose serum pepsinogen type I level and/or the types I/II ratio are lower than normal, the odds ratio of having gastric cancer is significantly high. Therefore, this enzyme assay is used for screening high-risk individuals for gastric cancer.

Table 9.1. Positive rates (%) of preoperative serum tumor markers in gastric cancers

| Marker | Cut-off value | Stage[a] | | | | BD[b] |
		I	II	III	IV	
CEA	>5 µg/l	5	7	18	52	2
CA19-9	>37 U/ml	3	11	37	67	3
CA72-4	>4.8 U/ml	0	5	19	57	2
NCC-ST-439	>4.5 U/ml	5	10	30	31	4
CA125	>35 U/ml	0	0	0	79	0
AFP	>20 µg/l	0	0.6	1	3	0

[a] TNM Classification; [b] benign gastric disease. (From the Gastric Surgery Division and Clinical Laboratory, National Cancer Center Hospital, Tokyo 1982–93.)

A subaerobic bacterium, *Helicobacter pylori*, is detected in gastric juice, gastric mucus, and in the apical surface of the gastric mucosa, which is highly associated with and thought to be a causative factor for gastric and duodenal ulcers, and acute and chronic gastritis. Parsonnet *et al.* (1991) have reported that the antibody against helicobacter is frequently found in the serum of gastric cancer patients, and in the general population of those countries who have a higher incidence of gastric cancer. Therefore, carriers of helicobacter are thought to have a higher risk for gastric cancer (Parsonnet *et al.* 1991) and for gastric lymphoma (Wotherspoon *et al.* 1991).

The diagnosis of gastric helicobacter infection is confirmed by detection of the bacteria or by positive culture from gastric juice or biopsied specimens obtained by endoscopy. Antihelicobacter antibodies are elevated in patients' serum. As helicobacter produces an enzyme, urease, urea is detected in the expiration or oral mucus of the carrier. Enzyme-linked immunoassays are also available for this enzyme.

4.7. Cytology

The cytology of gastric juice is not commonly undertaken because of the widespread use of endoscopy. However, it still has a value in those countries where trained radiologists or endoscopists are not available for gastric cancer screening. To obtain fresh cells from gastric mucosa, via the nasal or oral route, a gastric tube has to be swallowed by the patient. Moderate hand pumping and washing of the stomach with a syringe and 100–200 ml of cooled buffered saline, followed by immediate centrifugation, are recommended. Giemsa and Papanicolaou stains are used routinely.

If group III or more malignant cells are found, the patient should be sent for radiology and endoscopy.

4.8. Ultrasonograpy

There are two types of ultrasonography (US) for the supplemental diagnosis of gastric cancer but not for screening. The first is the routine external abdominal scan, ultrasonography or echotomography, for all the abdominal organs including stomach, liver, pancreas, and paraaortic lymph nodes. This linear scanning device is suitable as a routine preoperative test to determine the extent of gastric cancer. A skilled examiner can visualize the depth and range of invasion in the gastric wall and the involved paraaortic lymph nodes located deep in the retroperitoneal spaces. However, this test gives poor information when the examiner is not experienced, the patient is obese, or when gas remains in the GI tract.

The second is endoscopical ultrasonography (EUS) using a flexible endoscopic device (Caletti *et al.* 1993). This test can provide information on submucosal tissue, thickening, rigidity, and infiltration in the gastric wall, relationship to the surrounding tissues, extragastric invasions, and adjacent lymph node metastasis. A scirrhous-type carcinoma, or so-called 'linitis plastica' with diffuse submucosal infiltration can be diagnosed with an EUS. These tests are helpful for preoperative staging of gastric cancer (Akahoshi *et al.* 1992), but reported diagnostic accuracies are varied—from 95% to 69%. In a comparative study with peritoneoscopy (see below), for diagnosis of paraaortic lymph nodes metastasis and peritoneal invasion, EUS was found to be inferior to (laparoscopy) (Watt *et al.* 1989).

4.9.   X-ray CT scan

The X-ray computed tomography (CT scan) for the abdomen can give information on organs in the abdominal cavity (Balfe *et al.* 1981). This test is not suitable for screening and diagnosing gastric cancer. In advanced gastric cancer, a CT scan provides supplementary information on any possibility of resectability. Liver metastasis, perigastric invasion, lymph node involvement, and ascitic fluids can also be diagnosed by this method. In instances of non-surgical treatment, such as chemotherapy, the effectiveness of a therapy can be assessed by measuring the sizes of metastatic tumors. A rapid postcontrast view can visualize metastases as small as 1 cm in diameter.

4.10.   Peritoneoscopy (laparoscopy)

Recent developments in electronic and flexible fiberoptic peritoneoscopy, a number of accessory devices for peritoneoscopic surgery, and technical skill has revived this method. It can serve not only as a simple supplementary diagnostic method but also as an useful new therapeutic method for diseases of abdominal organs including the stomach. Peritoneoscopy is also useful in diagnosing serosal invasion, peritoneal dissemination, lymph node, and liver metastasis in patients with advanced gastric cancer. Superior accuracies are reported when compared to abdominal US, EUS, and CT scanning (Watt *et al.* 1989). Unnecessary exploratory laparotomy can be avoided by employing peritoneoscopy instead (Ajani *et al.* 1995). Some trials on peritoneoscopic regional gastrectomy for early gastric cancer are being carried out. However, a long-term evaluation of this surgery has not yet been reported.

REFERENCES

Ajani, J.A., Mansfield, P.F., and Ota, D.M. (1995). Potentially resectable gastric carcinoma; current approach to staging and preoperative therapy. *World J. Surg.* (*US*), **19**, 216–20.
Akahoshi, K., Misawa, T., Fujishima, H., Chijiiwa, Y., and Nawate, H. (1992). Regional lymph node metastasis in gastric cancer: evaluation with endoscopic US. *Radiology*, **182**, 559–64.
Balfe, D.C., Koehler, R.E., Karstaedt, N., *et al.* (1981). Computed tomography of gastric neoplasms. *Radiology*, **140**, 431–6.

Caletti, G., Ferrari, A., Brocci, E., and Barbara, L. (1993). Accuracy of endoscopic ultra-sonography in the diagnosis and staging of gastric cancer and lymphoma. *Surgery*, **113**, 14–27.

Haekkinen, I.P.T. *et al.* (1979). Clinical-pathological study of gastric cancers and precancer-ous states detected by fetal sulphoglycoprotein antigen screening. *Cancer Res.*, **40**, 4308–12.

Hallissey, M.T., Allum, W.H., Jewke, A.J., Ellis, D.J., and Fielding J.W. (1990). Early diag-nosis of gastric cancer. *Brit. Med. J.*, **301**, 513–15.

Hsing, A.W., Hansson, L.E., McLaughlin, J.K., Nyren, O., Blot. W.J., Ekbom A., *et al.* (1993). Pernicious anemia and subsequent cancer. A population-based cohort study. *Cancer*, **71**, 745–50.

Ichikawa, H. (1993). X-ray diagnosis and its latest progress. In *Gastric cancer*, (ed. M. Nishi and H. Ichikawa), pp. 232–45. Springer, Tokyo/Berlin.

Kagevi, I., Lofstedt, S., and Persson, L.G. (1989). Endoscopical findings and diagnosis in unselected dyspeptic patients at a primary health care center. *Scand. J. Gastroenterol.*, **24**, 145–50.

Lansdown, M., Quirke, P., Dixon, M.F., Axon, A.T., and Johnston, D. (1990). High grade dyspepsia of the gastric mucosa: a marker for gastric carcinoma. *Gut*, **31**, 977–83.

Lee, S., Iida, M., Yao, T., Shindo, S., Okabe H., and Fujishima, M. (1990). Long term follow-up of 2529 patients reveals gastric ulcers rarely become malignant. *Dig. Dis. Sci.*, **35**, 763–8.

Lundegardh, G., Hansson, L.E., Nyren, O., Adami, H.O., and Krusemo, U.B. (1991). The risk of gastrointestinal and other primary malignant diseases following gastric cancer. *Acta Oncol.*, **30**, 1–6.

Miki, K., *et al.* (1989). The significance of low serum pepsinogen levels to detect stomach cancer associated with extensive chronic gastritis in Japanese subjects. *Jpn. J. Cancer Res.* **80**, 111–14.

Parsonnet, J., Friedman, G.D., and Vandersteen, DP. (1991). *Helicobacter pylori* infection and the risk of gastric carcinoma. *N. Eng. J. Med.*, **325**, 1127–31.

Snooks, S.J., Cotter, M., and Payne, R.A. (1989). Gastric cancer: a continuing diagnostic challenge—a district general hospital's experience. *Br. J. Clin Pract.*, **43**, 454–7.

Yoshida, S., Sasako, M., Kato, H., and Moriya, N. (1992). Early detection of gastrointesti-nal cancers: recent progress in endoscopy and surgical results. In *Cancer diagnosis*, (ed. P. Bannasch), pp. 33–41. Springer, Berlin/Heidelberg.

Watt, I., Stewart, I., Anderson, D., Bell, G., and Anderson, J.R. (1989). Laparoscopy, ultra-sound and computed tomography in cancer of the oesophagus and gastric cardia: a prospective comparison for detecting intra-abdominal metastases. *Br. J. Surg.*, **76**, 1036–9.

Wotherspoon, A.C., Ortiz-Hidalgo, C., Falson, M.R., and Issacson, P.G. (1991). *Helico-bacter pylori*—associated gastritis and primary B-cell gastric lymphoma. *Lancet*, **338**, 1175–6.

10

Radiology

Masakazu Maruyama, Yasumasa Baba, and Norishige Takemoto

1. INTRODUCTION

In Japan, gastric cancer is still the leading cause of death (Hisamichi *et al.* 1991), although the mortality rate has recently been decreasing. The reduction of gastric cancer is currently a public health policy in Japan. In 1987, Ohta and associates reported that early gastric cancer accounted for one-third of all surgically resected cases in a period of 33 years from 1946 to 1978. In a recent study by Nakajima *et al.* (1994), at the same center, on early cancer comprised nearly a half or more of all resected cases in a period of 5 years between 1985 and 1990 (Fig. 10.1).

This tendency is observed in many Japanese institutions where there is specialization in gastroenterology. At present a considerable number of gastric cancers with favorable prognosis have been detected and treated. However, there are still many patients with advanced gastric cancer who visit hospital with symptoms, and are judged to have a poor prognosis.

Llorens and co-workers (1991) studied 86 cases with early cancer out of 1290 cases of gastric cancer which had been diagnosed over a period of 11 years from 1980. In their series, early cancer comprised only 6.7% of the total number of gastric cancers. This difference in the early/advanced cancer ratio should not merely be

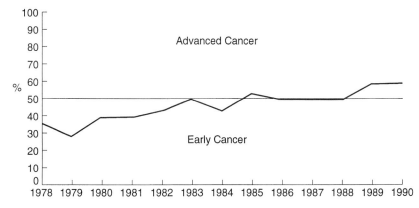

Fig. 10.1. The ratio of early to advanced cancer from 1978 to 1990 at the Cancer Institute Hospital, Tokyo. (by Nakajima, T. 1994).

attributed to the difference in the quality of diagnostic capability but to a variety of cultural situations between countries. In the author's experience, in some South American countries there is a considerable difference in their decision-making policies regarding screening, etc. Moreover, a religious element can play an important role in decision-making, compared to the Japan, where the population readily attends clinics when any symptoms appear. In addition, the health insurance system has assisted in motivating the Japanese to attend a clinic for an examination by radiology and endoscopy. Furthermore, mass screening for gastric cancer, regulated by the Health Insurance Law for Aged People, should not be underestimated. (Miller *et al.* 1991).

2. THE ROLE OF CLASSICAL RADIOLOGY IN THE MANAGEMENT OF GASTRIC CANCER

There are three major roles of classical radiology of the stomach using a barium meal suspension, these are: screening for gastric cancer, assessment of the invasive depth of cancer; and delineation of the lateral spread of cancer. Generally, in Japan, screening for gastric cancer is fundamentally distinguished from the other two roles. In screening, the diagnosis of a definite cancer is not required, but the presence of some abnormality is noted. The mass screening for gastric cancer with indirect radiographic examination is carried out for this purpose.

The assessment of the invasive depth and the delineation of the lateral spread of the cancer are the most important procedures which should be carried out before surgery. In double contrast radiography, diagnosis should be performed in conditions where gastric juice has been removed from the stomach and the volume of air controlled, in order to obtain a detailed information.

Following the routine diagnostic procedure employed in Japan, radiographic or endoscopic examination is usually done first, except when a mass is palpable in the abdomen. In this instance, computed tomography (CT) or ultrasound (US), or Magnetic resonance imaging (MRI) may be the first choice. The cumulative diagnosis by radiography and endoscopy examination can estimate the depth of the tumor.

The recent development of endoscopic ultrasound (EUS), however, has made it possible to assess the architecture of the gastric wall, including a cancerous lesion, and its relation to neighboring structures. CT or MRI is performed to visualize the thickness of the affected gastric wall and its relation to the neighboring structures and to detect lymph node and liver metastases. Liver metastases can also be investigated by US (Yoshinaka and Shimazu 1989).

3. SCREENING FOR GASTRIC CANCER

3.1. The present status of classical radiology in conjunction with endoscopy

It appears that the use of classical radiology using a barium meal seems to be decreasing both in Japan and in many other countries. However, there have been several publications discussing use of classical radiology with other diagnostic imaging modalities. It is not certain whether all radiologists would have abandoned classical radiology or whether they have been inevitably involved in modern diagnostic imaging techniques such as CT, US, and MRI.

Apparently, radiologists appear to believe that endoscopy is superior to radiology, as far as the detection of gastric cancer is concerned. As a general trend, it has been disclosed that the first screening for gastric cancer on an out-patient basis is done by forward-viewing endoscopy in most Japanese institutions (Maruyama 1990), and that radiology is performed as a detailed examination, before surgery in patients with gastric cancer. Also, too much reliance on endoscopy and biopsy for the final diagnosis has made making a comparative study of both diagnostic techniques very difficult.

In their early report, Shirakabe *et al.* (1972) described that the initial routine radiographic examination detected 86% of all gastric cancers, and the first endoscopic examination after the initial radiographic examination detected another 9%. In 1983, Shirakabe and Maruyama (1989) also reported that the routine radiographic examination missed 10.4% (72/695) of a single early cancer and 35.1% (39/111) of multiple lesions that were subsequently detected by endoscopic examination or examination of resected specimens. They stressed that 17 single lesions escaped detection by both radiographic and endoscopic examinations.

In 1986, Maruyama illustrated the efficiency of radiology and endoscopy in the diagnosis of gastric cancer with computer-controlled processing of diagnostic data, and described that diagnosed malignancy was confirmed in only 36.2% of all cases diagnosed as early cancer by the initial radiographic examination using remote-controlled X-ray television viewing equipment.

Furthermore, the histological examination after surgery disclosed that 64.3% of all cancers diagnosed as early actually were early cancer. Maruyama also reported that 1.5% of the cases diagnosed as normal in the initial radiographic examination were finally confirmed as cancer by subsequent endoscopy when the endoscopy group is regarded as a denominator. They account for 0.2% (11/5630) of all cases diagnosed as normal. In other words, these are 11 cases missed by the initial radiographic examination (Fig. 10.2a–d).

In Maruyama's series, the sensitivity of the initial radiographic examination was 97.1%, the specificity 32.3%, and the accuracy 46.2%. Only a minor difference was found in the sensitivity and specificity between radiology and endoscopy in the diagnosis of gastric cancer, including early and advanced cancers. This result indicates that there are a large number of false-positives, which can be attributed to the tendency of radiologists to avoid false-negatives. In addition, the production of many false-positives, by many radiologists, is because, there still remains a difference in image quality between the initial and the second detailed examination (Fig. 10.3a–c).

It is not infrequently experienced that the image quality of the initial radiographic examination is not sufficient to allow the diagnosis of early cancer. In particular, controlling the volume of air plays a decisive role for delineation of subtle mucosal abnormalities such as type IIc early cancer (Fig. 10.4a,b).

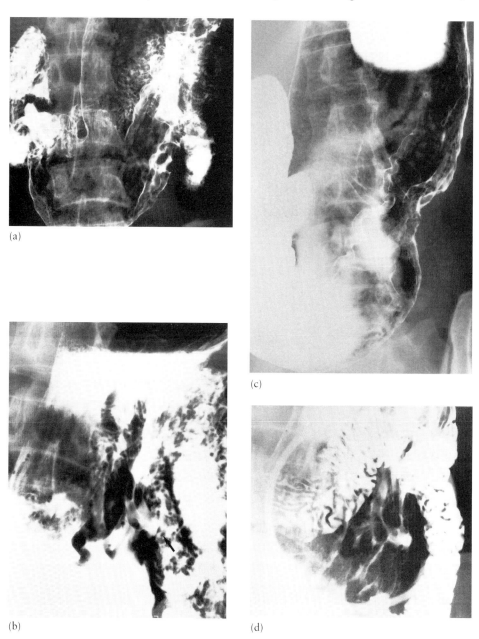

Fig. 10.2. Borrmann type 3 cancer involving the serosa missed in the screening. On a double contrast image taken in the screening the overlapped duodenal and jejunal loop interfered with the visualization of an advanced cancer located in the greater curvature of the lower gastric body (a). The presence of an abnormality was not noted in an compression image (b), and a small cancer crater (arrow) was pointed out by the review of this image after the cancer was detected endoscopically. A double contrast image in the second detailed study (c) revealed a filling defect and mass in the greater curvature of the lower gastric body, and the part of the cancer crater was clearly demonstrated in an compression image (d).

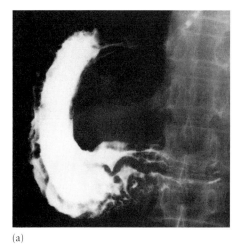

(a)

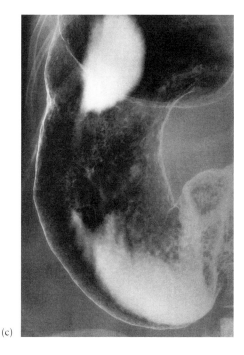

(c)

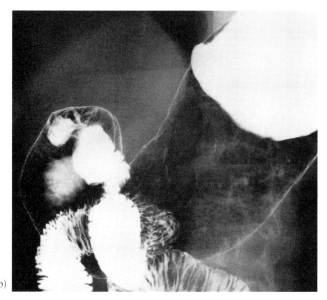

(b)

Fig. 10.3. Advanced cancer, Borrmann type 3, with metastases to the lung and supraclavicular lymph node. Prone mucosal relief image taken in the screening examination (a) revealed very slight poor lumen distention of the gastric body as compared to the lower portion of the stomach which was not recognized. A double contrast image in the left poster oblique position (b) shows only the irregularity of the lesser curvature of the gastric body (arrow line). A prone double contrast image disclosed an extensive cancerous erosion in the anterior wall of the gastric body (c).

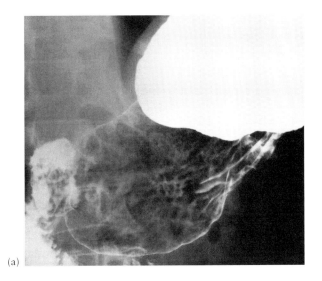

(a)

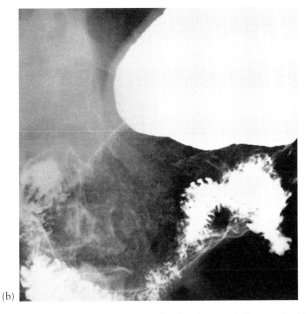

(b)

Fig. 10.4. A type IIc early gastric cancer was visualized rather precisely on a double contrast image in a slight lumen distention taken as the first step of the screening (a). However, the lesion is perceived with difficulty in a moderate lumen distention taken as the second step (b).

In 1988, Hamada and co-workers (1988) reported that only 73.6% of all early gastric cancer cases (72.2% of elevated-type cases and 74.1% of depressed-type cases) could be detected by the initial radiographic examination, even when cases of vague abnormalities were included. In 1987, Takasu (1988) reported that panendoscopy missed 10.1% of early cancers and 9.3% of advanced cancers in an 11-year-period from 1976.

In 1989, Otsuji and co-workers (1989), based on their 9-year experience of panendoscopy performed on an asymptomatic group aged 50 years and over, described that the oversight of gastric cancer occurred in 7.2%. They calculated the morbidity of gastric cancer in a age group of 50 years and over as 2.38% in males and 0.99% in females. Yao and associates (1990) stated that the degree of oversight of cancer by the initial radiographic examination was nearly equivalent to that of endoscopy, which was done as the first screening method. They stressed the importance of pursuing a high-quality, accurate radiographic examinations in order that any oversight is reduced to a minimum.

In 1990, Nishizawa and co-workers reported that in 306 cases of advanced cancers detected by the examination sequence in which radiology preceded endoscopy for a 10 year period, 7 cases (2%) were missed by radiology, and 2 cases (0.6%) were missed by endoscopy. Based on their experience, they stated that examination by radiology tends to overlook advanced cancers in the upper part and anterior wall of the stomach and type IIc early cancer, and that endoscopic examination is prone to overlook advanced cancers of the linitis plastica type.

It must be emphasized that using panendoscopy with a forward-viewing type of endoscope gives much less diagnostic information about cancer than do the other types of endoscopy. This even applies to the present situation where a videoendoscope provides a much better image quality than conventional equipment. If more stress was given to the importance of biopsy under these circumstances, the differences in efficacy of differing diagnostic methods might decline. The only factor that could improve the rate of diagnosis of EGC is the training of endoscopists in the biopsy techniques (Maruyama 1986).

3.2. Technical considerations in the screening for gastric cancer

In the basic approach to radiographic examination it is assumed that any lesion that can be visible macroscopically can be detected radiographically. Exact reproduction of macroscopic findings is the major requirement for achieving this purpose (Maruyama 1979).

The initial or routine radiographic examination in screening for gastric cancer consists of a combination of the various examination methods and includes: mucosal relief study, barium-filled film, double contrast study, and compression study. However, double contrast radiography is most important study as it forms the main frame of the examination.

Single contrast examination alone is never carried out in Japan. It could be proposed that double contrast radiography is only one of several techniques and that too much reliance on this method should be avoided. It may be true that the successful results achieved in the early days using double contrast radiography has set a precedent that it is superior to any other modalities. However, if it is carried out inadequately, this technique provides much less information than other methods (Fig. 10.5a–c). However, this awareness of its drawbacks does lead to considerable accuracy in the initial screening for gastric cancer.

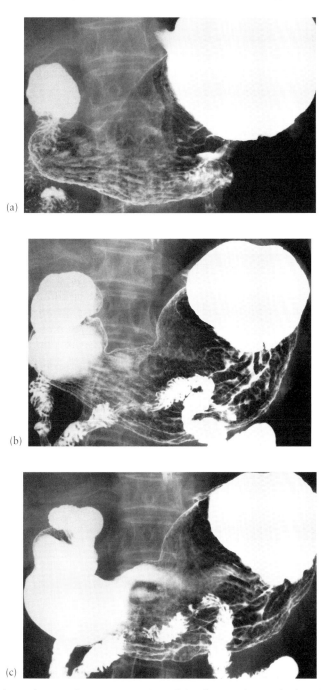

(a)

(b)

(c)

Fig. 10.5. Advanced cancer, Borrmann type 2 involving the propria muscle. A supine frontal double contrast image shows no abnormality (a). A faint barium collection and its surrounding raised wall is noted in a double contrast image that was taken to allow the barium remain in the depression, by controlling the position of the patient (b). The lesion was precisely demonstrated by collecting the barium in the cancer crater and around the raised wall (c).

The first radiographic examination begins with an exposure sequence shown in Table 10.1, although there are some variations in the positioning of the patient and the number of films used. For double contrast radiography of the stomach the principal requirements are an adequate volume of barium and gas, and frequent positional changes of the patient. More than 200 ml of barium is necessary except in some patients with a deformity of the stomach. Less than 200 ml of the barium meal suspension does not produce a good quality double contrast image, because the entire mucosal surface cannot be washed out with such a small volume. Consequently, the effects of mucus and gastric juice cannot be reduced to minimum. Unfortunately, there has been little experience in using a high-density barium suspension with low viscosity in Japan.

It is generally accepted that the ideal amount of gas might be that which makes it possible to obtain a double contrast an image of the middle portion of the body of stomach in the supine frontal position. This volume of gas may give the impression that the stomach is overdistended. Recently, however, the gaseous distension of the stomach is obtained in two steps even for the initial radiographic examination (Figs 10.4A,B). In the first step, the stomach is distended by a small volume of gas using 2 g of effervescent granules in order to obtain an optimal double contrast image from the gastric antrum to the incisura region (Fig. 10.4A).

The use of effervescent granules is unnecessary when a volume of gas is already present in the gastric fornix. The swallowed air during the intake of barium may sometimes allow an optimal distension of the gastric antrum and incisura region. However, a subtle mucosal abnormality of this area, like a small type IIc lesion (Fig. 10.4B), is often effaced by overdistension. Moreover, even a large advanced cancer may be missed due to the vertical dislocation of the gastric antrum which is caused by excessive gaseous distension.

In the second step, an additional 2–3 g of effervescent granules are given, and double contrast images of the lower gastric body to the fornix are obtained. However, lesions in this area, especially those in the upper gastric body and cardia, are frequently missed without adequate gaseous distension.

Table 10.1 Radiographic examination: Sequence of exposure in the routine examination of the stomach

---

 1. Mucosal relief image in the prone position
 2. Barium-filled image in the upright position
 3. Double contrast image in the supine frontal position
 4. Double contrast image in the supine left posterior oblique position
 5. Double contrast image in the supine right posterior oblique position
 6. Double contrast image in the semiupright, right decubitus, or steep right posterior oblique position
 7. Barium-filled image in the prone position
 8. Double contrast image in the upright frontal position
 9. Double contrast image in the upright left posterior oblique position (with barium passing through the cardia)
10. Compression images

Frequent positional changes should be made in order to wash out the mucosal surface with a rapid flow of barium. By shifting the contrast medium from the fundus to the antrum, adherent mucus is washed out and the gastric juice is mixed together with the barium, resulting in an optimal barium coating to the mucosal surface.

3.3.   Differences in image quality of the initial and subsequent detailed studies

Western radiologists may raise the question of whether detailed radiographic examination is necessary when a diagnosis of cancer has already been obtained by endoscopy and biopsy. However, one must recognize the difference in the image quality between the initial and radiographic examinations. It is not infrequently encountered that the extent of a depressed-type early cancer is defined equivocally in the initial radiographic examination (Figs 10.3A–3C). In particular, the precise distance from its proximal border to the esophagogastric junction should be made clear for subsequent surgery.

Moreover, an investigation to reduce the difference in image quality among the two examinations has long been continued. It should be noted that the presence of gastric juice is a decisive factor which interferes with the visualization of subtle mucosal abnormalities. For this reason, removal of gastric juice is the minimum requirement in the detailed radiographic examination, although there is some controversy concerning the necessity of aspirating gastric juice in order to show a lesion in the gastric cardia (Nishimata *et al.* 1987).

4.   ASSESSMENT OF THE INVASIVE DEPTH OF CANCER

4.1.   Diagnosis of polypoid early and advanced carcinoma

Theoretical basis

The radiographic diagnosis of early polypoid cancer is based essentially on the more detailed analysis of radiographic results, which leads to the recognition of the polypoid lesion (Maruyama *et al.* 1982*a*). The differential diagnosis is thus more easily ascertained. The analysis starts with the recognition of the size, form, and surface pattern of the polypoid lesion. These lesions typically range from 1 cm to 4 cm in their widest diameter, except in unusual cases. The height of a polypoid lesion is next estimated on a compression or double contrast image; the estimation of the height provides a rough distinction between type I and type IIa lesions when a polypoid lesion is interpreted to be malignant.

Most important for the differentiation between malignant and benign lesions is surface pattern. The surface pattern of a benign hyperplastic polyp is almost always smooth regardless of its size, whereas that of a malignant lesion is granulated or lobulated. This type of appearance, although irregular and enlarged, essentially has a similarity to the surrounding mucosa that bears the lesion (Fig. 10.6).

Radiographically, this condition is visible as a uniform granularity of various degrees recognized as the so-called 'areae gastricae'. Usually, it depends on the

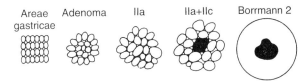

Fig. 10.6.   Surface pattern of polypoid lesions of the stomach. From Shirakabe and Maruyama, 1989, with permission.

intensity of the intestinal metaplasia. In most instances of early polypoid cancer, its surface pattern is comparable to that of the surrounding areae gastricae. In other words, a tendency to imitate the pattern of the areae gastricae is preserved in a polypoid cancer whose invasion is limited at least to the submucosal layer (Fig. 10.7a,b). This observation is the most reliable radiographic sign for establishing the diagnosis of early cancer of a polypoid lesion (Shirakabe and Maruyama 1989). Obviously, double contrast radiography is best suited for visualizing a background where polypoid cancer has developed.

As the cancerous infiltration extends deeper than the submucosal layer, this similarity of the surface pattern disappears and is usually replaced by erosion or ulceration in most cases. This condition is classified as advanced cancer, Borrmann type 2 (type 2 in the classification by the Japanese Research Society for Gastric Cancer), which comprises about 26.6% of all advanced cancers (Ohta *et al.* 1993). Sometimes, early cancer type IIa + IIc can be distinguished, but with difficulty,

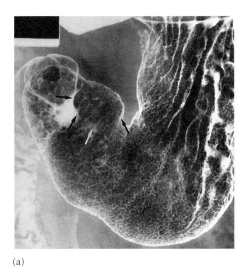

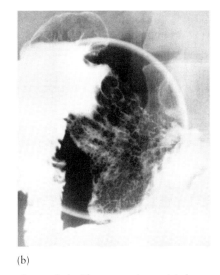

(a)   (b)

Fig. 10.7.   Type IIa early cancer limited to the mucosal membrane. A double contrast image (a) shows a localized portion of the mucosa with granularity in the gastric antrum that is nearly regular in size but larger as compared to the normal areae gastricae pattern surrounding it (arrows). The difference in size of granularity between the surface of the lesion and the normal areae gastricae was made more clear on a compression image (b).

from advanced cancer, Borrmann type 2 in the 2 cm level. In this case, the granular surface pattern is frequently a clue that suggests that the invasion is still limited to the submucosa (Fig. 10.8).

In some cases, erosion or ulceration does not occur on its surface as the size of a polypoid lesion becomes larger than 4 cm. This type of lesion develops into a large polypoid mass with an irregularly lobulated surface and is called advanced cancer, Borrmann type 1. This type accounts for approximately 2.2% of all advanced cancers (Ohta *et al.* 1993). Generally, it is the size (2 cm) that makes the distinction between early polypoid cancer and Borrmann type 1 cancer. In contrast, even a large polypoid cancer maintains a similarity to the surrounding mucosa (Maruyama and Hamada 1994). (*Alimentary tract radiology*). In any event, the surface pattern of early polypoid cancer reveals one of the developing phases of differentiated cancer.

Gross appearance of polypoid lesions

The gross appearance of types gastric polypoid lesions are basically defined as pedunculated, subpedunculated, and sessile. The sessile lesion is further divided into two subtypes: one with constriction at the base, and the other with gradual sloping. Most lesions of type IIa have a constriction at the base, whereas benign

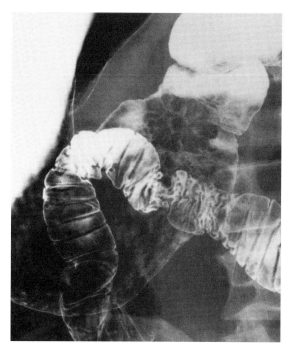

Fig. 10.8.   Type IIa + IIc early cancer with the involvement of the submucosa (prone double contrast image). The surface granularity of the raised wall is an indication suggesting that the invasive depth is no deeper than the submucosa, although the size of the lesion is greater than 2 cm. From Maruyama and Baba, 1994, with permission.

lesions, including epithelial and submucosal lesions, show a gradual sloping. The gross classification of gastric polypoid lesions by Yamada and Fukutomi (1966) (Fig. 10.9) has been widely used because it is simple and approximately defines the form of polypoid lesions endoscopically as well as radiographically.

Borrmann types 1 and 2

A Borrmann type 1 lesion is a large polypoid lesion, usually exceeding 3 cm at its greatest diameter, with large irregular lobulation. Sometimes, a slight surface depression may be present. A Borrmann type 1 lesion is seen as a large, irregular filling defect of the margin on radiographs of a barium-filled lesion and as an irregular tumor shadow with rough lobulation on double contrast and compression radiographs. Occasionally, a large pedunculated lesion may be an early carcinoma that also falls into the original classification of Borrmann type 1.

The Borrmann type 2 lesion is visible as a localized filling defect of the gastric wall on a radiograph obtained with the use of compression. Those obtained with the latter method demonstrate an irregular crater with a greatly raised margin sharply circumscribed from the normal surrounding mucosa (Fig. 10.5c) Its size usually exceeds 3 cm in its greatest diameter (Fig. 10.10a,b). The smaller Borrmann type is difficult to distinguish from early cancer type IIa + IIc with involvement of the submucosa (Fig. 10.8).

4.2.   Diagnosis of depressed and ulcerated cancer

Theoretical basis for the diagnosis of early cancer

The invasion pattern in early depressed cancer is regarded as two-dimensional and in advanced cancer as three-dimensional (Maruyama *et al.* 1976). In other words, the thickness of invasion can be disregarded in cases of early cancer, whereas the invasive depth and staging become important in advanced cancer. Consequently, the diagnosis of early depressed cancer is based on the analysis of a depression and converging fold (Fig. 10.11).

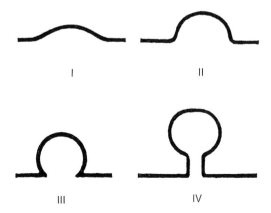

Fig. 10.9.   Classification of polypoid lesions of stomach. (From Yamada 1966, p. 45, 1996, with permission.)

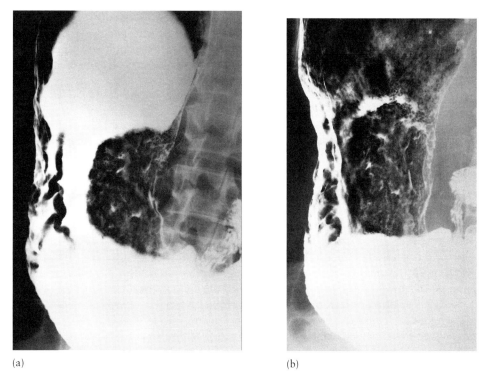

(a)   (b)

Fig. 10.10.   Large advanced cancer, Borrmann type 2 involving the serosa. Prone compression image reveals a sharply demarcated large mass and cancer crater in the gastric body (a). A prone double contrast image in the upright position indicates that the lesion is in the anterior wall (b).

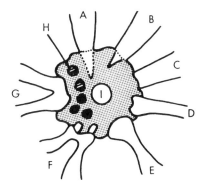

Fig. 10.11.   Various appearances of converging folds and unevenness in early depressed cancer. A, gradual tapering; B, abrupt tapering; C, abrupt interruption; D and E, clubbing; F, fusion with abrupt tapering; G, fusion (V-shaped deformity); H, unevenness; I, regenerative epithelium. From Shirakabe and Maruyama, 1989, with permission.

The depression is analysed in terms of its outline, surface, and depth. The depression is usually irregular and has a serrated or spiculated margin, whereas a benign ulcer usually has a sharp, straight margin. The irregular margin, however, is sometimes seen in cases of recurrent peptic ulcers and cannot be distinguished from that of an early depressed cancer. The margin of an early depressed cancer is usually distinct from the normal mucosal surface but sometimes shifts gradually, without distinction, to normal mucosa. The extent of early depressed cancer is therefore frequently difficult to define.

Types IIc, IIc + III, and III

The differences between types IIc and III is recognized radiographically by the thickness of the collected contrast medium in a depression. A thickness in the depression of a peptic ulcer indicates a type III lesion (Fig. 10.12), and a thinner collection of the contrast medium indicates a depression of type IIc (Fig. 10.13). Thus a combination of the two different depths is termed type IIc + III (Fig. 10.12), or III + IIc. Usually, the deeper part (type III) is in the centre of the depression surrounded by the shallow part. A type IIc lesion dose not reveal a uniform density of the contrast medium in the depression. A scar of an ulcer may sometimes be seen as a slight depression. The same depression may be seen in an erosion or in a healing peptic ulcer (Maruyama *et al.* 1982*b*). In these instances, however, the depression is more faint than that of a type IIc lesion, and a homogeneous density of the contrast medium is revealed.

The radiographic examination of a type IIc lesion is best demonstrated with the double contrast method. For the precise delineation of a type IIc lesion, postural maneuvers must be performed carefully during the double contrast examination so that the contrast medium dose not flow out of the depression (Maruyama 1979).

Type III lesions have depth, whereas type IIc lesions may be scarcely recognizable at the peripheral part of a deeper ulcer depression. In such cases the presence of cancer is

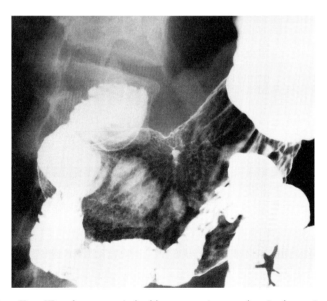

Fig. 10.12.   Type IIc + III early cancer. A double contrast image taken in the supine, left posterior oblique position delineates a small ulceration (III) and the surrounding shallow erosion (IIc).

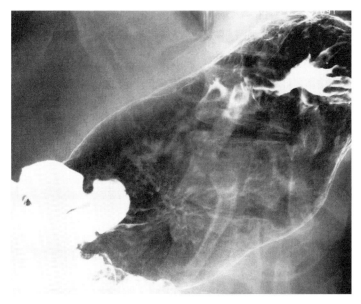

Fig. 10.13.   Type IIc early cancer. A double contrast image taken in the right posterior oblique position permits a frontal view of a typical type IIc lesion located in the posterior wall of the gastric body.

radiographically identified as the slightest change of a type IIc lesion or an irregularity of the niche itself (maruyama and Hamada 1994). This can surround the niche totally or partially (Kumakura *et al.* 1973*a,b*). Close observation may reveal the irregularity of the niche. Sometimes, the surrounding radiolucent defect of the niche may be prominent in a type III lesion when an acute peptic change has taken place.

Attention should be directed to a profile niche that does not show any irregularity. In type III + IIc lesions, the profile niche is so prominent that the surrounding type IIc lesion may be missed (Maruyama 1979) and the diagnosis of a benign peptic ulcer is made. Thus, the Hampton line alone cannot be a sign of a benign peptic ulcer. A frontal view of the niche and the surrounding mucosa is required to ensure that the lesion is type IIc. During follow-up studies the niche in type III lesions may decrease in size, and the surrounding type IIc lesion increases and is recognized clearly (Maruyama and Hamada 1994). The niche finally disappears, and a fairly large type IIc lesion then becomes evident (Maruyama 1979). This phenomenon has been called the 'malignant cycle' (Murakami 1967) and has been observed by many radiologists and endoscopists (Okabe 1968; Sakita *et al.* 1971).

The theoretical basis for the diagnosis of advanced cancer

The radiographic diagnosis of advanced gastric cancer can be established by demonstrating an evidence of tumor formation on radiographs. The tumor is demonstrated with the compression or double contrast method. The views of such an advanced cancer constantly reveal a filling defect, a surrounding raised margin, and shrinkage of the affected portion of the entire thickness of the stomach.

Sometimes, a lesion occurs with a slight to moderate involvement of the propria muscle which macroscopically simulates type IIc early cancer. It rarely reveals an invasion of the entire thickness of the gastric wall and a direct invasion of adjacent structures. This is called an advanced cancer simulating-type IIc, and is classified into Borrmann type 5 (7.4% including the other unclassifiable type) using the JRSGC (1981) classification.

Borrmann type 3

This type comprises about 42.8% of all advanced cancers (Ohta *et al.* 1993). Usually, the Borrmann type 3 lesion is larger than Borrmann type 2. Radiographs after barium filling reveal a filling defect and stiffening of the gastric wall (Fig. 10.14a,b). A compression radiograph shows a large, irregular crater and surrounding radiolucent defect which is not as well defined as that of the Borrmann type 2 lesion. Double contrast radiographs best demonstrate the whole aspect of the Borrmann type 3 lesion. Stiffening of the gastric wall extends beyond the range of a cancer crater because of the diffuse infiltration of the gastric wall.

Usually, the mucosal convergence is interrupted at the margin of the crater which is not as prominent as the one seen with a Borrmann type 2 lesion. Sometimes, a component of type IIc may surround the crater; in this case a greater or lesser deformity of the stomach resulting from extensive cancerous infiltration may be revealed.

Borrmann type 4

This type accounts for about 21% of all advanced cancers (Ohta *et al.* 1993). A Borrmann type 4 lesion is called a diffuse infiltrative carcinoma in Western literature (Borrmann called it diffuse carcinoma). Thickening of the gastric wall caused by diffuse cancerous infiltration and pronounced proliferation of fibrotic tissue are gross characteristics of this type. Linitis plastica is a Borrmann type 4 lesion in a broad sense of this classification.

The Borrmann type 4 lesion is seen on barium radiographs as a deformity of the stomach. The gastric antrum is the typical site of involvement and is greatly narrowed (Fig. 10.15a,b). A double contrast radiograph demonstrates poor distensibility of the gastric wall, and often the primary site as an erosion or ulceration (Fig. 10.16). In a late stage, this primary site is enlarged, giving a disturbed appearance of the mucosal surface. Finally the surface is extensively replaced by a large, irregular erosion. A pattern of malignant folds with enlargement and twisting is not prominent in most instances of Borrmann type 4 lesion. No definite tumor forms are present in this type. Sometimes, the proximal limit of infiltration may be difficult to define; double contrast radiography can be effective in this respect.

The linitis plastica type of carcinoma and its early phase

The linitis plastica type of carcinoma is typical seen in patients younger than 40 years of age. It is characterized radiographically by deformity and shrinkage involving the entire stomach. A pattern of malignant folds with enlargement and twisting is also seen. Careful radiographic examination shows a depressed lesion in the area where the mucosal folds are prominent, corresponding to the primary

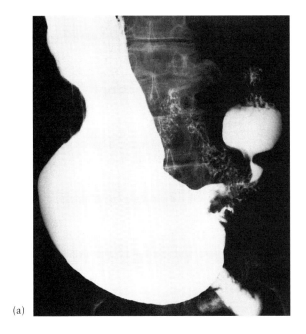

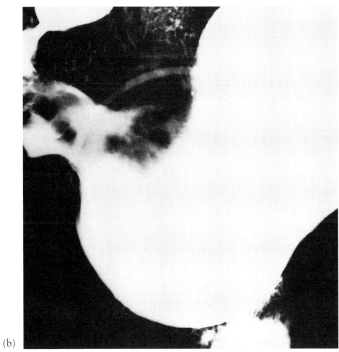

Fig. 10.14. Advanced cancer, Borrmann type 3 (infiltrating, ulcerating type) involving the serosa. A prone double contrast image reveals narrowing with filling defect of the gastric antrum (a). A compression image demonstrates the irregular cancer crater and surrounding raised wall with less sharp demarcation as compared to that of Borrmann type 2 (localized, ulcerating type) (b).

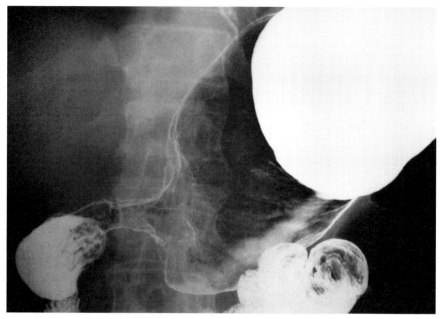

(a)

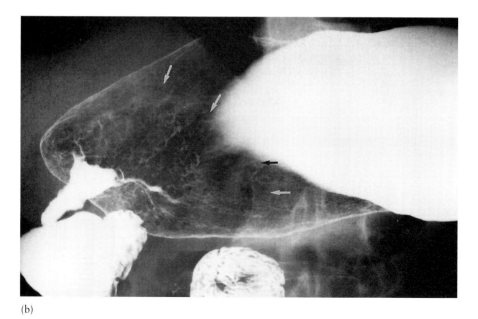

(b)

Fig. 10.15. Advanced cancer, Borrmann type 4 (diffuse type). A double contrast image in the supine frontal position (a) shows marked narrowing from the pylorus to the mid-gastric body. In the narrowed potion the mucosa is disturbed with irregular erosions. An additional double contrast image taken in the same position defines the proximal extension of the cancer (b, arrows).

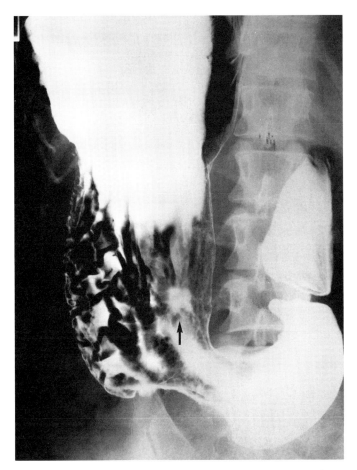

Fig. 10.16.   Linitis plastica type cancer. A prone double contrast image shows the primary focus of cancer (arrow) in the anterior wall of the lower gastric body. From Maruyama and Hamada, 1994, with permission.

focus of linitis plastica, which is most common in the gastric body (Nakamura *et al.* 1980).

In routine radiographic examinations a stomach that had been judged as normal may change into a 'leather bottle' structure within a few months. Retrospective studies of the first radiographic examination may reveal only the slightest abnormality of the gastric wall. Many efforts have been made to detect the early phase of linitis plastica; it is the only problem that remains unresolved in the diagnosis of gastric cancer, even now when the diagnosis of early gastric cancer has been well established.

Nakamura and co-workers (1980) estimated that the time required from the evolution of the cancer to the linitis plastica form may be 3–8 years, the mean being 6 years. With their hypothesis the early detection of linitis plastica was facilitated by the discovery of a type IIc lesion smaller than 2 cm in the mucosa of the fundus.

The radiographic diagnosis of early linitis plastica should include: (1) the detection of a pathologic condition of linitis plastica without shrinkage of the stomach (Fig. 10.17); and (2) the detection of early undifferentiated cancer in the mucosa of the fundic gland area (Fig. 10.18). Attention should be directed to the discovery of a type IIc lesion in this mucosa. Double contrast radiography, with as great a volume of gas as needed to provide separation of the prominent mucosal folds is required for this purpose.

The first condition is diagnosed by detecting abnormalities such as slight spiculation and stiffening of the mucosal folds. Accumulated experience with cases of linitis plastica in which the stomach does not shrink would be necessary to obtain clinical proof that type IIc lesions develop into linitis plastica.

Advanced cancer simulating-type IIc

Most lesions of this type are cancers which macroscopically are not definite advanced cancers. They raise a problem for estimating the invasive depth in depressed cancers. The radiographic analysis of the invasive depth in the depressed lesions aims not only

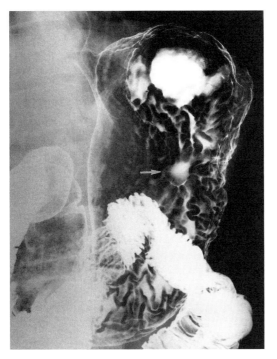

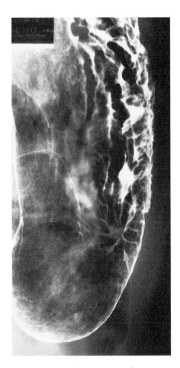

Fig. 10.17. Linitis plastica type cancer in a contracting phase. A double contrast image in the supine frontal position reveals a slightly poor distensibility of the greater curvature of the gastric body. However, the stomach is not totally shrunken. The primary focus (arrow) is surrounded completely in the fundic gland mucosa.

Fig. 10.18. Type IIc early cancer in the fundic gland area. A double contrast image in the left lateral position reveals a small IIc lesion (arrow) in the greater curvature of the lower gastric body.

at estimating the invading front, but also at recognizing the entire invasive pattern of the cancer based on the concept that invasion is continuous.

The submucosal involvement of an early cancer is, generally, slight and limited only to the central part. Consequently, the radiographic evidence of extensive submucosal involvement suggests the possibility of an advanced cancer simulating type IIc. Therefore, an involvement that is deeper than the submucosal layer is always considered when an extensive surrounding translucency is visible on the compression image (Maruyama 1979). Such a translucency, however, is not always seen in lesions with extensive submucosal involvement.

For the estimation of the invasive depth a change in the volume of gas can be useful. The changing aspect of the depression and the converging folds provide invaluable information on how to estimate the pattern of invasion as well as the invasive depth (Igarashi *et al.* 1977).

A mucosal cancer or a cancer with slight submucosal involvement does not produce a tumor shadow of a double contrast image even with a small volume of gas. However, a double contrast radiograph with a moderate to large volume of gas alone is not able to suggest an involvement deeper than the submucosal layer. In a lesion with an extensive involvement of the submucosa and slight to moderate involvement of the propria muscle a tumor shadow which is visualized on a double contrast image in a moderate to large grade of gaseous distension of the stomach is effaced by an excessive volume gaseous distension (Maruyama 1979).

A compression image always reveals a pronounced translucency of the tumor shadow. These observations make a distinction from radiographic images of the definite advanced cancer. In addition to the analysis of the radiographic findings already mentioned, EUS (Figs 10.20B, 10.21C) and CT are indispensable for assessing the thickness of the affected gastric wall.

4.3. The role of endoscopic ultrasonography in the assessment of invasive depth

It was anticipated that the invasive depth of cancer could be assessed much more accurately by endoscopic ultrasound (EUS), which provides substantial evidence of alterations in each layer of the gastric wall involved by cancer. However, results fell short of our expectations. At the author's institution, the invasive depth of cancer limited to mucosal membrane was diagnosed correctly in 66% of cases, and 34% of these were diagnosed as having cancer with submucosal involvement (Fig. 10.19). The invasive depth of cancer involving the submucosa was assessed correctly in 45% of cases, and another 41% were diagnosed as having cancer limited to the mucosal membrane. Some cases with the invasive depth of the propria muscle were diagnosed as having cancer involving the submucosa (Fig. 10.20a,b).

The presence of peptic ulceration in a lesion of depressed early cancer is a factor that makes the assessment of invasive depth difficult. Peptic ulceration is associated in 36.3% of depressed cancers, including early and advanced cancers, which are smaller than 3 cm (Takekoshi *et al.* 1990) and the rate of peptic ulceration complicating depressed cancers rapidly increases as their size become larger.

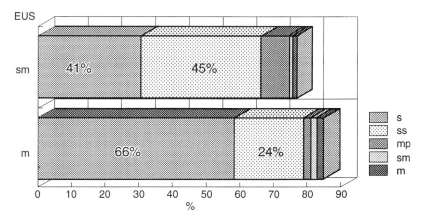

Fig. 10.19. Assessment of invasive depth by endoscopic ultrasound in early cancer. s: serosa, ss: subserosa, mp: muscularis propriae, sm: submucosa, m: mucosa. (From the Cancer Institute Hospital, Tokyo, 1989–90.)

In 1990, Chonan and associates (1990*a,b*) reported that in the depressed type of early cancer associated with ulceration, EUS could correctly assess the invasive depth in 50% of carcinoma with submucosal involvement. This reveals the difficulty in distinguishing cancerous invasion from fibrosis caused by ulceration. In other words, an EUS image reveals an area of fibrosis including cancer cells' hypo-echoic zone, and in the actual diagnosis the deeper front of the area is recognized as the invasive depth of cancer.

The indices for the estimation of invasive depth of early cancer associated with peptic ulceration are based on the grade of the interruption of the five-layer structure of the gastric wall which is caused by peptic ulceration. In a open ulcer co-existing with early depressed cancer the depth of ulceration is judged as being UI-II (tissue defect of mucosa and submucosa). When the fourth layer and beneath remain intact, it is judged as being UI-III (tissue defect from mucosa to propria muscle) and when the fifth layer is intact, and the interruption of the fifth layer is judged as UI-IV (propria muscle is penetrated).

In an ulcer scar complicating depressed early cancer, UI-IIs is referred to as a state in which the fourth layer and beneath remain intact. Fusion of the fourth layer is observed in UI-IIIs, and notching of the fifth layer is characteristic for UI-IVs in addition to fusion of the fourth layer. In early cancers associated with peptic ulceration UI-II and UI-IIs account for more than 80%.

The index for intramucosal carcinoma-associated peptic ulceration is a wedge-shaped low echoe in the third layer without alteration of fourth layer in UI-II and UI-IIs, and retraction of the third layer to the mucosal membrane in UI-III and UI-IIIs and their scars. Involvement of the submucosal layer is possible when those EUS signs become irregular (Kida *et al.* 1988).

Invasive depth of depressed advanced cancer is less accurately assessed by EUS than for early cancer. In the author's institution, EUS could correctly diagnose the invasive depth of advanced cancer involving the propria muscle in 33% of cases

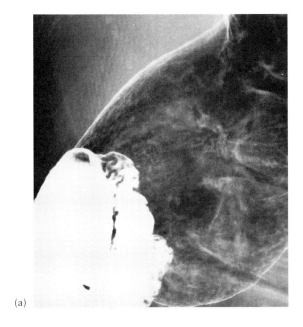

(a)

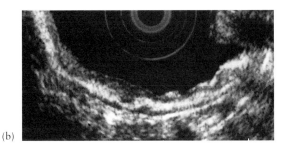

(b)

Fig. 10.20.   Advanced cancer simulating type IIc early cancer. The diagnosis of early cancer involving the submucosa was made radiographically (a). In the endoscopic ultrasound diagnosis, the involvement of the propria muscle was indicated by the presence of thickening and interruption of the fourth layer (b), and it was confirmed by the histologic examination after surgery.

(Fig. 10.21a–c), that involving the subserosa in 20%, and that involving the serosa in 63% (Fig. 10.22).

Chonan and associates (1990*a,b*) described that the correct diagnosis of invasive depth was made in 55.6% of the cancers involving the propria muscle (pm), in 50% of the cancers involving the subserosa (ss), in 83.3% of the cancers in which the serosa was exposed (se), and in 66.7% of the cancers with the invasion to the neighboring structures (sei).

These results were substantiated in a case meeting of 13 experts where depressed early and advanced cancers were presented (Yao 1990). The hit rate of the diagnosis among the 13 experts was 40.2% in early cancers, and 77% in advanced cancers.

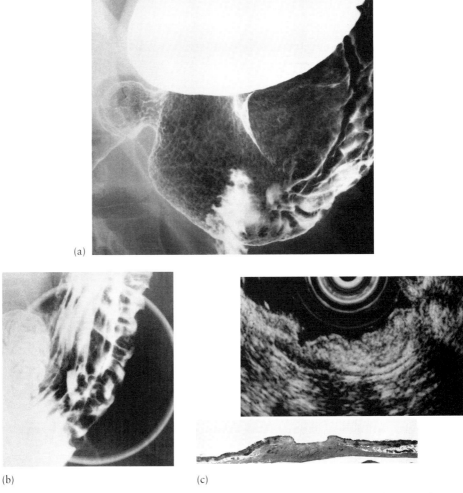

Fig. 10.21. Advanced cancer simulating type IIc early cancer. The diagnosis of advanced cancer involving the propria muscle was made radiographically, based on double contrast (a) and compression image (b). The endoscopic ultrasound diagnosis (c) was the same as that of radiology, and it was proved to be correct by histologic examination after surgery.

EUS correctly diagnosed the invasive depth in 57% of the presented cases. There is no doubt that EUS is useful for the assessment of the invasive depth of cancer. However, much more experience is required to know the limits, as well as to prove the merits, of EUS.

4.4. The role of computed tomography

In Japan computed tomography (CT) is not indicated for symptomatic patients as the first choice of examination, by which the operability of gastric cancer is deter-

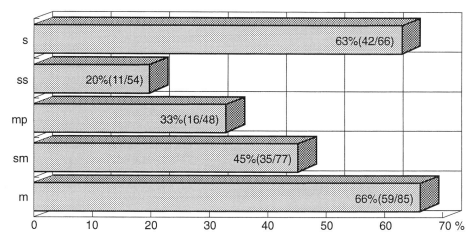

Fig. 10.22. Overall result in the assessment of invasive depth by endoscopic ultrasound. Abbreviations are same as in Fig. 10.19.

mined. In the majority of Japanese institutions, the screening for gastric cancer is performed by means of endoscopy and/or radiology. CT is effected in order to assess the involvement of the neighboring structures and node and liver metastasis. Accordingly, CT is indicated not only for cases of advanced cancer but also for early cancer.

Liver metastasis is investigated, particularly in case of differentiated adenocarcinoma. US is also implemented to estimate the liver metastasis. Sometimes, even intraoperative US is included when the possibility of solitary liver metastasis is suspected by the other imaging data before surgery.

In CT findings gastric cancer is visualized as thickening of the gastric wall or as tumor formation (Ohkura *et al.* 1984). CT, however, is not able to demonstrate the architecture of the gastric wall. Consequently, the invasive depth of cancer limited to the gastric wall cannot be diagnosed. CT can diagnose if the serosa is severely involved or if the contiguous structures are involved.

Komaki and Toyoshima (1983), however, claimed that diagnostic accuracy of CT in evaluating tumor invasion to the adjacent structures is not as high as has been reported.

Ohkuma and co-workers (1984) reported that CT could correctly diagnose the extent of serosal involvement in 80% of gastric cancers, peritoneal dissemination in only 20%, liver metastasis in 83%, and lymph node metastasis in 59%. In CT findings, a lymph node measuring more than 1 cm is judged to be metastatic. Sometimes, a metastatic node measures less than 1 cm (Hori *et al.* 1984), and CT is not able to diagnose lymph node metastasis. In addition, an enlarged lymph node is not always metastatic, but may be inflammatory. Consequently, the diagnosis of lymph node metastasis is reluctantly made in the case of early cancer, in which lymph node metastasis is reported to be 12.7% (Ohta *et al.* 1987), although an enlarged node is visualized on CT.

5. THE DELINEATION OF THE LATERAL SPREAD OF CANCER

This is of utmost importance especially when determining the proximal surgical resection line of the stomach bearing a depressed early cancer and an advanced cancer, Borrmann types 3 and 4. For this purpose, radiographic images are able to provide substantial information in terms of approximate distance from the esophagogastric junction.

The proximal border of a cancer can be defined without difficulty if it is sharply defined. If it is ambiguous, a meticulous evaluation of radiographic images is required. In this respect the concept of the histologic type should be considered for the delineation of, the lateral spread of a cancer itself and estimation of a distance between the proximal border and esophagogastric junction (Fig. 10.23). The extent of esophageal invasion is assessed also in terms of the histologic type of gastric cancer. The invasion pattern of the differentiated adenocarcinoma is different from that of undifferentiated adenocarcinoma.

5.1. Correlation of histologic-type and depressed early cancer

In most cases of early depressed cancer the surface of the depression is uneven because of an irregular proliferation of cancerous tissue (Figs 10.4a, 10.13). Sometimes an island-like nodule remains in the depression, and is more prominent than the unevenness of the cancer depression (Fig. 10.15). This nodule consists of regenerative epithelium. Its presence strongly suggests the possibility of early

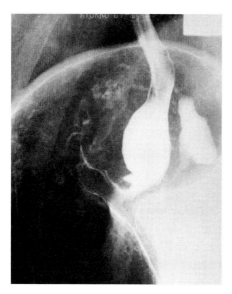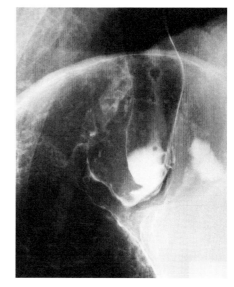

Fig. 10.23.   Cancer of the gastric cardia with the slight involvement of the esophagus. A double contrast image in the prone, semi-upright position shows narrowing of the distal esophagus with continuity from the esophagogastric junction. The main tumour (Borrmann type 2) is indicated by arrows.

cancer. The depth of the depression varies depending on the cancer erosion and associated peptic ulceration.

The converging folds in early depressed cancer reveal characteristic changes, such as tapering, clubbing, interruption, and fusion (Fig. 10.11). These abnormal patterns of folds are signs of early depressed cancer. Also, it was reported by Nakamura and Sugano (1968) that these abnormal patterns can be separated into differentiated and undifferentiated carcinomas, and that the difference between these two histologic types is visualized in well-documented radiographic investigations (Baba *et al.* 1977).

The radiographic characteristics of early depressed cancer are better understood when its histologic type is classified into the two basic types mentioned above. This is a major classification of gastric carcinoma, which is comparable to Lauren's intestinal and diffuse type (Lauren 1965). And Ming's expanding and infiltrative type (Ming 1977). The concept of poorly differentiated adenocarcinoma (por) by the JRSGC (Sakita *et al.* 1971) is not in the World Health Organization classification and typing (Watanabe *et al.* 1990). Clinically, however, this type is regarded as undifferentiated carcinoma.

As Baba and associates (1991) emphasized in 1991, the radiographic images of early depressed cancer are closely correlated with the two histologic types, undifferentiated and differentiated (Fig. 10.24). The significant differences are shown in radiographic images, and this recognition of the histologic type enables easier estimation of the invasive depth and extent of horizontal spread of early cancer.

In the radiographic characteristics of undifferentiated, early cancer a depression generally consists of irregular granularity (Fig. 10.12 and 10.13) or nodularity (Fig. 10.13), and the depression is sharply defined (Fig. 10.13). The abrupt interruption and tapering of the converging folds (Fig. 10.13), also form well-defined margin of the depression in the undifferentiated type. Intestinal metaplasia of the surrounding mucosa is less prominent in the undifferentiated type as a cancer focus becomes smaller.

In contrast to the above, in differentiated cancer, a depression lacks granularity or nodularity and shows a pattern similar to the normal surrounding mucosa in the differentiated type. Usually, the depression is outlined by subtle, but irregular

undifferentiated type	differentiated type

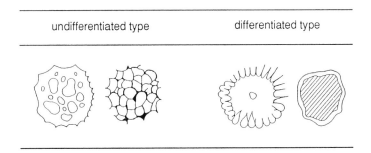

Fig. 10.24. Correlation of histologic type of early depressed cancer and radiographic images. (Modified from Baba *et al.* 1991, p. 1109, table 2, with permission).

spiculations (Fig. 10.19). The converging folds may be clubbed at the margin of depression, and gradually tapered in the depression (Fig. 10.19). In the differentiated type, moderate to severe intestinal metaplasia is observed in the surrounding mucosa although a lesion is small in size.

5.2.   The type IIb-like lesion

A type IIb lesion can be referred to as a cancerous lesion in its incipient phase. This concept was confirmed when pure type IIb lesions were discovered incidentally in the stomach during surgical procedures for other primary lesions; all were smaller than 0.5 cm (Nakamura and Sugano 1968). Many clinical cases that were not classified as pure type IIb, however, have simulated Type IIb lesions. A subtle difference was seen in the elevation or depression from the normal surrounding mucosa, and consequently the border of these lesions was not clearly defined.

This appearance has been called a type IIb-like lesion (Fig. 10.25) (Baba *et al.* 1991). The concept of the histologic type of cancer is also applied to this lesion. The surface pattern of a differentiated carcinoma may simulate the surrounding normal mucosa (Fig. 10.7), whereas that of an undifferentiated carcinoma is almost homogenous. In the undifferentiated carcinoma showing IIb-like spread a lesion is frequently covered with normal foveolar epithelium with scattered microerosions (Baba *et al.* 1977). The proximal limit of the type IIb-like lesion should be defined as precisely as possible in order to determine the line of surgical

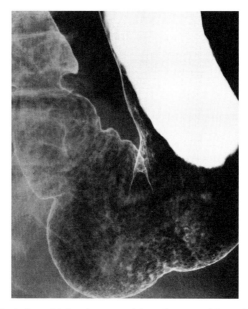

Fig. 10.25.   Type IIb-like lesion with involvement of the submucosa. The only abnormality visualized in a double contrast image (left posterior oblique view) is the irregular lesser curvature of the gastric antrum, and a very faint difference in barium coating in the vicinity of the irregular lesser curvature.

excision. The endoscopic approach, including the dye-spraying method and carbon ink injection, is indispensable for defining the proximal limit (Kumakura *et al.* 1972; Takekoshi *et al.* 1977).

5.3.   Superficial spreading carcinoma

The first record of superficial spreading carcinomas appears in the report by Stout (1942). He collected 15 cases of depressed cancer that spread along the mucosa and called them 'superficial spreading carcinomas.' The first case was an intra-mucosal carcinoma whose horizontal spread measured 9 × 6 cm in diameter. Stout did not offer any strict definition of superficial spreading carcinoma based on the extent of its horizontal spread; for example, the horizontal spread of the second case measured 3.2 × 3 cm in diameter. This spread is not significant enough to be defined as a superficial spreading carcinoma; rather, it should be classified as a typical type IIc or type IIc + III early carcinoma in the light of current Japanese experience.

In Japan, the strict definition of superficial spreading carcinoma has also not yet been established. The term is generally employed, however, for a superficial early carcinoma, that is, a type II early carcinoma. In this type of early carcinoma the product of its greatest diameter (a) and the diameter perpendicular to the greatest diameter (b) (S = a × b) is greater than 5 cm^2 (Yasui 1973).

The radiographic diagnosis of superficial spreading carcinoma is straight-forward except for type IIb-like lesions (Fig. 10.23), which are difficult to diagnose. A typical type IIa or IIc lesion with surface dimensions of 25–36 cm^2, is easily diagnosed by double contrast radiography (Maruyama and Hamada 1994). The diagnostic difficulty arises, however, when the surface dimensions are more than 36 cm^2 (Yasui 1973). In that event, the affected mucosa becomes so large that recognition of the mucosal abnormality in contrast to a small part of normal mucosa is difficult.

5.4.   Early cancer smaller than 1 cm

The detection of early carcinoma that is smaller than 1 cm is very difficult in the initial radiographic examination. In 1990, Hamada and co-workers described that a limit of radiographic detection was 0.6 cm in the polypoid early cancers, and 0.5 cm in the depressed early cancers. They also stated that the detection rate was 52% in the polypoid early cancers, 50% in the depressed early cancer less than 0.5 cm, and 56.9% of early depressed cancers measuring 0.6–1.0 cm.

Most depressed carcinomas smaller than 1 cm in diameter are not accompanied by ulceration (Takekoshi *et al.* 1990). Consequently, the detection of such a lesion is difficult regardless of its nature. Hamada and co-workers also reported that early cancers not associated with ulceration was detected in only 30.2% of cases whereas that associated with ulceration was detected in 82.4%. If a lesion is situated in an area in which double contrast radiography offers a good view of mucosal details, malignancy can be diagnosed by following the general principles of radiographic diagnosis (Fig. 10.26a,b).

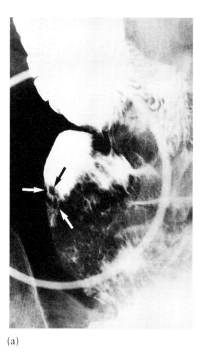 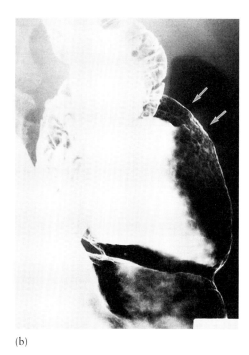

(a)   (b)

Fig. 10.26.   Early cancer smaller than 1 cm. A tiny irregular depression and its surrounding elevation in the greater curvature of the gastric antrum (arrows) (a) was demonstrated by compression. The lesion is visualized as localized rigidity of the greater curvature which may reflect the depression in a prone double contrast image (arrows) (b). From Maruyama and Baba, 1992, with permission.

A lesion associated with ulceration can be easily detected and diagnosed as malignant. The presence of mucosal convergence is also a particularly good clue for diagnosis.

When a lesion is smaller than 0.5 cm in its largest diameter (microcarcinoma) the radiographic diagnosis of malignancy is not always possible because the lesion is too small for the criteria of malignancy to be applied. Sometimes, an irregular surrounding translucency, which is unusual in cases of a benign ulcer, strongly suggests malignancy. In this case, double contrast radiography provides less possibility of detection than the compression method.

Endoscopy may be more effective than radiology for detection of microcarcinomas. At present, microcarcinomas have attracted the attention of endoscopists because they can be treated endoscopically. Even a type IIc lesion without ulcerative change can be excised by the endoscopic snare device.

5.5.   Esophageal invasion of gastric cancer

The esophagus is frequently involved because a cancer located in the gastric cardia or in the vicinity of the esophagogastric junction. Even an early cancer may involve the lower esophagus. Generally, the invasion pattern in the esophagus depends on the histologic type of gastric cancer mentioned above.

In the differentiated type, an affected portion of the esophagus usually shows obvious filling defects due to tumor formation, and cancerous invasion continually replaces the esophageal mucosa. However, there is no clear distinction from the normal esophagus in the undifferentiated type, and cancer diffusely invades the submucosa and beneath, not being exposed to the mucosal surface. It is not unusual to that a smooth enlarged fold is the only sign of esophageal involvement (Maruyama and Hamada 1994).

REFERENCES

Baba, Y., *et al.* (1977). A comparative study between radiologic and macroscopic findings of early gastric carcinoma with IIb-like intramucosal spread: with special reference to radiologic definition of proximal boundary. *I-to-Cho (Stomach and Intestine)*, **12**, 1087–1103.

Baba, Y., *et al.* (1991). Histological classification of gastric cancer related to radiological and endoscopic manifestations. *I-to-Cho (Stomach and Intestine)*, **26**, 1109–24.

Chonan, A., *et al.* (1990*a*). Clinical evaluation of endoscopic ultrasonography (EUS) on estimation of the depth of invasion in advanced gastric cancer with depressed lesion. *Gastroenterol. Endoscopy*, **32**, 493–500.

Chonan, A., *et al.* (1990*b*). Clinical evaluation of endoscopic ultrasonography (EUS) on the diagnosis for depressed type early gastric cancer associated with ulceration. *Gastroenterol. Endoscopy*, **32**, 1081–91.

Hamada, T., *et al.* (1988). Detectability of gastric cancer by radiology as compared to endoscopy. In *Review of clinical research in gastroenterology*, (ed. M. Maruyama and K. Kimura). Igakushoin, Tokyo.

Hamada, T., *et al.* (1990). Detection of early gastric cancer less than 1 cm in diameter during routine radiological examination. *I-to-Cho (Stomach and Intestine)*, **25**, 39–48.

Hisamichi S., *et al.* Evaluation of mass screening programme for stomach cancer in Japan. In *Cancer screening*, (ed. A.B. Miller, J. Chamberlain, N.E. Day, M. Hakama, and P.C. Prorok). Cambridge University Press.

Hori, M., *et al.* (1984). Detection of lymph nodes of the stomach cancer with computed tomography. *Rinsho Geka (J. Clin. Surg.)*, **39**, 543–6.

Igarashi, T., *et al.* (1977). Estimation of the depth of invasion in Type IIc cancer: from the view of dynamic observations by double contrast study. *I-to-Cho (Stomach and Intestine)*, **12**, 433–8.

JRSGC (Japanese Research Society for Gastric Cancer) (1981). The general rules for the gastric cancer staging in surgery and pathology. Part I. Clinical classification. Part II. Histological classification of gastric cancer. *Jpn. J. Surg*, **11**, 127–39.

Kida, M., *et al.* (1988). Endoscopic ultrasonography in diagnosis of the degree of gastric cancer invasion. *J. Med. Ultrason.*, **52**, 441.

Komaki, S. and Toyoshima, S. (1983). CT's capability in detecting gastric cancer. *Gastrointest. Radiol.*, **8**, 307–13.

Kumakura, K., *et al.* (1972). Radiological diagnosis of type IIb and IIb-like lesions of the stomach. *I-to Cho (Stomach and Intestine)*, **7**, 21–36.

Kumakura, K., *et al.* (1973*a*). Limitation in radiological diagnosis of malignant ulcer of the stomach. *I-to-Cho (Stomach and Intestine)*, **8**, 1183–99.

Kumakura, K., *et al.* (1973*b*). X-ray diagnosis of superficial spreading carcinoma of the stomach. *I-to-Cho (Stomach and Intestine)*, **8**, 1313–26.

Lauren, P. (1965). The two histological main types of gastric carcinoma: Diffuse and so-called intestinal type carcinoma. An attempt at a histoclinica classification. *Acta Pathol. Microbiol. Scand.*, **64**, 31–49.

Llorens, P., *et al.* (1991). Dignsotico del cancer gastrico y terapeutica endoscopica de las leiones gastricas incipientes. *Gastroenterologia Latinoamericana*, **1**, 29–44.

Maruyama, M. (1979). Early gastric cancer. In *Double contrast gastrointestinal radiology with endoscopic correlation*, (ed. I. Laufer). Saunders, Philadelphia.

Maruyama, M. (1986). Comparison of radiology and endoscopy in the diagnosis of gastric cancer. In *Cancer of the stomach*, (ed. P.E. Preece, A. Cushieri, and J.M. Wellwood). Grune & Stratton, San Diego.

Maruyama, M. (1990). Present status of examination of the upper gastrointestinal tracts, the total result of inquiry. *I-to-Cho (Stomach and Intestine)*, **25**, 59–61.

Maruyama, M. and Baba, Y. (1992). Gastric cancer. In *Double contrast gastrointestinal radiology*, (2nd edn). (ed. Laufer, I. and Levine, M.S.). pp. 517.

Maruyama, M. and Baba, Y. (1994). Gastric carcinoma. In *The radiologic clinics of North America*, (ed. Ott, D.J. and Gelfand, D.W.), pp. 1242.

Maruyama, M. and Hamada, T. (1994). Diagnosis of gastric cancer in Japan. In *Alimentary tract radiology*, (5th edn). (ed. P. Freeny and G.W. Stevenson), Vol. I, pp. 399–428. Mosby, St. Louis

Maruyama, M., *et al.* (1976). Radiodiagnostic possibility of gastric carcinoma involving the proper muscle layer. *I-to-Cho (Stomach and Intestine)*, **11**, 855–68.

Maruyama, M., *et al.* (1982*a*). Theoretical basis for the radiographic diagnosis of polypoid early cancer. In *Atlas of x-ray diagnosis of early gastric cancer*, (ed. H. Shirakabe *et al.*). Igaku-Shoin, Tokyo.

Maruyama, M. *et al.* (1982*b*). Radiographic diagnosis of peptic ulcer. In *Atlas of x-ray diagnosis of early gastric cancer*, (ed. H. Shirakabe *et al.*). Igaku-Shoin, Tokyo.

Miller, A.B., *et al.* (1991). State of the art on screening for stomach cancer. In *Cancer screening*, (ed. A.B. Miller, J. Chamberlain, N.E. Day, M. Hakama, and P.C. Prorok). pp. 355. Cambridge University Press.

Ming, S.C. (1977). Gastric carcinoma: A pathobiological classification. *Cancer*, **39**, 2475–85.

Murakami, T. (1967). New concept for an ulcer-cancer of the stomach. *Juntendo Igaku Med. J.*, **13**, 157.

Nakajima, T., *et al.* (1994). Progress of treatment of gastric cancer in Cancer Institute Hospital, Tokyo. *Jpn. J. Cancer Chemother.*, **21**, 1810–5.

Nakamura, K. and Sugano, H. (1968). Carcinoma of the stomach in incipient phase: Its histogenesis and histological appearances. *Gann*, **59**, 251–8.

Nakamura, K., *et al.* (1980). Growing process to carcinoma of linitis plastica type of the stomach from cancer development. *I-to-Cho (Stomach and Intestine)*, **15**, 225–34.

Nishimata, H., *et al.* (1987). Diagnostic ability of screening x-ray examination to pick-up type IIc early gastric cancers in the fundic gland area-Early detection of linitis plastica type gastric cancers. *I-to-Cho (Stomach and Intestine)*, **22**, 1027–36.

Nishizawa, M., *et al.* (1990). Methodology to avoid missing advanced gastric cancer. *I-to-Cho (Stomach and Intestine)*, **25**, 49–58.

Ohkuna, K., *et al.* (1984). Computed tomography staging of gastric cancer. *I-to-Cho* (*Stomach and Intestine*), **19**, 1313–19.

Ohta, H., *et al.* (1987). Early gastric carcinoma with special reference to macroscopic classification. *Cancer*, **60**, 1099–1106.

Ohta, K., *et al.* (1993). Update of gastric cancer surgery. *Karkinos*, **6**, 25–32.

Okabe, H. (1968). Analysis of gastric cancer followed up under the diagnosis of benign ulcer. *I-to-Cho* (*Stomach and Intestine*), **3**, 705–10.

Otsuji, M., *et al.* (1989). Assessment of small diameter panendoscopy for diagnosis of gastric cancer: comparative study with follow-up survey data. *I-to-Cho* (*Stomach and Intestine*), **24**, 1291–7.

Sakita, T., *et al.* (1971). Observations on the healing of ulcerations in early gastric cancer: the life cycle of the malignant ulcer. *Gastroenterology*, **60**, 835–44.

Shirakabe, H. and Maruyama, M. (1989). Neoplastic diseases of the stomach. In *Alimentary tract radiology*, (eds. A. Margulis and H.J. Burhenne), pp. 595–625. Mosby, St. Louis.

Shirakabe, H., *et al.* (1972). Comparison of x-ray and biopsy examinations for the diagnosis of early gastric cancer. *Jpn. J. Clin. Oncol.*, **12**, 93–8.

Stout, A.P. (1942). Superficial spreading type of carcinoma of the stomach. *Arch. Surg*, **44**, 651–7.

Takasu, Y. (1988). Detection of early cancer by panendoscopy, Recent progress in diagnosis of cancer and treatment of digestive diseases. *J. Jpn. Soc. Int. Med.*, **77**, 1651–4.

Takekoshi, T., *et al.* (1977). Significance of endoscopic carbon ink injection method in recognition of boundary of gastric carcinoma, with special reference to defining proximal boundary. *I-to-Cho* (*Stomach and Intestine*), **6**, 1031–41.

Takekoshi, T., *et al.* (1990). Radical endoscopic treatment of early gastric cancer. In *Endoscopic approaches to cancer diagnosis and treatment*, Gann Monograph on Cancer Research, No. 37, (ed. Y. Oguro and K. Takagi), pp. 111–26. Japan Scientific Societies Press, Tokyo London.

Watanabe, H., *et al.* (1990). Histological typing of esophageal and gastric tumors. In *WHO international, histological classification of tumors*, (2nd edn). Springer, Berlin.

Yamada, T. and Fukutomi, H. (1966). Polypoid lesions of the stomach. *I-to-Cho* (*Stomach and Intestine*), **1**, 145–50.

Yao, T. (1990). Advanced cancer simulating early cancer (Introduction, a brief summary on the case conference on the estimation of invasive depth of gastric cancer). *I-to-Cho* (*Stomach and Intestine*), **25**, 1381–1413.

Yao, T., *et al.* (1990). Failure to detect gastric cancer at the initial examination and measures against it. *I-to-Cho* (*Stomach and Intestine*), **25**, 27–37.

Yasui, A., *et al.* (1973). Pathology of superficial spreading type of gastric carcinoma. *I-to-Cho* (*Stomach and Intestine*), **8**, 1305–10.

Yoshinaka, H. and Shimazu, H. (1989). The diagnosis of lymph node metastasis gastric cancer by ultrasound. *Rinshoi*, **15**, 1840–4.

11

Endoscopy

Shigeaki Yoshida

1. CONVENTIONAL ENDOSCOPY: INSTRUMENTS AND PRINCIPAL TECHNIQUES

1.1. Instruments

Many types of endoscope are prepared for gastroscopy. The lateral-view type is the most commonly used for detailed observation of the stomach, because it allows optimal viewing. However, it does not satisfactorily screen the esophagus and duodenum, and the direct-view type is most commonly used as a panendoscope for screening the upper gastrointestinal (GI) tract. There is also an oblique-view type, but is not generally used because of the necessity of expert manipulation. However, it is better than the direct-view type for screening the posterior wall of the stomach and taking a biopsy from this area.

The diameter of the endoscope is determined by the pain or distress patients experience during the examination. The narrow version is less stressful, but imaging is inferior to that of the wide type. In Japan, hence, the narrow version is mainly used for upper GI screening, and the wide one for precise viewing, such as for the final preoperative examination.

1.2. Standard methods of observation and recording

Endoscopic observation can start from the oral cavity, observing first the tongue then the uvula, larynx, pharynx, and vocal cord. The scope is then placed on the esophageal orifice behind the vocal cord, and pushed gently into the esophagus. In the esophagus, the compression sign of the left main bronchus is seen on the left upper view field at the distance of 25 cm from a foretooth, and this can be a good marker for identifying the location. After precise observation of the esophago-cardiac junction, the scope is inserted into the stomach.

In the stomach, the location of the scope should first be identified. Usually, the scope lies on the posterior wall of the gastric fundus and the so-called 'gastric canal' named after the canal-like appearance from the upper to the lower gastric body, is seen in the left view field. With air inflation, the location becomes much clearer and the scope is gently inserted along the canal, checking any abnormalities. The incisura angularis is next seen at the upper view field (lesser curvature side), then the pyloric ring. Through the ring, the scope finally reaches the duodenal bulb. At this point, the scope is pulled back slowly, checking any duodenal and gastric abnormalities. At the level of the upper gastric body, the scope is reinserted in the lower gastric body, and then inverted and gently pulled back for checking any abnormality on the gastric fundus and lesser curvature of the body. During this procedure endoscopic images are taken serially, not only of lesions but also of normal areas by rotating the scope and any lesions are checked on the lesser curvature, anterior wall, greater curvature, and posterior wall sides of the stomach to avoid any possibility of error. Without doubt, the value of endoscopy rests on accurate observation, which is essential for macroscopic typing, location and extension of cancer invasion, and for planning a treatment strategy. In addition, having serial images allows for postoperative analysis of lesions diagnosed as benign endoscopically, or of those overlooked as being non-specific in the previous endoscopy, because, unlike the colon, the location of lesions can be identified according to the various anatomical markers, such as the cardiac orifice, folds on the greater curvature, incisura angularis, or pyloric ring of the stomach.

For this reason, gastroscopic images are taken serially of each case examined, even when no abnormality is detected. By assembling a store of images, early diagnosis has developed remarkably due to the retrospective analysis of early expression of cancerous lesions, particularly for those seen as less malignant endoscopically (Yoshida *et al.* 1984).

2. RECENT DEVELOPMENTS IN EARLY DIAGNOSIS

2.1. Chronological trends in early gastric cancer

In Japan, the detection of early gastric cancer (EGC) began by defusing and classifying, by endoscopy, the various types of cancer. This was effected by the Japanese Gastroenterological Endoscopy Society in 1962 (Tasaka 1962). In those early days, EGC was uncommon and most lesions were identified from the differential diagnosis of deeply ulcerated (type III) or polypoid (type I) lesions, which are easily detected. In the 1970s, early diagnosis progressed and it became possible to detect those lesions showing the appearance of an ulcer scar (type IIc) and a plateau-like elevation (type IIa).

In the 1980s, early diagnosis of gastritis-like malignancy (IIb-like type) has occurred because of results from retrospective studies of rapidly growing cancer. Two examples (cases 1 and 2) are shown in Figs 11.1 and 11.2. In the first case, the small redness on the lesser curvature of the antrum, detected at the initial examination (four years before the final: Fig 11.1a) became more rough-surfaced and enlarged by the time of the second examination (two years before the final: Fig. 11.1b), and rapidly developed into a Borrmann type 3 advanced cancer, as shown in Fig. 11.1c. In the second case, a shallow and faintly reddish depression was seen on the posterior wall of the body (Fig. 11.2a) at the initial endoscopy, and it developed into a Borrmann type 4 advanced cancer (Fig. 11.2b), only 40 days after the previous examination. These examples indicate the importance of diagnosis for non-ulcerative and superficial (gastritis-like) malignancies seen as faint mucosal irregularities (Yoshida *et al.* 1981).

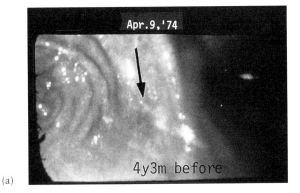

(a)

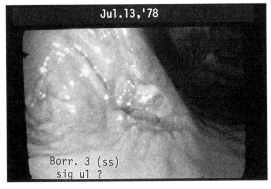

(b)

(c)

Fig. 11.1. (a) An endoscopic image of tissue in a 49-year-old male, taken about 4 years before the final examination. A small reddish area is seen on the lesser curvature of the antrum. (b) An endoscopic image of the same patient, taken about 2 years before the final examination. The small reddish area has become larger and its color pattern deeper, in association with a slight mucosal depression. (c) The final endoscopic image of the same patient. A tumorous lesion with a deep central excavation with a surrounding elevated wall (Borrmann type 3 advanced cancer) appeared on the lesser curvature of the antrum. The resected specimen revealed a signet-ring cell carcinoma (sig) invading to subserosa (ss) histologically. The presence or absence of peptic ulceration within the lesion could not be confirmed (ul?). See also colour plate section.

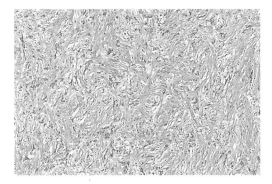

Fig. 4.9 Poorly differentiated
adenocarcinoma (scirrhous type).

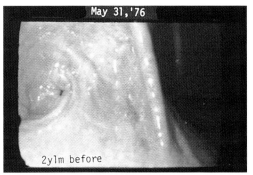

Fig. 11.1(b) (see page 170 for caption)

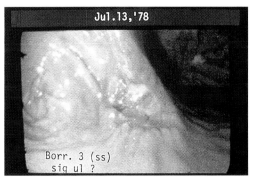

Bormann type 3 advanced cancer.
Fig. 11.1(c) (see page 170 for full caption)

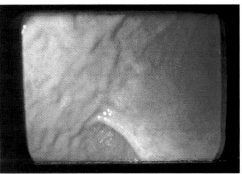

Gastritis-like EGC, subclassified as 'flat
discolored type'.
Fig. 11.4 (see page 176 for full caption)

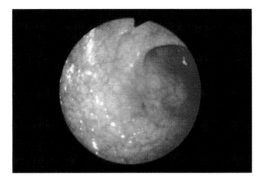

Gastritis-like EGC, subclassified as 'flat hyperemic type'.

Fig. 11.5 (see page 176 for full caption)

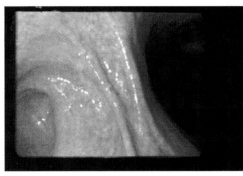

Gastritis-like EGC, subclassified as 'superficial uneven type'.

Fig. 11.6 (see page 176 for full caption)

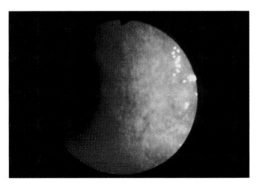

Conventional endoscopy of gastritis-like EGC.

Fig. 11.7(a) (see page 178 for full caption)

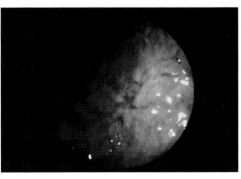

Dye-sprayed gastritis-like EGC.

Fig. 11.7(b) see page 178 for full caption)

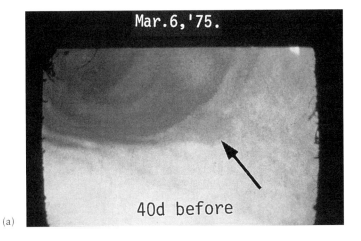

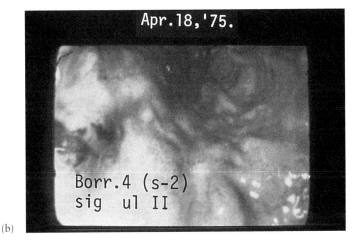

Fig. 11.2. (a) An endoscopic image of tissue in a 57-year-old female, taken only 40 days before the final examination. A shallow and non-ulcerative depression is indicated on the posterior wall of the gastric body. (b) The final endoscopic image of the same patient. The superficial gastric lesion rapidly changed into scirrhous-type cancer with penetrating serosal invasion (S2) and a shallow peptic ulceration within the submucosal layer (ul II) was detected from the cancerous area.

Between 1962 and 1991, there were more than 2400 surgical cases of EGC at the National Cancer Center Hospital. Figure 11.3 shows chronological trends in gross endoscopic appearance of the well-documented 1864 solitary EGCs, subclassified into four types endoscopically: polypoid, ulcerative, gastritis-like, and advanced cancer-like types. The polypoid type is defined as EGC showing obvious protrusion, the ulcerative one as that showing ulceration and/or fold convergence, the gastritis-like one as that showing a superficial non-ulcerative appearance and advanced cancer-like ones that evidently show advanced cancer-like appearance

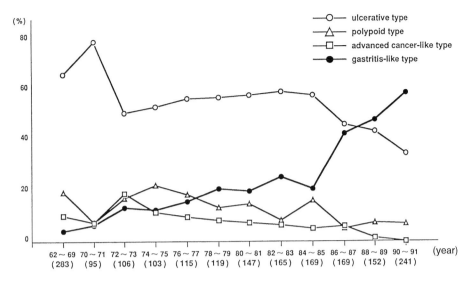

Fig. 11.3.   The chronological trend in the endoscopic appearance of early gastric cancer (EGC).

endoscopically. As shown in Fig. 11.3, the incidence of the gastritis-like type has been increasing considerably in recent years, particularly since 1984, until finally reaching 59% in 1990 and 1991.

Table 11.1 shows the incidence of EGC and the five-year survival rate. The survival rate has improved remarkably in recent years in proportion to the increase in incidence of EGC, and during 1985–9, the incidence of EGC reached 53% (639/1211) and the five-year survival rate was calculated as 71% (860/1211). The chronological trend of the five-year survival rate by stage of gastric cancer is shown in Table 11.2. The five-year survival rate steadily improved annually for each stage, except stage III (1985–9) which decreased slightly. The chronological trend in EGC and surgical results apparently indicates the contribution of the recent early detection to the survival of cancer patients, and also the importance of early detection based on the differentiation of gastritis-like malignancy.

Table 11.1.   Chronological trends in gastric cancer: incidence of 5-year survival in early cancer and surgical cases

Period	No. of surg. cases	No. of 5-yr survivors (%)	No. of early cancer cases (%)
1962–9	1628	684 (42)	358 (22)
1970–4	1020	571 (56)	325 (32)
1975–9	967	561 (58)	330 (34)
1980–4	1165	757 (65)	502 (43)
1985–9	1211	860 (71)	639 (53)

Data from the National Cancer Center Hospital, Tokyo (1962–89).

Table 11.2. Chronological trends in 5-year survival rate (%) by stage of gastric cancer

Stage	Period 62–9	70–4	75–9	80–4	85–9	Total
I	88 (429)	89 (390)	91 (396)	91 (536)	94 (647)	91 (2398)
II	59 (279)	69 (134)	72 (94)	80 (125)	81 (130)	68 (762)
III	34 (380)	43 (244)	46 (235)	57 (247)	53 (201)	44 (1307)
IV	4 (534)	11 (245)	13 (221)	11 (234)	15 (233)	9 (1467)
Total	42% (1622)	56% (1020)	58% (967)	65% (1165)	71% (1211)	56% (5991)

Figures in parentheses are the number of cases.
Data from the National Cancer Center Hospital, Tokyo (1962–89).

2.2. Diagnostic findings of gastritis-like EGC

Table 11.3 shows the endoscopic appearance (colour patterns and surface structure) of the 132 cases of gastritis-like EGC diagnosed endoscopically as benign. Their colour patterns were subclassified into discoloured, hyperemic, and normocoloured, and their surface structures into flat well-demarcated, flat poorly demarcated, and uneven groups. The 132 cases were further classified endoscopically into flat discoloured (27 cases of group *a* in the table), flat hyperemic (63 cases of

Table 11.3. Color and surface patterns in endoscopic appearance of gastritis-like EGCs diagnosed as benign endoscopically[*]

Surface pattern	Color pattern Discolored	Hyperemic	Normocolored	Total
Flat				
Well-demarcated	19 (a)	9 (b)		28
Poorly demarcated	8	54	1[**]	63
Uneven	2	20	19 (c)	41
	29	83	20	132

Cases of groups *a*, *b* and *c* can be subclassified into flat discolored, flat hyperemic, and superficial uneven types, respectively.
[**] One case of type IIb EGC without any diagnostic findings.

group *b*), and superficial uneven types (41 cases of group *c*), endoscopic characteristics of each type could be summarized as follows. In the flat discoloured type well-demarcated lesions are dominant (19/27: 70%), whereas the greater part (45/53: 83%) of the flat hyperemic type shows poorly demarcated lesions. In the superficial uneven type, discoloured lesions are few, and most of them (39/41: 95%) are normocoloured or hyperemic.

Table 11.4 shows the histological and endoscopic types of the 132 gastritis-like EGCs. The histological types were divided into intestinal and diffuse types, according to Lawrence's classification. The incidence of intestinal type was 30% in the flat discoloured, 62% in the flat hyperemic, and 93% in the superficial uneven types, indicating that this endoscopic subclassification is correlated to the histological characteristics of gastritis-like EGCs. Table 11.5 shows size distribution of the three subtypes. There was a wide range in the flat discoloured and the hyperemic types, whereas small lesions less than 1 cm were dominant (19/41: 47%) in the superficial uneven type. Site distribution is shown in Table 11.6. In the flat discoloured type, most (21/27: 78%) of the lesions were located in the upper (*C*) and middle (*M*) one-third third of the stomach. The incidence of location in the lower one-third (*A*) of the stomach was more frequent (38%) in the flat hyperemic type than in the flat discoloured type (22%), and it was dominant (60%) in the superficial uneven type.

These results may indicate the possibility of screening gastritis-like EGCs as follows. When evaluating the upper two-thirds of the stomach (cardia and gastric body), we should pay attention mainly to color changes of the mucosa, in particular to the well-demarcated discoloration or the poorly demarcated redness, and for the lower one-third of the stomach (antrum), be alert to superficial unevenness of the mucosa, such as a tiny depression surrounded with hyperemic or normocolored hyperplastic mucosa. Representative cases of gastritis EGCs are shown in Figs 11.4–11.6).

Table 11.4. Histological and endoscopic types of gastritis-like EGCs diagnosed as benign endoscopically[*]

Endoscopic subtype	Histological type		Total
	Intestinal	Diffuse	
Flat discolored	8	19	27
	(30)	(70)	(100)
Flat hyperemic	39	24	63
	(62)	(38)	(100)
Superficial uneven	38	3	41
	(93)	(7)	(100)
Total	85	46	131[*]

[*] One case of type IIb was excluded.
Figures in parentheses are percentages.

Table 11.5. Size distribution of endoscopic subtypes of gastritis-like EGCs diagnosed as benign endoscopically[*]

Endoscopic subtype	Size (max. diam. cm)				Total
	≦1	<1–≦2	<2–≦5	<5	
Flat discolored	7	9	8	3	27
	(26)	(33)	(30)	(11)	(100)
Flat hyperemic	16	15	24	8	63
	(25)	(24)	(38)	(13)	(100)
Superficial uneven	19	7	12	3	41
	47)	(17)	(29)	(7)	(100)
Total	42	31	44	14	131[*]

[*] One case of type IIb was excluded.
Figures in parentheses are percentages.

Table 11.6. Site distribution of flat discolored, flat hyperemic, and superficial uneven subtypes of gastritis-like EGCs diagnosed as benign endoscopically[*]

Endoscopic subtype	Stomach region			Total
	C	M	A	
Flat discolored				
Anterior wall		4	2	6 (22)
Lesser curv.		10	1	11 (40)
Posterior wall	2	4	2	8 (30)
Greater curv.		1	1	2 (8)
Total	2 (8)	19 (70)	6 (22)	27 (100)
Flat hyperemic				
Anterior wall	1	8	4	13 (21)
Lesser curv.	2	20	10	32 (51)
Posterior wall	1	5	4	10 (16)
Greater curv.		2	6	8 (12)
Total	4 (6)	35 (56)	24 (38)	63 (100)
Superficial uneven				
Anterior wall		2	4	6 (15)
Lesser curv.	1	9	10	20 (49)
Posterior wall		2	6	8 (20)
Greater curv.		2	5	7 (16)
Total	1 (2)	15 (37)	25 (61)	41 (100)

[*] C, upper; M, middle; A, lower one-third of the stomach, respectively.
Figures in parentheses are percentages.

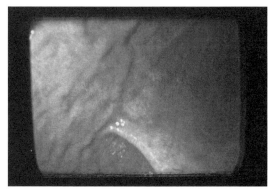

Fig. 11.4. An endoscopic image of a case of gastritis-like EGC, subclassified as 'flat discolored type'. A well-demarcated discolored area is seen on the anterior wall of the lower gastric body without fold convergence. The final diagnosis was a mucosal cancer of signet-ring cell carcinoma, 12 mm in diameter. See also colour plate section.

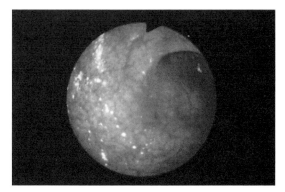

Fig. 11.5. An endoscopic image of a case of gastritis-like EGC, subclassified as 'flat hyperemic type'. A ill-demarcated faint reddish area is seen on the anterior wall near the greater curvature of the lower body. The final diagnosis was a EGC with submucosal invasion and its histological type was well-differentiated tubular adenocarcinoma. See also colour plate section.

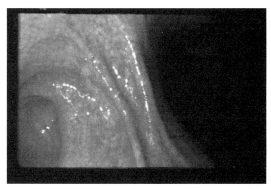

Fig. 11.6. An endoscopic image of a case of gastritis-like EGC, subclassified as 'superficial uneven type'. Irregularities in the mucosal structure are seen on the lesser curvature of the antrum. With precise observation, the margin of shallow depression including the uneven mucosa are distinguishable. See also colour plate section.

Table 11.7.   Grade distribution of findings suggesting malignancy in 'gastritis-like' EGCs observed by conventional and dye-spraying endoscopy

Conventional endoscopy	Dye-spraying endoscopy (grade)				Total
	0[a]	1[b]	2[c]	3[d]	
Grade 0[a]	3	4	7	9	23
	(13)	(17)	(31)	(39)	(100)
Grade 1[b]	0	4	17	19	40
		(10)	(42)	(48)	(100)
Total	3	8	24	28	63
	(5)	(13)	(38)	(44)	(100)

[a] Undetectable malignancy; [b] Rather benign; [c] Rather malignant; [d] Definitely malignant.
Figures in parentheses are percentages.

2.3.   Dye-spraying endoscopy for detecting EGCs

Even with the most precise observation it is occasionally difficult to detect the definitive diagnostic findings of gastritis-like malignancy showing faint, mucosal irregularities. A dye-spraying technique, particularly the 'contrast method' using 0.1% of indigocalmin (Tsuda 1967), is indispensable for detecting such fine mucosal irregularities. Table 11.7 shows results of a comparative study of 63 gastritis-like EGCs using conventional and dye-spraying endoscopy. The clarity of malignant findings is divided into the following four grades: grade 0 (undetectable malignancy); grade 1 (rather benign); grade 2 (rather malignant); and grade 3, (definitely malignant).

All of 63 cases was evaluated as grade 0 or grade 1 by conventional endoscopy. After dye-spraying, increase of grade was seen in 87% (20/23) of the cases in grade 0, and in 90% (36/40) of those in grade 1. In particular, 39% (9/23) of grade 0 and 48% (19/40) of grade 1 have changed dramatically, grade 3, clearly indicating the diagnostic utilities for detecting gastritis-like EGCs. Examples are shown in Fig. 11.7a,b.

2.4.   Biopsy in borderline lesions

Histological diagnosis by biopsy is indispensable for detecting EGCs with a less malignant appearance. It is, however, not always ideal, particularly with regard to a cancer with scattered invasion (Yoshida *et al.* 1990*a*). The limitations of biopsy are mostly caused by the tiny size of specimens and heterogeneity of atypism within a cancerous invasion. In our series, biopsies performed three months prior to the final examination failed to reveal malignancy in a case of ulcerative EGC of nearly 2 cm in size. In borderline lesions, the possible malignancy is greater, because of the difficulties in histological differentiation between adenoma and the carcinoma with less cellular atypism ('very well-differentiated tubular adenocarcinoma': Fujii *et al.* 1994).

Table 11.8 shows the final diagnosis of the 243 lesions resected after the initial biopsy result of group III (adenoma or borderline: 'group classification' by the

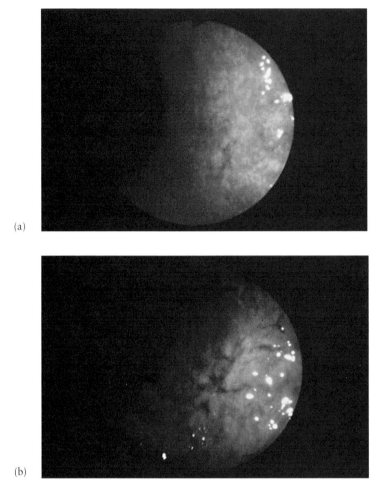

(a)

(b)

Fig. 11.7. Endoscopic images of a case of gastritis-like EGC, taken by conventional and dye-spraying endoscopy. A submucosal cancer is located on the lesser curvature of the lower gastric body. However, with conventional endoscopy (a), it is difficult to detect the lesion. After dye-spraying (b) the malignant findings of moth-eaten appearance (encroachment) at the tip of weakly converging folds or irregular margin of the depression can be easily detected. See also colour plate section.

JRSGC 1981). Of the 243 lesions, 35 (14%) were malignant, in which 25 were cancers, and the remainder were 10 focal cancers in adenomas. In addition, malignant potential was significantly greater in the lesions with a depressed component (8/25: 32%) than those without depression (27/218: 12%) ($P < 0.01$). With respect to the endoscopic appearance of the 243 lesions, malignancy was dominant in those greater than 2 cm, and showed a polypoid or gastritis-like form and a reddish color (see Table 11.9). The multivariate analysis of the 243 lesions examining the correlation of the endoscopic findings to the malignancy of lesion, revealed that: (1) the colour of the lesion showed the highest partial coefficient, and

Table 11.8. Endoscopic evidence of presence or absence of depressed component and final diagnosis of group III resected lesions[*]

Depressed component	Final diagnosis			Total
	C	F	A	
Presence	6	2	17	25
	(32)			(100)
Absence	19	8	191	218
	(12)			(100)
Total	25	10	208	243
	(14)			(100)

[*] C, cancer without adenoma; F, focal cancer with adenoma; A, adenoma.
Figures in parentheses are percentages.

Table 11.9. Endoscopic appearance and malignant potential of group III lesions; examined for their macroscopic type, size, and color[*]

	Final diagnosis			Total
	C	F	A	
Macroscopic type				
Polypoid	7 (16)	3 (7)	35	45 (100)
Flat polypoid	7 (8)	8 (9)	72	87 (100)
Small polypoid	0	1 (2)	41	42 (100)
Fold-like	2 (15)	1 (8)	10	13 (100)
Gastritis-like	3 (12)	7 (28)	15	25 (100)
Depressed	2 (40)	0	3	5 (100)
Total	21 (10)	20 (9)	176	217 (100)
Size of lesion (cm)				
$\geqq 1$	0	3 (4)	76	79 (100)
$> 1 - \geqq 2$	9 (11)	6 (7)	67	82 (100)
> 2 cm	12 (21)	11 (20)	33	56 (100)
Total	21 (10)	20 (9)	176	217 (100)
Color of lesion				
Discolored	5 (5)	2 (2)	90	97 (100)
Normocolored	4 (6)	7 (10)	62	73 (100)
Hyperemic	12 (26)	11 (23)	24	47 (100)
Total	21 (10)	20 (9)	176	217 (100)

[*] C, cancer without adenoma; F, focal cancer with adenoma; A, adenoma.
Figures in parentheses are percentages.

followed by (2) size, (3) macroscopic appearance, and (4) combination with depressed component (see Table 11.10). Because these four variables have a high statistical significance of $P < 0.01$, the group III lesions demonstrating any of (1) to (4) above by endoscopy can be regarded as at high risk for malignancy.

Table 11.10.   Partial coefficient and its statistical significance obtained from multivariate analysis of Hayashi's quantification theory (no. 2), examining correlation between endoscopic and clinicopathological features and malignancy of the group III lesion

Feature	Partial coefficient	Statistical significance (p)
Color	0.3562	< 0.01
Size	0.2800	< 0.01
Macroscopic type	0.2448	< 0.01
Depressed component	0.2001	< 0.01
Sex	0.1735	< 0.05
Location	0.1726	< 0.05
Histology (tub[a] vs. pap[b])	0.0134	n.s.

n.s., not significant; [a] tubular adenoma; [b] papillary adenoma.

The above results clearly indicate the limitations of biopsy and the importance of detailed endoscopic investigation of the lesion in order to make an accurate early diagnosis. Blind acceptance of biopsy results may compromise the patient's, prognosis. When there is a questionable diagnosis by biopsy, the endoscopic appearance of the lesion should be studied in detail and a rebiopsy should be made without hesitation.

Recently, many oncogenes and suppressor genes have been disclosed to be related to gastric cancer progression. Gene analysis on biopsy specimens for early diagnosis is now ongoing, particularly by examining the mutation on the p53 suppressor gene. In our data, no mutation of p53 was detected from 17 adenomatous lesions, whereas 36% (10/28) of EGC were positive: (unpublished data). Concerning lymphomatous lesions, gene analysis of immunoglobin heavy-chain rearrangement on biopsy specimens is now applied to clinical use for differentiating the benign and malignant gastric lymphomas (Ono *et al.* 1993). These results may indicate that gene analysis can not only support histological diagnosis but also reveal the nature of premalignant conditions.

3.   NEW ENDOSCOPIC INSTRUMENTS

3.1.   Electronic endoscopy

Recent advances in optoelectronics provides us with a new technique—electronic endoscopy—in which the optical image is converted into electronic signals, corresponding to digital colour values of red (R), green (G), and blue (B) by a charged coupled device (CCD) at the tip of the scope. These digital RGB signals are transmitted to an image processor (videosystem center), and reproduced into visual color information by frame memory. They are finally transmitted, after electronic reconversion into analog signals, to a broadcasting monitor.

Videoimage endoscopy has several advantages, such as providing high-resolution color images, and the possibility of monitoring by several diagnosticians, etc. Perhaps the most valuable advantage is that of easy handling of image processing and filing with the aid of a computerized system, because of the transformation of optical images into electronic RGB signals (Yachida and Ohyama 1989). Furthermore, videoimage endoscopy can be applied to the quantification of images, and our preliminary studies have indicated that it can be used as colorimeter (Kawai *et al.* 1988). As shown in Fig. 11.8, our newly developed endoscopy, which takes the digital endoscopic image directly into the computer system, shows the spectroscopic colour values of a random sampling area and gives its measurements on the chromaticity diagram.

The easy handling of image processing has a further use in measuring size (distance) endoscopically by stereoimage videoendoscopy. Fundamentally, this comprises two scopes, which are set in one shaft, and two light and image guides, as shown in Fig. 11.9. There are two lenses (CCDs) containing 35 000 pixels on the tip of the scope with a focal distance of 5.8 mm (the diameter of the scope is 13 mm). In the image processor, a three-dimensional measurement is performed on the anastigmatic image by computer calculation. Figure 11.10a shows two dye-spraying images of type IIa (elevated) EGC taken by the stereoscope, which are shown as two kinds of three-dimensional image with an image-processing program, as shown in Fig. 11.10b. The error rate of measuring size by this scope was less than 10%, which is allowable for clinical use.

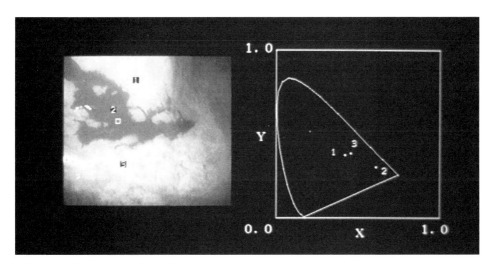

Fig. 11.8. Images showing results of spectroscopic analysis in a case of gastric bleeding by electronic endoscopy. Sampling points are shown in the white open square in the endoscopic image. In this case, two samples (nos 1 and 3) were taken from the surrounding mucosa and one (no. 2) from the bleeding point. The color value of each point is expressed quantitatively on the chromaticity diagram. The position of no. 2 in the diagram is very close to the pure red area and those of nos 1 and 3 are slightly different from each other (no. 1 is shifted to the more whitish area), although they are seen as almost the same endoscopically.

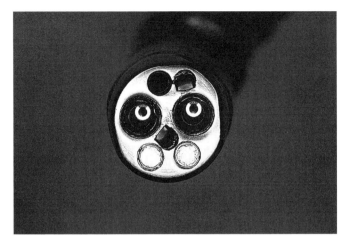

Fig. 11.9.   An image showing the tip of the stereoscopic electronic endoscope, these are two lenses (CCDs) each with a focal distance of 5.8 mm. The maximum diameter of the scope is 13 mm.

For diagnosing gastritis-like malignancy, the ability of viewing the differentiation of faint mucosal irregularity is indispensable. However, there can be a tendency to be subjective rather than empirical than in cases of ulcerative or polypoid lesions. Computed endoscopy measuring color value and size, therefore, is expected to screen the faint mucosal irregularity more quantitatively.

3.2. Endosonography

Instruments and technique

Recent technology has provided us with another new instrument:—endosonography—which makes it possible to visualize inner structures in lesions of the GI tract or adjacent organs by direct scanning with ultrasonic waves from within the tract. Its diagnostic accuracy has been improving year by year because of developments in the scanning device. Endosonography has two methodologies: those performed with a radial transducer, and those with an ultrasonic microprobe.

In the former, using a specialized endoscope, examination begins with a conventional (lateral-viewed) observation to identify the location of the lesion, and then, after removal of the air, more than 300 ml of deaerated water is passed through the endoscope channel in order to transmit ultrasonic waves generated from the mechanical radial sector located at the distal end of the scope (deaerated water immersion method). The area examined rapidly revolves around the axis of the scope (420 rpm) generating both ultrasonic waves and capturing mucosal reflexes through 360 degrees. A balloon technique can be used for scanning lesions located in difficult areas, for water retention. In this case, ultrasonic scanning is carried out from the inside the balloon which is expanded with deaerated water which covers the scanning sector. The advantage of these methods is the ability of obtaining the

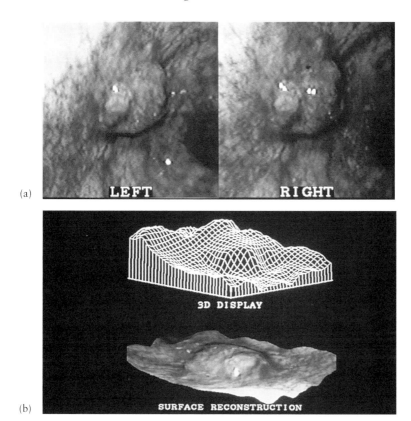

Fig. 11.10. (a) Dye-spraying endoscopic images of a type IIa (plateau-like elevated) EGC taken by a stereoscope. The position of the lesion is slightly shifted between the two images taken by the right and left lenses. (b) A color image and line drawing showing the three-dimensional appearance of the lesion, produced by the image processing program.

image as a round slice of the lesion and its background at the same time. The latest model of Olympus GF-UM20 is equipped with two kinds of scanning wavelengths, 7.5 MHz and 12 MHz, for obtaining a high resolution image in both deep (with 7.5 MHz) and shallow (with 12 MHz) areas.

Only recently, has the ultrasonic microprobe been improved in its image quality and put to practical use. In this procedure, the microprobe is inserted in the endoscope channel and ultrasonic scanning is carried out by placing the probe on the lesion which is immersed in deaerated water. The advantage of this procedure is that it provides a linear scanning image (profile appearance) of the lesion with good correspondence to the endoscopic appearance, although the image quality is not as good as that provided by a radial transducer mechanism. An example is shown in Fig. 11.11.

Endosonography has two uses in cancer diagnosis. One is differential diagnosis and the other the estimation of vertical invasion in gastric malignancy (T-staging).

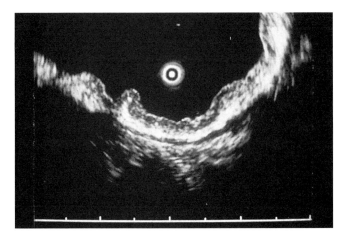

Fig. 11.11. An endosonographic image of EGC type IIc taken by ultrasonic microprobe (20 MHz). A shallow depressed area is seen with a boundary echo pattern limited within the third layer, indicating the limit of invasion within the mucosal layer.

The following section discusses the results obtained by endosonographs together with a radial transducer mechanism.

Differential diagnosis

With endosonography, most of non-scirrhous-type advanced cancers revealed thickening of the gastric wall and a nodular hypoechoic mass replacing the original layer structure (Fig. 11.12). However, in cases of scirrhous-type cancer, the affected area was only seen as a marked thickening of the gastric wall, preserving the layer structure of the stomach (Fig. 11.13). Malignant lymphomas (ML) showed similar findings to those observed in non-scirrhous-type cancers, (i.e. thickening of the gastric wall and destruction of layer structures). But their echo levels were mostly lower than those of carcinoma (Fig. 11.14a), and the echo patterns of spotty and/or multinodular feature which can be regarded as pathognomonic (Boku *et al.* 1994), was noted in those having follicular formation histologically (Fig. 11.14b).

It was, however, not easy to differentiate between some early (shallow invasive) malignancies and benign epithelial lesions such as adenoma ulcers and polyps. In particular, in deep ulceration, it was very difficult to differentiate between benign peptic ulcers and cancerous lesions, including ulceration. This is the most weak aspect of endosonography and may limit its use.

Diagnosis of depth of cancerous invasion

Table 11.11 shows our results of ultrasonic estimation for the vertical degree of cancerous invasion (Yoshida *et al.* 1990*b*). The accuracy was high among the lesions which were diagnosed as mucosal or beyond subserosal by endosonography. Misdiagnosis of vertical invasion was mostly caused by technical inadequacy which failed to reveal the deepest point of the lesions except for ulcerating

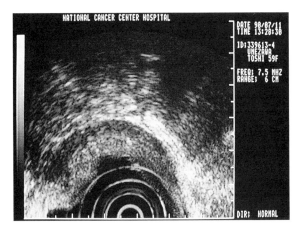

Fig. 11.12. An endosonographic image of non-scirrhous-type advanced gastric cancer, taken by a radial transducer mechanism. A nodular hypoechoic mass appearance replaces the original layer structure with thickening of the gastric wall.

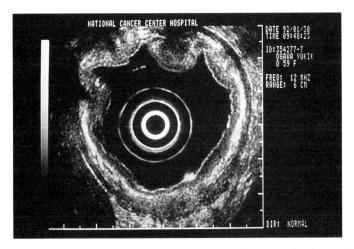

Fig. 11.13. An endosonographic image of scirrhous-type stomach cancer, taken by a radial transducer mechanism. The affected area can be seen as a marked thickening of the gastric wall, preserving the layer structure of the stomach.

carcinomas where exact differentiation of cancerous invasion from fibrous tissue induced by ulceration was almost impossible. The diagnostic accuracy of estimating the depth of cancer invasion was 69%, being particularly poor in lesions with submucosal or muscularis propria invasion. Other Japanese papers have reported similar percentages, submucosa and muscle layer from fibrosis due to ulceration within the cancerous area.

Although there is a certain measure of diagnostic in accuracy, gastric endosonography is applicable in general, and particularly for differential diagnosis between

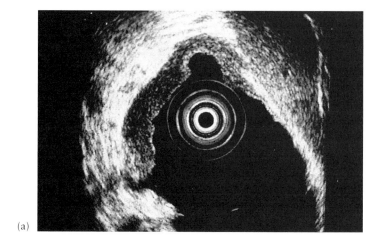

(a)

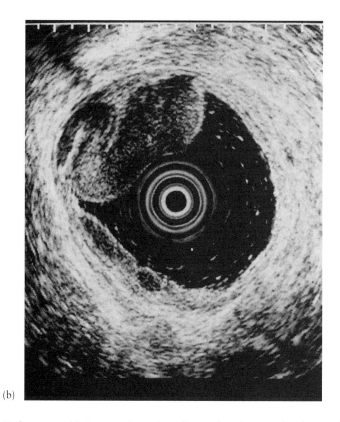

(b)

Fig. 11.14. Endosonographic images of gastric malignant lymphoma, taken by a radial transducer mechanism. A similar mass appearance to non-scirrhous-type cancer is seen, but its echo level is more lower than that of cancer (a) and granular or nodular echo patterns are noted in the lesions combining with follicular formation histologically (b).

Table 11.11. Accuracy of preoperative endosonographic diagnosis for estimating the degree of vertical invasion of the gastric wall

Ultrasonic diagnosis	Histological diagnosis				
	m	sm	pm	beyond ss	Total
m	21 (91)	2 (9)	0	0	23 (100)
sm	12 (41)	15 (52)	1 (3)	1 (3)	29 (100)
pm	1 (7)	3 (20)	7 (47)	4 (27)	15 (100)
Beyond ss	0	2 (5)	7 (18)	29 (76)	86 (100)
Total	34	22	15	34	105

Figures in parentheses are percentages.

scirrhous and non-scirrhous cancers. However, its use is limited in differential diagnosis between cancerous and lymphomatous lesions and for exact estimation of the degree of vertical invasion of cancer.

ACKNOWLEDGEMENTS

This work was supported in part by Grants-in Aid for Cancer Research from the Ministry of Health and Welfare of Japan, and for the Comprehensive 10-year Strategy of Japan.

REFERENCES

Boku, N., Yoshida, S., Ohtsu, A., Fujii, T., Abe, K., Hijikata., A., *et al.*, (1994). The differential diagnosis of malignant lymphoma and reactive lymphoreticular hyperplasia of the stomach using endoscopic ultrasonography. *Digestive Endoscopy*, 6, 163–9.

Fujii, T., Yoshida, S., Abe, K., Saito, D., Yamaguchi, H., Oguro, Y., *et al.* (1994). 'Very well differentiated tubular adenocarcinoma' of the stomach: Its endoscopic and histopathological characteristics. *Jpn J. Clin. Oncol.*, 24, 128–34.

JRSGC (Japanese Research Society for Gastric Cancer) (1981). The general rules for the gastric cancer study in surgery and pathology. *Jpn. J. Surg.*, 11, 127–45.

Kawai, M., Yamaguchi, H., Yoshida, S., Saito, D., Hijikata, A., Miyamoto, K., *et al.* (1988). Application of electronic endoscope to colorimeter; and evaluation of clinical utilities (in Japanese with English summary). *Prog. Digest. Endosc.*, 32, 69–72.

Ono, H., Kondo, H., Saito, D., Yoshida, S., Shirao, K., Yamaguchi, H., *et al.* (1993). Rapid diagnosis of gastric malignant lymphoma from biopsy specimens: Detection of immunogloblin heavy chain rearrangement by polymerase chain reaction. *Jpn. J. Cancer Res.*, 84, 813–17.

Tasaka, S. (1962). National questionnaire of early gastric cancer of Japan (in Japanese). *Gastroenterol. Endosc.*, 4, 4–19.

Tsuda, Y. (1967) Endoscopic observation of gastric lesions with dye spraying technique (in Japanese). *Gastroenterol Endosc.*, **9**, 189–95.

Yachida, M. and Ohyama, N. (1989). Color image restoration using synthetic method. *Opt. Commun.*, **72**, 22–6.

Yoshida, S., Yoshimori, M., Hirashima, T., Yamaguchi, H., Tajiri, H., Nakamura, K., *et al.* (1981). Nonulcerative lesion detected by endoscopy as an early expression of gastric malignancy. *Jpn. J. Clin. Oncol.*, **11**, 495–506.

Yoshida, S., Yamaguchi, H., Tajiri, H., Saito, D., Hijikata, A., Yoshimori M., *et al.* (1984). Diagnosis of early gastric cancer seen as less malignant endoscopically. *Jpn. J. Clin. Oncol.*, **14**, 225–41.

Yoshida, S., Tsuji, Y., Saito, D., Yamaguchi, H., Boku, N., Oguro, Y., *et al.* (1990*a*). Clinical and histological issues of endoscopic biopsy in diagnosing gastric cancer (in Japanese with English summary). *Stomach and Intestine*, **25**, 959–69.

Yoshida, S., Miyamoto, K. and Hijikata, A. (1990*b*). Endosonography: its diagnostic utilities for gastric cancer. In *New trends in gastric cancer*, (ed. P.I. Reed, M. Carboni, B.J. Johnston, and S. Guadagni), pp 79–86. Kluwer, Dordrecht.

Part V: Prevention

12

Primary prevention

Suketami Tominaga

1. INTRODUCTION

The decreasing trend of the mortality rate in stomach cancer is a global pheno-menon (Tominaga 1987). This declining trend was observed earlier in Western industrialized nations than in less developed countries (Figs 12.1, 12.2) (Aoki *et al.* 1992; Kuroishi *et al.* 1994). The reason for the common declining trend of stomach cancer is not yet clear, but it is likely that changes in dietary habits, including methods of food preservation and processing, may have brought beneficial effects unintentionally. This could be regarded as 'a natural experiment', 'unintentional prevention', or 'passive primary prevention' (Tominaga 1987). It is unlikely that improved diagnosis (decreased overdiagnosis of stomach cancer) or stomach cancer screening has brought such a marked decrease in stomach cancer mortality, because a similar declining trend was observed in the incidence rate in the United States (Devesa and Silverman 1978; Pollack and Horn 1980; Miller 1983; Swanson and Young 1983) and Scotland (Sedgwick *et al.* 1991), where stomach cancer screening has not been conducted. The main cause of the marked reduction in the mortality rate in stomach cancer and incidence in the United States is not clear, but it has been regarded as largely due to improvements in food storage and preservation, with the consequent reduction of various carcinogenic substances normally present in food (Miller *et al.* 1980).

2. LESSONS FROM EMIGRANT STUDIES

It is a well-known fact that the Japanese living in Hawaii and the western coast of the United States show a much lower incidence and mortality rate from stomach cancer compared to native Japanese (Buell and Dunn 1965; Tominaga 1985). The main reason for this has been considered to be the effects of environmental factors, especially Westernized dietary habits. Kolonel *et al.* (1983) compared Japanese and Caucasian dietary patterns and found that the Japanese were consuming pickled vegetables and dried/salted fish more frequently and were also eating larger amounts of animal protein, total and saturated fat, and cholesterol than Caucasians. Hankin *et al.* (1975) compared dietary patterns of Issei (born in Japan and emigrated to Hawaii), Nisei (born in Hawaii), and Kibei (born in Hawaii and raised in Japan) and found that Issei and Kibei were taking larger amount of

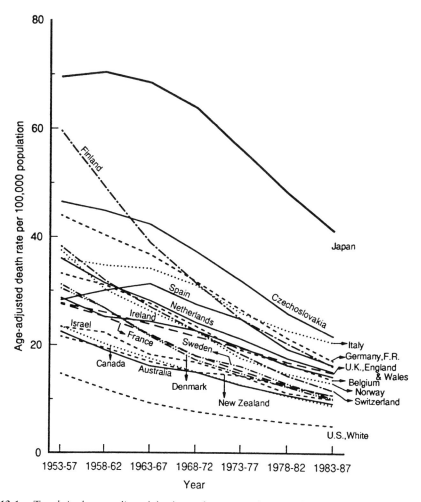

Fig. 12.1. Trends in the age-adjusted death rate from stomach cancer for selected countries (1953–87, males). (From Kuroishi *et al.* 1994.)

Japanese-style foods (rice, tofu, miso soup, fish, kamaboko, pickled vegetables, etc.) than Nisei, and body weight, subscapular skinfold thickness, and serum cholesterol levels were higher in Nisei than in Issei and Kibei.

3. LESSONS FROM ECOLOGICAL STUDIES

Tominaga (1987) examined chronological correlations between the trends in the stomach cancer mortality rates and trends in some dietary patterns in Japan and found that the stomach cancer mortality rate was positively related to rice and salt intake and inversely related to consumption of vitamins C, A, and milk and milk-

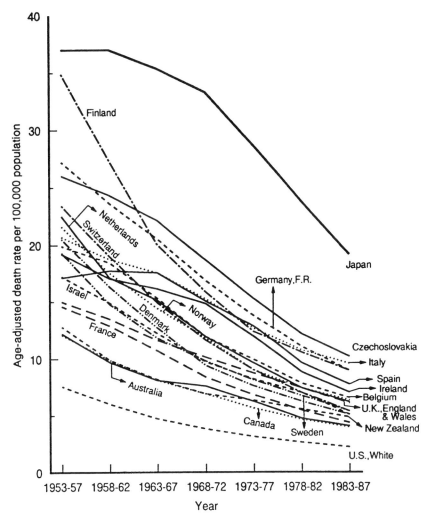

Fig. 12.2. Trends in the age-adjusted death rate from stomach cancer for selected countries (1953–87, females). (From Kuroishi *et al.* 1994.)

products, plus the availability of refrigerators (Fig. 12.3). Dietary patterns and methods of food preservation and processing have been gradually Westernized in the past and will continue in Japan and probably in other non-Western countries. These may have brought a decrease of stomach cancer incidence and may bring about a future decrease.

Several investigators have studied correlations between the incidence or mortality from stomach cancer and consumption of selected food in some selected countries or regions. Tominaga *et al.* (1982) examined correlations (from 22 countries) between the age-adjusted mortality from stomach cancer in 1972 and average per

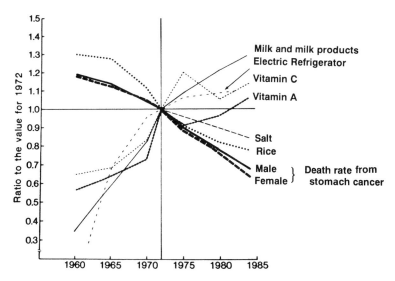

Fig. 12.3.   Comparisons of relative trends (values in 1972 = 1.0) of the age-adjusted death rate from stomach cancer and dietary factors in Japan. (From Tominaga 1987.)

capita food intake in 1960–3, alcohol consumption in 1964, and tobacco consumption in 1965. They found that consumption of fish and cereals was positively related to stomach cancer mortality, whereas consumption of meat, milk and milk-products, oils and fats, and sugar was inversely related. (Consumption of tobacco and alcohol was not closely related to the mortality rate in this study). These results from international correlation analyses suggest that cereals and fish could play a role as risk factors, and food items related inversely to stomach cancer mortality may well act as protective factors in its aetiology. However, there is a possibility that these apparently significant correlations are spurious and that such food items are simply indices of other causal factors. Other chronological and spacial correlation analyses also suffer from problems. Although correlation analyses may give some important clues as to the aetiology of diseases for which marked time trends and large geographical variations are observed, the causal relationship must be confirmed by analytical epidemiology and experimental studies (Tominaga *et al.* 1982).

4. MAJOR RISK FACTORS FOR STOMACH CANCER

From many epidemiological and experimental studies several risk factors for stomach cancer have been identified (Kono and Hirohata 1996). Of these, salt and salt-preserved food are regarded as the most important environmental risk factors, and raw vegetables and fruits are regarded as important protective factors. Correa and co-workers postulated several aetiological hypotheses of stomach cancer, especially the intestinal-type, based on previous epidemiological and experimental studies (Correa *et al.* 1975, 1982, 1985; Correa 1988). Of these, salt and salt-preserved food are likely to cause chronic damage to the stomach mucosa (Correa *et al.* 1975). This hypothesis can be supported by both epidemiological studies (Haenszel *et al.* 1972, 1976; Correa *et al.* 1985; Tajima and Tominaga 1985; Kato *et al.* 1990; Tsugane *et al.* 1991) and experimental studies (Tatematu *et al.* 1975; Takahashi *et al.* 1983). The effect may be due to salt itself and/or nitrite, nitrate, and exogenous or intragastric-formed nitrosamine.

From many epidemiological studies, fresh vegetables and fruits have consistently been found to be protective factors against stomach cancer (Higginson 1966; Graham *et al.* 1967, 1972; Haenszel *et al.* 1972; Correa *et al.* 1985; Risch *et al.* 1985; Tajima and Tominaga 1985; Trichopoulos *et al.* 1985; Jedrychowski *et al.* 1986; Buiatti *et al.* 1989; Chyou *et al.* 1990). Vitamins C, A, beta-carotene, and some other unknown factors in vegetables and fruits can exacerbate gastric carcinogenesis through various mechanisms.

In recent years, the association between infection with *Helicobacter pylori* and stomach cancer has been studied by many investigators (Forman *et al.* 1990, 1991; Correa *et al.* 1990; Nomura *et al.* 1991; Parsonnet *et al.* 1991; Talley *et al.* 1991). The IARC Working Group on the Evaluation of Carcinogenic Risks to Humans (IARC 1994) evaluated carcinogenic risks of *H. pylori* to gastric cancer and concluded that there was inadequate evidence in animal models but adequate evidence in humans for the carcinogenicity of infection with *H. pylori*. Their overall evaluation was that infection with *H. pylori* was carcinogenic to humans (group 1). However, it is not yet certain that stomach cancer could be prevented by eradication of *H. pylori*.

5. INTERVENTION TRIAL

Intervention trials to test the efficacy of chemoprevention in reducing the risk of stomach cancer in high risk populations have been conducted by only a few researchers. Muñoz *et al.* (1996) have been conducting a double-blind randomized trial in San Cristobal, Venezuela, to evaluate the efficacy of treatment for *Helicobacter pylori* infection and antioxidant treatment (beta-carotene, vitamins C, and E) in blocking the progression of precancerous stomach lesions. The major points of their research plan were as follows. The study subjects are 2000 individuals aged 35–69 who participate in the stomach cancer screening programme. At study entry, a detailed dietary questionnaire is administered, and gastroscopy performed with the collection of four antral and one corpus biopsies. In the original protocol, two treatment phases were considered. In phase I, study subjects were to be randomized to receive anti-*H. pylori* treatment or placebo during the two weeks and one month after termination of this treatment. In phase II, subjects were to be randomized to antioxidant treatment or placebo and to receive the assigned treatment for three years. Several end-points will be used to assess the effect of the treatment: progression or regression of the precancerous lesions, changes in the mucins, and proliferating cell nuclear antigens. The biochemical markers will be defined later. They have completed pilot studies to test the efficacy of anti-*H. pylori* drugs (metronidazole, bismuth subcitrate, amoxycillin) and to compare the ability of raising the levels of ascorbic acid in plasma or gastric juice with two antioxidant regimes: slow release vitamin C or standard vitamin C. In view of the results obtained from the pilot studies (Buatti *et al.* 1994; de Sanjose *et al.* 1996), the main trial has started with phase II treatment only; subjects are being randomized to antioxidants or placebo. The main intervention trial is still ongoing and the results are not yet published. Correa *et al.* (personal communication), in Colombia, are also conducting an intervention trial of stomach cancer on 700 subjects with a histological diagnosis of atrophic gastritis or intestinal metaplasia by using ascorbic acid (2 g/day) or beta-carotene (25 mg/day), but the trial is still ongoing and details of this study are not yet published.

6. GUIDELINES FOR PRIMARY PREVENTION

Based on current knowledge of the aetiology of stomach cancer, the following guidelines can be recommended for primary prevention of stomach cancer:

1. To avoid salt and salt-preserved food as much as possible.
2. To take vitamin C and/or beta-carotene-rich fresh vegetables and fruits as frequently as possible.

It is not certain how much stomach cancer could be prevented by observing the above guidelines. However, based on the results of previous epidemiological studies, some 30–50% of stomach cancers might be prevented, especially in high-risk populations.

REFERENCES

Aoki, K. *et al.* (ed.) (1992). *Death rates for malignant neoplasms for selected sites by sex and five year age group in 33 countries*. University of Nagoya Coop Press, Nagoya.

Buell, P. and Dunn, J. (1965). Cancer mortality among Japanese Issei and Nisei of California. *Cancer*, **18**, 656–64.

Buiatti, E., *et al.* (1989). A case-control study of gastric cancer in Italy. *International Journal of Cancer*, **44**, 611–16.

Buiatti, E., *et al.* (1994). Difficulty in eradicating *Helicobacter pylori* in a population at high risk for stomach cancer in Venezuela. *Cancer Causes and Control*, **5**, 249–54.

Chyou, P.-H., *et al.* (1990). A case-control study of diet and stomach cancer. *Cancer Research*, **50**, 7501–4.

Correa, P. (1988). A human model of gastric carcinogenesis. *Cancer Research*, **48**, 3554–60.

Correa, P., *et al.* (1975). A model for gastric cancer. *Lancet*, **2**, 58–60.

Correa, P., *et al.* (1982). Epidemiology of gastric carcinoma: review and future prospects. *Journal of the National Cancer Institute Monograph*, **62**, 129–34.

Correa, P., *et al.* (1985). Dietary determinants of gastric cancer in South Louisiana inhabitants. *Journal of the National Cancer Institute*, **75**, 645–53.

Correa, P., *et al.* (1990). *Helicobacter pylori* and gastric cancer: serum antibody prevalence in populations with contrasting cancer risks. *Cancer*, **66**, 2569–74.

de Sanjose, S., *et al.* (1996). Antioxidants, *Helicobacter pylori* and stomach cancer in Venezuela. *European Journal of Cancer Prevention*, **5**, 57–62.

Devesa, S.S. and Silverman, D.T. (1978). Cancer incidence and mortality trends in the United States: 1935–74. *Journal of the National Cancer Institute*, **60**, 545–71.

Forman, D., *et al.* (1990). Geographic association of *Helicobacter pylori* antibody prevalence and gastric cancer mortality in rural China. *International Journal of Cancer*, **46**, 608–11.

Forman, D., *et al.* (1991). Association between infection with *Helicobacter pylori* and risk of gastric cancer: evidence from a prospective investigation. *British Medical Journal*, **302**, 1302–5.

Graham, S., *et al.* (1967). Dietary and purgation factors in the epidemiology of gastric cancer. *Cancer*, **20**, 2224–34.

Graham, S., *et al.* (1972). Alimentary factors in the epidemiology of gastric cancer. *Cancer*, **30**, 927–38.

Haenszel, W., *et al.* (1972). Stomach cancer among Japanese in Hawaii. *Journal of the National Cancer Institute*, **49**, 969–88.

Haenszel, W., *et al.* (1976). Stomach cancer in Japan. *Journal of the National Cancer Institute*, **56**, 265–78.

Hankin, J.H., *et al.* (1975). Dietary patterns among men of Japanese ancestry in Hawaii. *Cancer Research*, **35**, 3259–64.

Higginson, J. (1966). Etiological factors in gastrointestinal cancer in man. *Journal of the National Cancer Institute*, **37**, 527–45.

IARC (International Agency for Research on Cancer) (1994). IARC Monographs on the Evaluation of Carcinogenic Risks to Humans. *Schistosomiasis, liver flukes and Helicobacter pylori*, Vol. 61, pp. 177–220. IARC Lyon.

Jedrychouwski, W., *et al..* (1986). A case-control study of dietary factors and stomach cancer risk in Poland. *International Journal of Cancer*, **37**, 837–42.

Kato, I., *et al.* (1990). A comparative case-control analysis of stomach cancer and atrophic gastritis. *Cancer Research*, **50**, 6559–64.

Kolonel, L.N., *et al.* (1983). Role of diet in cancer incidence in Hawaii. *Cancer Research*, **43** (suppl.), 2397–402.

Kuroishi, T., *et al.* (1994). World cancer mortality in 33 countries (1953–1987). In *Cancer mortality and morbidity statistics: Japan and the World—1994*, (ed. S. Tominaga, *et al.*). Japan Scientific Societies Press, Tokyo.

Kono, S. and Hirohata, T. (1996). Nutrition and stomach cancer. *Cancer Causes and Control*, **7**, 41–55.

Miller, A.B., (1983). Trends in cancer mortality and epidemiology. *Cancer*, **51**, 2413–18.

Miller, A.B., *et al.* (1990). Nutrition and cancer. *Preventive Medicine*, **9**, 189–96.

Muñoz, N. *et al.* (1996). Chemoprevention trial on precancerous lesions of the stomach in Venezuela: summary of study design and baseline data. In *Principles of chemoprevention* (IARC Scientific Publication, No. 139), (ed. B.W. Stewart, D. McGregor, and P. Kleihues). IARC Lyon.

Nomura, A., *et al.* (1991). *Helicobacter pylori* infection and gastric carcinoma among Japanese Americans in Hawaii. *New England Journal of Medicine*, **325**, 1132–6.

Parsonnet, J., *et al.* (1991). *Helicobacter pylori* infection and the risk of gastric carcinoma. *New England Journal of Medicine*, **325**, 1127–31.

Pollack, E.S. and Horn, J.H. (1980). Trends in cancer incidence and mortality in the United States, 1969–76. *Journal of the National Cancer Institute*, **64**, 1091–1103.

Risch, H.A., *et al.* (1985). Dietary factors and the incidence of cancer of the stomach. *American Journal of Epidemiology*, **122**, 947–59.

Sedgwick, D.M., *et al.* (1991). Gastric cancer in Scotland: changing epidemiology, unchanging workload. *British Medical Journal*, **302**, 1305–7.

Swanson, G.M. and Young, J.L. Jr. (1983). Trends in cancer incidence in metropolitan Detroit, 1937–1977: leads for prevention. *Preventive Medicine*, **12**, 403–20.

Tajima, K. and Tominaga, S. (1985). Dietary habits and gastrointestinal cancers: a comparative case-control study of stomach and large intestinal cancers in Nagoya, Japan. *Japanese Journal of Cancer Research (Gann)*, **76**, 705–16.

Takahashi, M., *et al.* (1983). Effect of high salt diet on rat gastric carcinogenesis induced by N-methyl-N′-nitro-N-nitrosoguanidine. *Gann*, **74**, 28–34.

Talley, N.J., *et al.* (1991). Gastric adenocarcinoma and *Helicobacter pylori* infection. *Journal of the National Cancer Institute*, **83**, 1734–9.

Tatematsu, M., *et al.* (1975). Effects in rats of sodium chloride on experimental gastric cancers induced by N-methyl-N′-nitro N-nitrosoguanidine or 4-nitroquinoline-1-oxide. *Journal of the National Cancer Institute*, **55**, 101–5.

Tominaga, S. (1985). Cancer incidence in Japanese in Japan, Hawaii, and Western United States. *National Cancer Institute Monograph*, **69**, 83–92.

Tominaga, S. (1987). Decreasing trend of stomach cancer in Japan. *Japanese Journal of Cancer Research*, **78**, 1–10.

Tominaga, S., *et al.* (1982). Usefulness of correlation analyses in the epidemiology of stomach cancer. *National Cancer Institute Monograph*, **62**, 135–40.

Trichopoulos, D., *et al.* (1985). Diet and cancer of the stomach: a case-control study in Greece. *International Journal of Cancer*, **36**, 291–7.

Tsugane, S., *et al.* (1991). Urinary salt excretion and stomach cancer mortality among four Japanese populations. *Cancer Causes and Control*, **2**, 165–8.

You, W.-C. *et al.* (1988). Diet and high risk of stomach cancer in Shandong, China. *Cancer Research*, **48**, 3518–23.

13

Secondary prevention: screening methods in high-incidence areas

Akira Oshima

1. INTRODUCTION

According to estimates of the world-wide incidence of major cancers in 1985, stomach cancer is the second most frequent, accounting for 9.9% of all new cancer cases (Parkin *et al*. 1993). The age-standardized incidence rate of stomach cancer is higher in Japan than anywhere else in the world.

Cancer screening is the only reliable method left for cancer prevention when primary prevention is not feasible. Although the risk factors of stomach cancer have gradually been elucidated, there are still no primary prevention measures, as there are for lung cancer (tobacco control programs), or for liver cancer (vaccination programs against hepatitis-B virus for infants).

In this chapter, the history of the screening program for stomach cancer in Japan is briefly described and screening methods are outlined. Evaluative studies are then introduced on the diagnostic validity of the screening test and on the efficacy and effectiveness of the screening program.

2. HISTORY AND CURRENT STATUS OF THE STOMACH CANCER SCREENING PROGRAM IN JAPAN

2.1. Outline of the history of the screening program

In the 1960s, the proportion of stomach cancer deaths among total cancer deaths was as high as about 40% in Japan, although it decreased to about 20% in 1993. Stomach cancer was then one of the most serious public health problems facing the nation and required an urgent solution. At that time, the risk factors for stomach cancer had not been clearly established, but excellent diagnostic techniques, such as double contrast radiology and endoscopy were being developed. However, most of the patients who came to hospitals with symptoms were in an advanced stage of cancer. Many experienced clinicians concluded, therefore, that it was essential to screen apparently healthy people outside the hospital environment and offer proper diagnostic tests to those with positive screening test results, in order to detect stomach cancer at an early stage. Around 1960, screening tests began to be studied diligently.

Photofluorography turned out to be an appropriate screening test for stomach cancer because it was more accurate and efficient than the fecal occult blood test, gastric juice analysis, physical examination, or other tests available at that time. In Japan, there was already an established system using mobile units, for early detection of pulmonary tuberculosis with photofluorography.

A special mobile unit with a photofluorographic apparatus for stomach cancer screening was developed by clinicians for the first time in 1960. This mobile unit made it possible to screen larger numbers of people outside the hospital environment (i.e. near their home or place of employment). Shortly thereafter, mass screening tests using mobile units began to be offered in many regions throughout Japan.

National government subsidies to prefectures for this screening program began in 1966 and, subsequently, the number of screened individuals increased rapidly. According to the Japanese Society of Gastric Mass Survey, the number of screened persons was about 2 million in 1970.

In February 1983, the Health and Medical Services Law for the Aged was put into force and the screening program for stomach cancer was integrated into the health service. Since then, municipalities have taken the responsibility for conducting cancer screening programs under national and prefectural subsidies. The subsidies were increased to include full-sized X-ray tests as well as miniature photofluorography. The target population are residents of each municipality aged 40 years and over who are unable to obtain a cancer screening test at their places of employment or elsewhere.

2.2. Outline of the current status of the cancer screening program

In 1993, about 4.4 million screening tests for stomach cancer were conducted as health services covered by the Health and Medical Services Law for the Aged. Although the Ministry of Health and Welfare has set the goal of annually screening 30% of the target population, the coverage still remained at the low level of 14%. It costs about (¥3500, equivalent to $35) to screen one person by photofluorography. Each individual screened pays about (¥500) and the remaining cost is equally divided between the national government, prefectures, and municipalities.

Mass screening tests for stomach cancer are also carried out at places of employment. The tests are similar to those covered by the Law for the Aged, and are made available to employees with no charge at most companies and institutions. Multiphasic health check-up programs are also common in Japan. Almost all programs cover stomach cancer screenings, usually by full-sized X-rays and sometimes by endoscopy. Fees for this type of health check-up are usually paid by screened persons themselves, but they are sometimes subsidized by their employers or health insurance organization. In addition, stomach X-rays or endoscopy are commonly offered to those patients who visit the hospital or clinic with slight epigastric symptoms. In these cases, 70–90% of the cost is covered by health insurance.

Mass screening programs offer opportunities for many people to undergo stomach cancer tests. According to a national survey conducted by the Ministry of Health and Welfare in 1985, about 60% of the general population, aged over 30, had had a stomach cancer screening test (Table 13.1). Although this is somewhat dated, there has been no subsequent national survey covering a large random sample since 1986. The proportion of those who had had stomach cancer tests was higher in the 35–74 year age group than in the under 34 or over 75 age group for both sexes. About 20% of the tests were offered as mass screenings in mobile units or in health centers by municipalities. Another 15% were offered as mass screenings in places of employment by companies. Thus, mass screening programs had an important role in providing the general population with the opportunity of having tests for stomach cancer.

According to a survey conducted in Tokyo for a random sample in 1990, the proportion of those who had had stomach cancer screening tests during the previous year was estimated to be about 48% in males and about 37% in females over the age of 40. Similar results were obtained by a survey conducted in Miyagi Prefecture. However, the proportion of mass screening tests conducted by municipalities, as health services covered by the Law for the Aged, was about 65% in rural areas within Miyagi Prefecture, much higher than that in the Tokyo metropolitan area (i.e. 7.5%).

3. SCREENING METHODS

3.1. Miniature photofluorography

According to the Japanese Society of Gastrointestinal Mass Survey (JSGMS), about 6.5 million people were screened in 1993. About 90% of the screening tests were

Table 13.1. Proportion of individuals who had stomach cancer tests, by sex and age group (1985, Japan)

			% of those who had tests	
Sex	Age (yrs)	No. of subjects	Ever	Regularly
Male	30–34	1722	46.3	10.5
	35–44	3908	62.7	18.8
	45–54	3193	71.1	27.4
	55–64	2374	73.6	24.9
	65–74	1344	70.2	16.8
	75–	683	57.8	11.6
Female	30–34	1739	36.2	4.3
	35–44	3991	49.4	8.4
	45–54	3309	62.6	15.9
	55–64	2711	64.7	16.7
	65–74	1854	60.1	11.5
	75–	1091	48.7	6.8
Total		27 919	59.8	15.6

From the Ministry of Health and Welfare, Japan.

conducted using a photofluorographic apparatus, and the remaining 10% were conducted with full-sized X-ray apparatus. In 1993, there were 1997 photo-fluographic machines, including 788 mobile units in Japan. Thus, a majority of the screening tests were conducted using photofluography in mobile units.

Since 1960, many improvements have been made both in the hardware and soft-ware involved in photofluorographic screening. In 1993, about 99% of photo-fluorographic machines used high-resolution image-intensifiers and 10×10 cm miniature film. In 1983, the JSGMS recommended a standard examination method using photofluorography. According to this method, seven consecutive photo-fluorograms of the stomach are taken routinely for each screened person in the following order:

(1) mucosal view in prone position or double contrast view of the anterior wall;
(2) barium-filled view in a prone position;
(3) double contrast view in a supine position;
(4) in a left anterior oblique position;
(5) in a right anterior oblique position;
(6) in a left anterior oblique with a semi-upright position; and
(7) a barium-filled view in an upright position (Fig. 13.1).

By 1990 about 86% of the screening institutions had adopted methods utilizing the standard seven or more exposures.

Usually, about 50 people are screened by an experienced technician during one screening session lasting three hours in a mobile unit. All the photofluorographic images are interpreted by experienced radiologists or gastroenterologists. In order

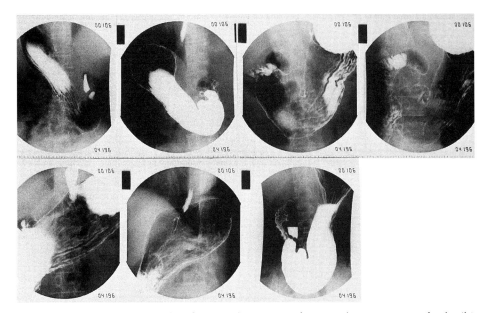

Fig. 13.1.   Standard methods of photofluorographic screening for stomach cancer (see text for details).

to decrease the number of false-negative results, cross-checking by two doctors has been systematically adopted in recent years. By 1993, about 83% of the screening institutions had adopted cross-checking methods.

Table 13.2 shows the results of a 1993 national survey by the JSGMS of the mass screening program using photofluorography. About 5.8 million people were screened and 12.7% of these were recommended for diagnostic work-up tests. Out of these, 76.6% underwent diagnostic testing by direct X-ray and/or endoscopy and 6248 stomach cancer cases were detected. The cancer detection rate was 0.11% and about 60% of cases detected by screening were early gastric cancer cases.

The stomach cancer screening test by photofluorography costs about ¥3500 for each screened person and a diagnostic work-up test by X-ray or endoscopy costs about ¥15 000. Therefore, it costs about ¥5 million to detect one stomach cancer case and about ¥10 million to detect one early gastric cancer case by photofluoro-graphic screening. Although many early gastric cancer cases can be detected by photofluorography, few screening programs using this technique have been applied in countries other than Japan. This is partly because of poor efficiency, financial problems, and/or difficulties in the maintenance of the apparatus. It costs about ¥45 million to construct one mobile unit with a photofluorographic machine.

3.2. Other screening tests

Full-sized X-ray testing and endoscopy are established techniques for work-up diagnosis of stomach cancer, but they can also be applied to screening. The difficulties in applying them to screening are problems of cost and the lack of trained personnel for performing the tests.

According to the JSGMS, about 667 000 people were screened in 1993 by full-sized X-ray tests, which constituted only 10% of the total stomach cancer screening tests conducted in that year. However, this is the number of screening tests conducted independently of multiphasic health check-ups, which were not included. In large cities, where there are many hospitals and clinics, stomach cancer screenings with full-sized X-ray tests began to be adopted as part of the health services covered by the Law for the Aged. There is a tendency for photofluorographic screenings to be con-ducted in rural areas and for full-sized X-ray screenings to be used in urban areas.

Table 13.2. Results of the mass screening program for stomach cancer using photofluorography, (1993, Japan)

	No.	(Percentage)	
Total screened	5817 078	(100.0)	
Diagnostic work-up tests recommended	737 249	(12.7)	(100.0)
Diagnostic work-up tests performed	564 972		(76.6)
Stomach cancer detected	6 248	(0.11)	

From the Japanese Society of Gastrointestinal Mass Survey.

Endoscopic screening is not as common, because the test is expensive and causes some discomfort, and also because there are only a limited number of physicians available to carry out this procedure.

In Japan, many cases of early gastric cancer have been diagnosed as a result of the progress of diagnostic techniques and due to the wide application of screening programs. Early gastric cancer is not a specific type of cancer that occurs only in Japan. The number of early gastric cancer cases has increased in countries, such as the United Kingdom (Fielding *et al.* 1980), Sweden (Ohman *et al.* 1980), and the United States (Green *et al.* 1981), in parallel with the application of double contrast radiology, fibreoptic endoscopy, and endoscopic biopsy. Hallisey *et al.* (1990) reported that the investigation of dyspeptic patients, aged over 40, by endoscopy on their initial visit to general practitioners could increase the proportion of early gastric cancer cases to 26%. According to reports by participants from Chile, Italy, Korea, and China at the fourth general meeting of WHO-Collaborating Center for Primary Prevention, Diagnosis and Treatment of Gastric Cancer, held in June 1990 in Tokyo, the proportion of early gastric cancer has increased in recent years. Sue-Ling *et al.* (1993) concluded, based on their experiences, that stomach cancer could be a curable disease in Britain with earlier diagnosis through a more widespread use of endoscopy.

Stomach cancer screening by blood testing has long been anticipated. The candidate screening method is measurement of the blood pepsinogen level and *Helicobacter pylori* antibodies. In 1982, a radioimmunoassay kit of serum groups I and II pepsinogens was developed (Ichinose *et al.* 1982). Clinical studies of stomach cancer screening using this test are now under way (Miki *et al.* 1993). Preliminary data suggest that this method might serve as a screening test to detect a person for endoscopy in the diagnosis of early gastric cancer

The association between *H. pylori* and stomach cancer is now being confirmed from an epidemiological point of view. However, it will take more time to determine whether the immunological techniques for *H. pylori* can be used as a screening test to select high-risk group. It is also important to observe whether irradiation of *H. pylori* will decrease the risk of stomach cancer, when this is verified, people with *H. pylori* infection will have a standard irradiation therapy to prevent the occurrence of stomach cancer.

4. DIAGNOSTIC VALIDITY OF PHOTOFLUOROGRAPHY

Miniature photofluorography is not as valid as the full-sized X- ray test because of the physical limitations of resolution. Shiga *et al.* (1991) examined the diagnostic validy of miniature photofluography by performing small-diameter panendoscopy tests on 17 976 randomly selected screened individuals. The results were as follows:

(1) 93% of 80 advanced cancer cases detected by small-diameter panendoscopy could be detected by photofluorography;

(2) 39% of 207 early gastric cancer cases detected by small-diameter panendoscopy could be detected by photofluorography. In the case of small early
gastric cancer (<2.0 cm), the detection rate by photofluorography was only
22%.

These results suggest that small early gastric cancer cannot be detected by
photofluorography. The point is, however, not whether screening with photofluorography can detect stomach cancer in the very early stage, but whether screening with photofluorography can detect cancer in the preclinical, curable stage.

Murakami *et al.* (1990) followed-up a large number of screened individuals in
order to estimate diagnostic validity. In estimating the validity of screening tests, a
key factor is to follow-up all screenees and to note all cancer cases diagnosed after
screening. Murakami *et al.* (1990) followed-up the screenees by means of a record
linkage to the population-based Osaka Cancer Registry.

Table 13.3 shows the results of a follow-up study of screenees after photofluorography. In addition to 96 stomach cancer cases detected by screening, 13
cases were diagnosed within one year after negative screening tests. When stomach
cancer cases diagnosed within one year of screening were regarded as cancer positives at the time of screening, the sensitivity was estimated to be 88.5% and the
specificity to be 92.0%. In 5 out of 13 false-negative cases shown in Table 13.3,
abnormal findings could be checked by again reviewing the miniature photofluorograms. No abnormal findings could be checked in the remaining 8 cases, in which
rapidly growing cancers, such as linitis plastica, were included.

In reviewing X-ray miniature films used in screening, almost all abnormal
findings are checked and recommended for diagnostic work-up tests in order not to
overlook early gastric cancer. Table 13.4 shows the results of diagnostic work-up
tests according to the results of screening miniature films. These data come from
screening tests conducted by the Osaka Cancer Prevention and Detection Center

Table 13.3. Stomach cancer cases diagnosed after screening tests

Results of test	No. of subjects	No. of stomach cancer cases[a]		
			Diagnosed during follow-up period	
		Detected by screening	< 1 year[b]	≧1 year
Positive	6903	96 (52)	4 (2)	36 (16)
Negative	78 202	–	13 (1)	220 (85)

[a] Number of early gastric cancer cases are shown in parentheses.
[b] When stomach cancer cases diagnosed within 1 year after screening were regarded as cancer positives
at the time of screening, then:

sensitivity = (96 + 4) / (96 + 4 + 13) = 0.885.
specificity = (78202 − 13) / (78202 − 13 + 6903 − 96 − 4) = 0.920.

From Murakami *et al.* (1990).

Table 13.4. Stomach cancer cases detected among individuals recommended for diagnostic work-up tests by findings on screening photofluorograms

Findings at screening	No. of subjects	Work-up tests performed	GC[a] detected	EGC[b] detected	Proportion of EGC in total cancers
A. Cancer	152 (100.0) (0.3)	147 (96.7)	112 (73.7) (16.8)	37 (24.3) (9.0)	33.0
B. Suspicion of cancer	359 (100.0) (0.8)	351 (97.8)	72 (21.4) (10.8)	39 (10.9) (9.5)	50.6
C. Cancer cannot be ruled out	2702 (100.0) (6.0)	2550 (94.4)	113 (4.2) (17.0)	68 (2.5) (16.5)	60.2
D. Benign diseases	34 958 (100.0) (77.6)	33 100 (94.7)	331 (0.9) (49.8)	239 (0.7) (58.2)	72.2
E. Probably normal, but recommended for work-up tests to confirm	6884 (100.0) (15.3)	6563 (95.3)	32 (0.5) (4.8)	28 (0.4) (6.8)	87.5
Total	45 055 (100.0) (100.0)	42 711 (94.8)	665 (1.5) (100.0)	411 (0.9) (100.0)	61.8

[a] GC, gastric cancer. [b] EGC, early gastric cancer.
Note: These subjects come from 429 830 screening tests conducted by the Osaka Cancer Prevention and Detection Center during 1987–91. The proportion of those recommended for diagnostic work-up test was 10.5%. From the Osaka Cancer Prevention and Detection Center. Figures in parentheses are percentages.

during 1987–91. Findings which clearly indicated the possibility of cancer (i.e. A, B, or C categories in Table 13.4) could be identitied in about half of the screen-detected stomach cancer cases. For early gastric cancer (EGC) cases, about one-third could be identified by screening fluorophotograms. Figure 13.2 shows the miniature X-ray films, taken as routine screening tests, which show definite EGC lesions.

Compared with the results of a study on the validity of other cancer screening tests by similar methods (Chamberlain 1982), stomach cancer screening by photofluorography is almost as sensitive as cervical cancer screening with the Pap smear test or breast cancer screening with mammography, but it is considerably less specific than either of these. This means that the predictive value of positive tests is lower than that of other cancer screening tests. However, it should be taken into account that many benign lesions, such as gastric ulcers, are also diagnosed by the program.

5. EFFICACY OF PHOTOFLUOROGRAPHY

When it was shown that stomach cancer could be detected at an early stage, screening programs were implemented in many areas without an appropriate epidemiological evaluation. This situation was very similar to that of cervical cancer screening programs found in many other countries. However, the optimistic assumption made by clinicians that early detection would always be beneficial is now considered to be incorrect (Cole and Morrison 1980). Following the wide

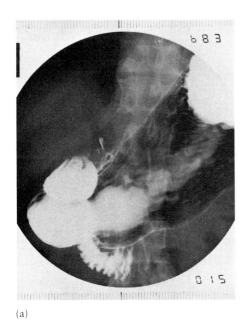
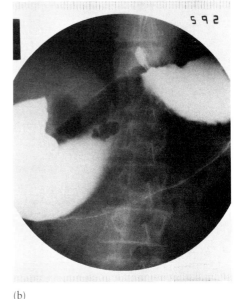

(a)   (b)

Fig. 13.2. Photofluorograms which show definite lesions of early gastric cancer: (a) type IIc; (b) type IIa.

implementation of screening programs in Japan, many studies have been conducted to evaluate their efficacy (Oshima 1988).

The five-year survival rate of cases of stomach cancer detected by screening is about 70%, which is much higher than that of those diagnosed under usual medical care (i.e. about 40% in Japan). In a comparison of survival rates, lead time bias, length bias and selection bias should be taken into consideration. Yamazaki *et al.* (1989) conducted a long-term follow-up study of 1139 patients with stomach cancer detected by screening. The 5-, 10-, and 15-year relative survival rates were 70.1%, 69.1%, and 70.3%, respectively. The relative survival rates continued to drop for five years from the start of observation, but there was no decline beyond five years. This means that the prognosis of cases detected by screening is much better even when considering lead time. However, length bias and selection bias cannot be corrected even in this comparison.

Table 13.5 shows a summary of evaluative studies on the efficacy of stomach cancer screening programs in Japan. Tsukuma *et al.* (1983) conducted a prospective study of EGC and showed that, if untreated, it will progress to advanced cancer and will finally result in stomach cancer death.

Table 13.5.   Summary of evaluative studies on the efficacy of the stomach cancer screening programs in Japan

Study	Type of study	Results of study
Tsukuma *et al.* (1983)	Natural history of early gastric cancer	Half of 56 untreated early gastric cancer cases progressed to advanced cancer in 37 months and died from gastric cancer 77 months after the diagnosis of early cancer
Kuroishi *et al.* (1986)	Geographical comparison of decrease in stomach cancer mortality rate	In 42 areas with high coverage rate (> 30%, average: 37.9%), the decrease of age-standardized stomach cancer mortality rate in the 40–69 age group from 1969–72 to 1973–7 was 12.8%, which was larger than that of 6.6% in 84 control areas (average of coverage rates: 11.7%)
Oshima *et al.* (1986)	Case-control study of stomach cancer screening	Odds ratio of screened vs. unscreened was calculated as 0.60 (90% confidence interval: 0.34–1.05) among males and 0.38 (90% CI: 0.19–0.79) among females
Fukao *et al.* (1995)	Case-control study of stomach cancer screening	Odds ratio of screened vs. unscreened during the 5 years prior to the date of diagnosis was estimated as 0.41 (95% CI: 0.28–0.61)

Kuroishi *et al.* (1986) surveyed the change in stomach cancer mortality rates from 1969–72 to 1973–7 in areas with different screening coverage rates but similar stomach cancer mortality rates between 1969 and 1972. In 42 areas with a high coverage rate (>30%), decrease of age-standardized mortality rate in the 40–69 age group was 12.8%, which was larger than that of 6.6% in 84 control areas.

Oshima *et al.* (1986) conducted a case-control study in Nose Town, Osaka, Japan. The case series consisted of all stomach cancer deaths during the period 1969–81. For each case, three controls of the same sex and the same precinct, born within five years of the case's birth year, were randomly selected from a statistical file of Nose Town residents alive at the date of death of the relevant case. Screening history was compared between the 91 cases and 261 controls before the date of cancer diagnosis. The odds ratio was estimated to be 0.60 (90% confidence interval: 0.34–1.04) among males and 0.38 (0.18–0.78) among females. In this study, only those screening tests by the Center for Adult Diseases, Osaka, which were provided by Nose Town public health services, were examined. Data from stomach X-ray tests carried out in hospitals and clinics and/or screening tests conducted at places of employment, where there were usually more males than females, could not be included in the analysis. This methodological limitation might have diluted the efficacy of screening among males, and this may have contributed to the difference between the odds ratios of males and females.

Recently, Fukao *et al.* (1995) conducted a similar case-control study in Miyagi Prefecture, which involved 188 stomach cancer deaths in 61 muncipalities. Cases were selected from those insured under the national health insurance system, which covers self-employed persons and employees of small businesses, who had no opportunity of being screened at their places of employment. Their screening history during the five years prior to the date of diagnosis was compared with that of the 577 matched neighborhood controls. The odds ratio was estimated to be 0.41 (95% confidence interval: 0.28–0.61). The odds ratio was lower in males (0.32) than in females (0.63), suggesting that screening was more effective in males. However, the 95% confidence interval for females was wide because the number of female cases was small.

Although these are observational studies and their results should be interpreted carefully, it can be said that the efficacy of stomach cancer screening programs is fairly well established when the results of the above evaluative studies are combined. These evaluative methodologies for stomach cancer screening are almost the same as those for cervical cancer screening.

6. THE ROLE OF THE JAPANESE SCREENING PROGRAM

Figure 13.3 shows trends of the age-standardized stomach cancer incidence rate and mortality rate in Osaka, Japan. The mortality rate declined almost in parallel with the incidence rate. Recently, however, the gap between the incidence and mortality rates has become more defined (i.e. the slope of decline of the mortality rate

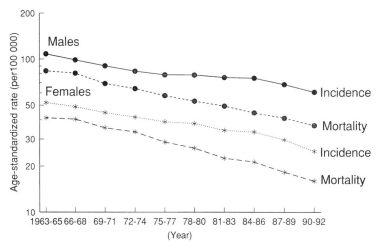

Fig. 13.3.   Trends in age-standardized incidence and mortality rates in stomach cancer, Osaka, Japan.

has become sharper than that of the incidence rate). This gap is more prominent in those age groups who undergo more intensive screening tests. Similar results were obtained from the Miyagi Prefecture study (Hisamich *et al.* 1991).

These data show that the decline in the mortality rate for stomach cancer in Japan is mainly due to factors such as change in dietary habits, but that it can be explained partly by efforts made in early detection. It can be reasonably estimated that the stomach cancer mortality rate will decrease more rapidly with efforts to expand the screening program. The key element is to enhance the level of coverage within the program. In addition to screening tests by photofluorography in mobile units, screening tests utilizing full-sized X-ray film in clinics and hospitals should be expanded, particularly in urban areas.

In addition to offering opportunities for large numbers of people to have stomach cancer tests, mass screening programs have had a role in distributing new and proved diagnostic techniques throughout Japan. It has been demonstrated by many screen-detected early gastric cancer cases that stomach cancer is a curable disease when diagnosed in the early stage. Currently, not only medical profession-als but also the general population in Japan realize that the key element of stomach cancer prevention is to have stomach X-ray tests and/or endoscopy tests regularly. Double contrast radiology and endoscopy tests can be conducted in many clinics and almost all hospitals in Japan.

In countries other than Japan, too, screening trials can play a similar role in demon-strating that stomach cancer can be detected at an early stage by advanced diagnostic techniques. For this purpose endoscopy is considered to be a more suitable screening modality than photofluorography, which requires a large initial investment. In this case, however, high-risk groups should be targeted. Hallissey *et al.* (1990) demon-strated that endoscopic investigation of dyspeptic patients aged over 40, following their initial consultation with their general practitioner can considerably increase the proportion of early gastric cancer cases. Similar trials are expected to be conducted in many countries where stomach cancer is still common. Serum tests for pepsinogen levels and/or *H. pylori* may also be useful in screening for high-risk groups.

REFERENCES

Chamberlain, J. (1982). Screening for cancer of various sites. In *The prevention of cancer*, (ed. M. Alderson), pp. 259–83. Edward Arnold, London.

Cole, P. and Morrison, A.S. (1980). Basic issues in population screening for cancer. *J. Natl. Cancer Inst.*, **64**, 1263–72.

Fielding, J.W.L, Ellis, D.J., Jones, B.G., Power, D.J., Waterhoese, J.A.H., and Brookes, V.S. (1980). Natural history of 'early' gastric cancer: results of a 10-year regional survey. *Br. Med. J.*, **281**, 965–7.

Fukao, A., Tsubono, Y., Tsuji, I., Hisamichi, S., Sugahara, N., and Takano, A. (1995). The evaluation of screening for gastric cancer in Miyagi Prefecture, Japan: a population-based case-control study. *Int. J. Cancer*, **60**, 45–8.

Green, P.H.R., O'Toole K.M., Weinbery, L.M., and Goldtarb, J.P. (1981). Early gastric cancer. *Gastroenterology*, **81**, 247–56.

Hallisey, M.T., Allum, A.J., Ellis, D.J., and Fielding, J.W. (1990). Early detection of gastric cancer. *Br. Med. J*, **301**, 513–15.

Hisamichi, S., Fukao, A., Sugawara, N., Nishikouri, M., Komatsu, S., Tsubono, Y., *et al.* (1991). Evaluation of mass screening programme for stomach cancer in Japan. In *Cancer screening*, (ed. A.B. Miller, J. Chamberlain, N.E. Day, M. Hakama, and P.C. Prorok), pp. 357–70. Cambridge University Press.

Ichinose, M., Miki, K., Furihata, C., Kageyama, T., Hayashi, R., Niwa, H., *et al.* (1982). Radioimmunoassay of serum group I and group II pepsinogens in normal controls and patients with various disorders. *Clin. Chimica Acta*, **126**, 183–91.

Kuroishi, T., Hirose, K., and Tominaga, S. (1986). An epidemiological evaluation of the efficacy of mass screening for stomach cancer in Japan—with special reference to the comparison of the trend in the age-specitic death rate from cancer of the stomach between high coverage-rate and conrol areas. *J. Gastroenterol. Mass Survey*, **73**, 33–40. (In Japanese with tables and figures in English)

Miki, K., Ichinose, M., Ishikawa, K.B., Yahagi, N., Matsushima, M., Kakei, N., *et al.* (1993). Clinical application of serum pepsinogen I and II for mass screening to detect gastric cancer. *Jpn. J. Cancer Res.*, **84**, 1086–90.

Murakami, R., Tsukuma, H., Ubukata, T., Nakanishi, K., Fujimoto, I., Kawashima, T., *et al.* (1990). Estimation of validity of mass screening program for gastric cancer in Osaka, Japan. *Cancer*, **65**, 1255–60.

Ohman, U., Emas, S., and Rubio, O. (1980). Relation between early and advanced gastric cancer. *Am. J. Surg.*, **140**, 351–5.

Oshima, A. (1988). Screening for stomach cancer: the Japanese program. In *Screening for gastrointestinal cancer*, (ed. J. Chamberlain and A.B. Miller), pp. 65–70. Hans Huber, Toronto.

Oshima, A., Hirata, N., Ubukata, T., Umeda, K., and Fujimoto, I. (1986). Evaluation of a mass screening program for stomach cancer with a case-control study design. *Int. J. Cancer*, **38**, 829–33.

Parkin, D.M., Pisani, P., and Ferlay, J. (1993). Estimates of the worldwide incidence of eighteen major cancers in 1985. *Int. J. Cancer*, **54**, 594–606.

Shiga, T., Nishizawa, M., Hosoi, K., Okada, T., Yamada, K., Okura, Y., *et al.* (1991). Evaluation of gastric mass survey from the point of view of the prevalence of gastric cancer among seemingly healthy individuals. *I-to-Cho* (*Stomach and Intestine*), **26**, 1371–87. (In Japanese with English abstract)

Sue-Ling, H.M., Johnston, D., Martin, I.G., Dixon, M.F., Lansdown, M.R.J., *et al.* (1993). Gastric cancer: a curable disease in Britain. *Br. Med. J.*, **307**, 591–6.

Tsukuma, H., Mishima, T., and Oshima, A. (1983). Prospective study of 'early' gastric cancer. *Int. J. Cancer*, **31**, 421–6.

Yamazaki, H., Oshima, A., Murakami, R., Endoh, S., and Ubukata, T. (1989). A long-term follow-up study of patients with gastric cancer detected by mass screening. *Cancer*, **63**, 613–17.

14

Secondary prevention: screening methods in low-incidence areas

John W.L. Fielding

1. INTRODUCTION

The excellent results achieved by treating early gastric cancer demands that every effort should be made to facilitate this diagnosis. The resources targeted at early diagnosis must be related to need. Clearly, in countries of high incidence, detection is an important priority, in countries of low incidence the need may not be so great for overall health-care policy, but the requirements of an individual should be preserved.

The method of detection has resource implications. Targeting an entire population is often expensive and is difficult to achieve: the Japanese mass screening programmes have only managed to screen about 14% of the population (Hisamichi *et al.* 1976). To maximize cost–benefits of any diagnostic programme, attempts should be made to identify high-risk groups. In many parts of the world, the incidence of gastric cancer is reducing. Despite this, gastric cancer still remains the most common cause of death from malignant disease in the world.

Our knowledge of the disease should be utilized to hasten the reduction of mortality world-wide. In high-incidence countries, programmes for early detection need to be tailored to the resources available. In most of Europe, the mortality from gastric cancer is in the order of 20 per 100 000 deaths per annum. In the United States, it is less than 10 per 100 000 per annum. These are areas for targeted programmes for high-risk groups.

2. HIGH-RISK GROUPS

Groups of individuals can be identified who have a higher risk than the normal population for developing the disease (Table 14.1).

Table 14.1. High-risk groups for developing stomach cancer

Patient groups	Premalignant condition	Premalignant lesions
Dyspeptic patients	Postoperative stomach	Chronic atrophic gastritis
Familial	Pernicious anaemia	Intestinal metaplasia
Occupational (e.g. coal-miners)		Dysplasia

2.1.   Dyspeptic patients

A feature common to most patients with gastric cancer is the development of specific symptoms. Over 75% of patients with advanced gastric cancer will have symptoms referable to the upper gastrointestinal tract (Swynnerton and Truelove 1952; Lundh/ *et al.* 1974; Cassell and Robinson 1976). The screening studies from Japan have demonstrated that 48% of patients with early gastric cancer detected in the screening programme do, in fact, have symptoms (Hisamichi *et al.* 1976). Two studies in the Western world have shown that the difference between symptom profiles of early and advanced gastric cancer is that the early lesions do not usually have the non-specific symptoms of advanced malignancy. A particular feature is the absence of weight loss in early lesions (Green *et al.* 1981; Fielding *et al.* 1980).

2.2.   Genetic preposition

A genetic predisposition to gastric cancer has been established. In populations that have moved from Japan to Hawaii, it has been demonstrated that within a generation, the incidence falls towards that of the local population (Buell and Dunn 1965). However, the incidence remains higher than that of the normal population, indicating that genetic factors may be important. Data from insurance companies also demonstrate this genetic risk (Videbaeck and Mosbecb 1954).

2.3.   Occupational risk

In addition to the genetic influences, enrivonmental factors can play a role, and certain occupations have been demonstrated to be at an increased risk of gastric cancer, the most notable group being coal-miners (Fielding *et al.* 1989).

2.4.   Premalignant conditions

Individuals who have had a previous gastric resection and those with pernicious anaemia have an increased risk of gastric cancer. The association with pernicious anaemia is well established. Patients with this condition now survive longer and the number developing a gastric carcinoma is higher than in the general population (Zamcheck *et al.* 1955). The risk of malignancy has been estimated to be 4–6 times the general population and appears to be related to age.

The data related to the role of gastric surgery for benign gastroduodenal disease are less conclusive (Domellof *et al.* 1977; Nicholls 1979; Farrands *et al.* 1983; Pickford *et al.* 1984). The variations in these studies can be explained by small numbers. However, Caygill *et al.* (1986) reported the follow-up of 4446 patients operated on for benign peptic ulceration more than 20 years previously, and demonstrated a 3.7-fold increase following gastric resection and a 7.9% increased risk following vagotomy. For gastric ulceration, the risk is a 3-fold increase over

20 years, rising to 5.5-fold after this. The risk is reported to be higher for Billroth II (8.6) than Billroth I (4).

2.5.   Premalignant lesions

Mucosal abnormalities: chronic atrophic gastritis; intestinal metaplasia; gastric dysplasia; and gastric polyps may be associated with increased risk of malignancy.

Atrophic gastritis has been classified into two major groups: autoimmune type A, which is associated with pernicious anaemia; and environmental type B (Imai 1971; Strickland and Mackay 1973; Correa 1980). The changes in type A occur in the fundus and body and may be found in patients who do not have overt pernicious anaemia. Type B gastritis is seen with greatest frequency in areas with the highest incidence of gastric cancer. It is a multifocal disease, usually starting at the incisura and involving the antrum and body.

The risk of developing cancer in the presence of atrophic gastritis is 10% over 10 years (Siurala *et al.* 1966; Strickland and mackay 1973).

Intestinal metaplasia has been classified into three groups depending on morphology and mucin histochemistry. Type I shows mature absortive cells and neutral mucins. Type II has no mature absorbtive cells but neutral mucins; in type III, the morphology is similar to II but the mucins are sulphated. From retrospective data, type III metaplasia appears to carry the highest risk of malignant transformation (Jass 1980).

There is no doubt of an association between dysplasia and cancer but quantifying this risk depends on the identification of true dysplasia which can often be difficult for the histopathologist. A study of 247 gastric biopsies, which were assessed by interested pathologists unaware of initial diagnosis, showed that of 26 cases where the diagnosis of dysplasia was made by either initial or review pathologists, there was concordance between two assessments in only three (Hallissey *et al.* 1990*b*). The results of a prospective study of high-grade dysplasia demonstrated an associated gastric cancer in 80% of cases while in low-grade dysplasia, an associated carcinoma was found in 20% (de Dombal *et al.* 1990).

Gastric polyps have been classified into two major groups (hyperplastic/regenerative and adenomas). Hyperplastic polyps account for 75–90% of gastric polyps: they arise from excessive regeneration of foveolar epithelium with no distinct border between the polyp and normal gastric mucosa; and malignant transformation is rare (Ming and Goldman 1965; Morson *et al.* 1979). However, an associated independent carcinoma may be seen in between 6.5% and 25% of cases (Tomasulo 1971; Laxen 1981; Seifert 1981). Adenomas account for between 8.2% and 25% of gastric polyps (Marshak and Feldman 1965; Tomasulo 1971; Harju 1986). True neoplasms have a distinct margin from surrounding mucosa with associated intestinal metaplasia and frequent mitotic figures. Malignant transformation is seen in 6–75%, with a lower incidence in small flat adenomas and an increased risk in adenomas over 2 cm in diameter.

3. DIAGNOSTIC TESTS

The best test for investigating the stomach is gastroscopy which affords visualization and biopsy of lesions. Radiology is often employed and the method of choice is the double contrast barium meal.

Although these tests are appropriate to symptomatic individuals, other tests may be more effective in a screening programme of asymptomatic populations. The Japanese have used mass radiography. This programme has screened nearly 10% of persons between the ages of 40 and 69 and achieved a detection rate of 1.2 per 100 000. These good results achieved in the Japanese programme have been as a result of radiology combined with endoscopy in selected patients. This is the trend that is likely to be maintained in screening programmes. Gastroscopy and biopsy are the investigations of choice in selected groups.

Other tests may be as valuable as double contrast radiology in determining the high-risk patient. The potential screening test can be either markers in gastric juice, serum markers, or clinical groups. The markers in gastric juice include fetal sialoglycoprotein, lactic dehydrogenase, beta-glucoronadase, and acid production.

Long-term follow-up of patients with reduced acid secretion has confirmed the increased risk of gastric cancer but it has also demonstrated that hypochlorhydria or achlorhydria is often a reflection of tumour bulk decreasing its value as a screening test (Misaki and Kawai 1981). Fetal sialoglycoprotein identified 42% of all gastric cancers, half of them being early (Hakkinen 1981). However, this work has not been repeated elsewhere and its value has not been confirmed. Lactic dehydrogenase and beta-glucoronidase are sensitive markers of gastric cancer but are abnormal in 5% of normal patients and 25% of patients with mild gastritis (Rogers *et al.* 1981). The markers in serum include gastrin and pepsinogens I and II. These are able to identify 60% of cancers and 75% of those with high-risk mucosal changes (Nomura *et al.* 1980; Westerveld *et al.* 1985; Hallissey and Fielding 1989). The tumour-specific antigen, CEA 72/4, has been shown to correlate with tumour bulk and may have a role in screening (Byrne *et al.* 1990).

4. DYSPEPTIC PATIENTS

The majority of patients with gastric cancer become symptomatic during the course of the disease. The Japanese have reported that 48% of screen-detected early cancers are symptomatic (Hisamichi *et al.* 1976). In the United Kingdom, the Registrar General produces figures which indicate general practitioner (GP) consultation rates by diagnosis. In a population of 100 000, 1590 patients present each year with dyspepsia. Of these, the diagnosis is made of disorders of function of the stomach in 1130, benign peptic ulcer disease in 430, and gastric cancer in 30. Thus, 1 in every 53 patients presenting with dyspepsia will have gastric cancer (OPCS 1972).

Open access endoscopy has been made widely available. This has not been shown to influence the stage of disease at the time of diagnosis. The availability of these programmes has not changed the time between the first visit to the GP and the referral for assessment. The delay for referral by GPs to open access endoscopy (21 ± 32 weeks) was similar to that for referral to out-patients (22 ± 40 weeks), (Holdstock and Bruce 1981). This approach has resulted in an increase in the number of patients undergoing investigation. To decrease the number of endoscopies without missing significant disease, profiles based on symptoms and age and sex of patients have been used (Mann *et al.* 1983; Davenport *et al.* 1985). The problem with profiles is that they are based on patients referred by GPs and the number of diagnosed early cancers is small.

Using an age limit of 40 in patients presenting with a history of more than two weeks of epigastric discomfort or weight loss and anorexia, 70% of gastric cancers within a population were diagnosed by investigating 1% of the population. The early gastric cancer rate in this study was 22.2% (Mollmann 1981). This has been investigated in the United Kingdom. General practitioners, from 10 practices, were asked to refer all new patients aged over 40 presenting with dyspepsia for investigation at the time of their first attendance. These patients were offered endoscopy within two weeks of presentation. At this endoscopy, biopsies were taken from any gastric abnormality. In addition, those demonstrated to have chronic atrophic gastritis, intestinal metaplasia, dysplasia, or gastric polyps were put into a surveillance programme of annual endoscopy. Those with benign gastric ulcers were endoscoped every two months until the ulcer was healed. Using this technique, 26% of the cancers diagnosed in the patients referred were early and 62% were resected for cure (Hallissey *et al.* 1990*a*). This study was conducted in two centres. From one, it has been possible to identify all patients who were registered to the study GPs that developed gastric cancer in five years before and the five years of the study. The proportion of early gastric cancers rose from 2% in the prestudy period to 18% during the study and the proportion resected for cure rose from 21% to 50%.

Further studies have been carried out, employing screening in high-risk groups, particularly coal miners. Using a symptomatic questionnaire, coal miners have been shown to be a suitable group for gastric premalignancy screening using an upper gastrointestinal symptom questionnaire and upper gastrointestinal endoscopy (Harrison *et al.* 1993).

5. POTENTIAL SCREENING PROGRAMMES FOR LOW-RISK POPULATIONS

It is now possible to initiate programmes that would select populations for endoscopic screening and for the detection of not only cancers but also premalignant lesions, who would then be entered into surveillance programmes. The possible methods that could be employed are outlined in Fig. 14.1. The test that could be employed would depend on economics and the ability to service an entire population. Conversely, selected groups of the population known to be at high risk could be selected for either the nonspecific test or go straight into an endoscopic programme.

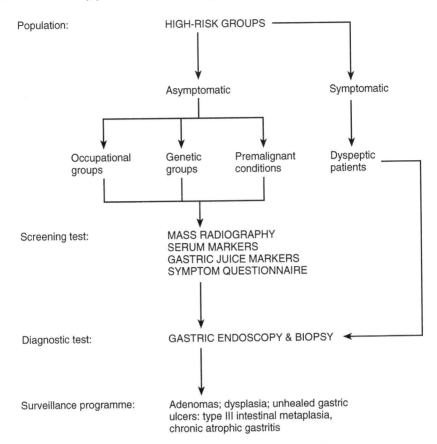

Fig. 14.1.   Possible screening programmes for low-risk areas.

REFERENCES

Buell, P. and Dunn, J.E. Jr. (1965). Cancer mortality amoung Japanese Issei and Nisei of California. *Cancer*, **18**, 656–64.

Byrne, D.J., Browning, M.C.K., *et al.* (1990). CA72-4: a new tumour marker for gastric cancer. *Br. J. Surg.*, **77**, 1010–13.

Cassell, P. and Robinson, J.O. (1976). Cancer of the Stomach: a review of 854 patients. *Br. J. Surg.* **63**, 603–7.

Caygill, C., Hill, M.J., *et al.* (1986). Mortality from gastric cancer following gastric surgery for peptic ulcer. *Lancet*, **i**, 929–31.

Correa, P. (1980). The epidemiology and pathogenesis of chronic gastritis: three aetiologic entities. In *Frontiers of gastrointestinal research. The stomach*, (ed. L. Van der Reis). pp. 98–108. Karger, Basel.

Davenport, P.M., Morgan, A.G., *et al.* (1985). Can preliminary screening of dyspeptic patients allow more effective use of investigational techniques. *Br. Med. J.*, **290**, 217–20.

de Dombal, F.T., Price, A.B., *et al.* (1990). The British Society of Gastroenterology early gastric cancer/dysplasia survey: An interim report. *Gut*, **31**, 115–20.

Domellof, L., Eriksson, S., *et al.* (1977). Carcinoma and possible precancerous changes of the gastric stump after Bilroth II resection. *Gastroenterology*, **73**, 462–8.

Farrands, P.A., Blake, J.R.S., *et al.* (1983). Endoscopic review of patients who have had gastric surgery. *Br. Med. J.*, **286**, 755–8.

Fielding, J.W.L.F., Ellis, D.J., Jones, B.G., *et al.* (1980). Natural history of early gastric cancer; results of a 10-year regional survey. *Br. Med. J.*, **281**, 965–7.

Fielding J.W.L.F., Powell, J., *et al.* (1989). *Carcinoma of the stomach: clinical cancer monograph*, Vol. III. MacMillan, Basingstoke.

Green, P., O'Toole, K., *et al.* (1981). Early gastric cancer. *Gastroenterology*, **81**, 247–56.

Hakkinen, I.P.T. (1981). Application of serum and gastric juice tumour markers to early diagnosis and screening of gastric cancer. In *Gastric cancer*, pp. 85–94. Pergamon Press, Oxford.

Hallissey, M.T. and Fielding, J.W.L. (1989). Pepsinogen I and gastrin: a screening tool for gastric cancer. *Gut*, **30**, A711.

Hallissey, M.T., Jewkes, A.J., *et al.* (1990*a*). Early detection of gastric cancer. *Br. Med. J.*, **301**, 513–15.

Hallissey, M.T., Newbold, K.M., *et al.* (1990*b*). Gastric biopsies. Difficulties in assessment. *Gut*, **31**, A615.

Harju, E. (1986). Gastric polyposis and malignancy. *Br. J. Surg.*, **73**, 532–3.

Harrison, J.D., Morris, D.L., and Hardcastle, J.D. (1993). Screening for gastric carcinoma in coal miners. *Gut*, **34**, 494–8.

Hisamichi, S., Nozaki, K., *et al.* (1976). Evaluation of mass screening program for stomach cancer. *Tohoku J. Exp. Med.*, **118**, (suppl.), 69–77.

Holdstock, G. and Bruce, S. (1981). Endoscopy and gastric cancer. *Gut*, **22**, 673–6.

Imai, T. (1971). Chronic gastritis in Japanese with reference to high incidence of gastric carcinoma. *J. Natl. Cance. Inst.*, **47**, 179–95.

Jass, J.R. (1980). Role of intestinal metaplasia in the histogenesis of gastric carcinoma. *Jpn. J. Surg.*, **11**, 127–45.

Laxen, F. (1981). Gastric polyps and gastric carcinoma. *Ann. Clin. Res.*, **13**, 154–5.

Lundh, G., Burn, J.I., *et al.* (1974). A co-operative international study of gastric cancer. *Ann. RCS, Eng.* **54**, 219–28.

Mann, J., Holdstock, G., *et al.* (1983). Scoring system to improve the cost-effectiveness of open access endoscopy. *Br. Med. J.*, **287**, 937–40.

Marshak, R.H. and Feldman, F. (1965). Gastric polyps. *Am. J. Dig. Dis.*, **10**, 909–35.

Ming, S.-C. and Goldman, H. (1965). Gastric polyps: a histogenetic classification and its relation to carcinoma. *Cancer*, **18**, 721–7.

Misaki, F. and Kawai, K. (1981). Acid secretion in different stages of gastric carcinoma. *Gut*, **22**, A877.

Mollmann, K.-M. (1981). Early diagnosis of gastric cancer. The possibility of delimiting high risk groups. *Dan. Med. Bull.*, **28**, 89–92.

Morson, B.C., Dawson, I.M.P., *et al.* (ed.) (1979). *Gastrointestinal pathology*. Blackwell, Oxford.

Nicholls, J.C. (1979). Stump cancer following gastric surgery. *World J. Surg.*, **3**, 731–6.

Nomura, A., Stemmermann, G.N., *et al.* (1980). Serum pepsinogen I as a predictor of stomach cancer. *Ann. Intern. Med.*, **93**, 537–40.

OPCS (Office of Population Census and Surveys) (1972). *Mortality statistics for general practice. Second national study 1970–1972.* HMSO, London.

Pickford, I.R., Craven, J.L., *et al.* (1984). Endoscopic examination of the gastric remnant 31–39 years after gastrectomy for peptic ulcer. *Gut*, **25**, 393–7.

Rogers, K., Roberts, G.M., *et al.* (1981). Gastric juice enzymes—an aid to the diagnosis of gastric cancer. *Lancet*, **i**, 1124–5.

Seifert, E. (1981). Gastric polyps In *Early gastric cancer*, pp. 56–63. Smith Klein and French, Welwyn Garden City.

Siurala, M., Varis, K., *et al.* (1966). Studies of patients with atrophic gastritis: a 10–15 year follow-up. *Scand. J. Gastroenterol.*, **1**, 40–8.

Strickland, R.G. and Mackay, I.R. (1973). A re-appraisal of the nature and significance of chronic atrophic gastritis. *Am. J. Dig. Dis.*, **18**, 426–40.

Swynnerton, R.F. and Truelove, S.C. (1952). Carcinoma of the stomach. *Br. Med. J.*, **i**, 287–92.

Tomasulo, J. (1971). Gastric polyps; histologic types and their relationship to gastric carcinoma. *Cancer*, **27**, 1346–55.

Vidaback, A. and Mosbech, J. (1954). The aetiology of gastric carcinoma elucidated by a study of 302 pedigrees. *Acta Med. Scand.*, **149**, 137–59.

Westerveld, B.D., Pals, G., *et al.* (1985). Qualitative and quantitative determinations of pepsinogen I in gastric cancer and premalignant changes of the stomach. In *Pepsinogen in Man: Clinical and genetic advances*, pp. 201–12. Liss, New York.

Zamcheck, N., Grable, E., *et al.* (1955). Occurrence of gastric cancer among patients with pernicious anaemia at the Boston City Hospital. *N. Eng. J. Med.*, **252**, 1103–10.

Part VI: Surgical treatment

15

Radical surgery

Mitsuru Sasako, Takeshi Sano, Hitoshi Katai, and Keüchi Maruyama

1. SURGICAL STRATEGY FOR GASTRIC CANCER

1.1. Gastric lymphatic drainage

The lymphatic system surrounding the stomach (see Figs 15.1 and 15.2) is divided into three layers, each of which might obstruct the passage of cancer cells into the systemic circulation. The reason for this complex system may be that, physiologically, the stomach has to face the challenge of many ingested bacteria. On the basis of this classification it is proposed that gastric cancer remains a localized disease confined to the stomach and local lymph nodes and that spread usually occurs in a stepwise manner from the first to the third tier of lymph nodes.

The general rules of the Japanese Research Society for Gastric Cancer (JRSGC 1993) are widely accepted and adopted in many countries. In these rules, lymph nodes are classified into 16 stations by location (Fig. 15.3). By recording the spread

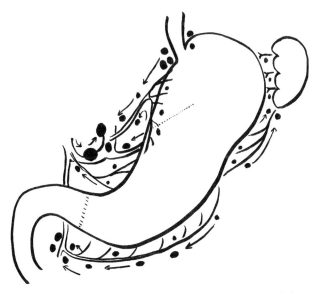

Fig. 15.1. Lymph drainage from the stomach flows into perigastric nodes and then to the second tier nodes (i.e. left gastric artery nodes, common hepatic artery nodes, coeliac artery nodes or splenic artery nodes).

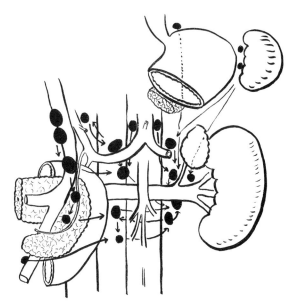

Fig. 15.2.   Further lymph drainage from the stomach. Flow from the common hepatic artery nodes feeds either directly or via nodes in the hepatoduodenal ligament or retropancreatic nodes into the paraaortic nodes. Flows from the coeliac, splenic hilus, or splenic artery nodes feed directly into the paraaortic nodes. There is a short pathway from the left cardial nodes to the paraaortic area along the inferior phrenic vessels.

Fig. 15.3.   From perigastric to paraaortic nodes, the regional lymph nodes are classified into 16 stations, defined in this figure. No. 4 nodes are subclassified into three groups, 4sa, 4sb, 4d. No. 8 station is also subclassified into two groups, 8a and 8p. No. 14 is subclassified into two groups, 14a and 14v. No. 1, right cardial nodes; No. 2, left cardial nodes; No. 3, nodes along the lesser curvature; No. 4, nodes along the greater curvature; No. 4sa, nodes along the short gastric vessels; No. 4sb, nodes along the left gastroepiploic vessels; No. 4d, nodes along the right gastroepiploic vessels; No. 5, suprapyloric nodes; No. 6, infrapyloric nodes; No. 7, nodes along the left gastric artery nodes; No. 8, nodes along the common hepatic artery, No. 8a, anterosuperior group; No. 8p, posterior group; No. 9, nodes around the coeliac artery; No. 10, nodes at the splenic hilum; No. 11, nodes along the splenic artery; No. 12, nodes in the hepatoduodenal ligament; No. 13, nodes on the posterior surface of the pancreatic head; No. 14a, nodes along the superior mesenteric artery; No. 14v, nodes along the superior mesenteric vein; No. 16, nodes around the abdominal aorta.

   Abbreviations: APIS, arteria phrenica inferior sinistra; AHC, arteria hepatica communis; AGB, arteriae gastricae breves; AGES, arteria gastroepiploica sinistra; AGP, arteria gastrica posterior; ACM, arteria colica media; AJ, arteria jejunalis; TGC, truncus gastrocolicus; VCD, vena colica dextra; VCDA, vena colica dextra accessoria; VCM, vena colica media; VGED, vena gastroepiploica dextra; VJ, vena jejunalis; VL, vena lienalis; VMS, vena mesenterica superior; VP, vena portae; VPDIA, vena pancreaticoduodenalis inferior anterior.

   Adapted from the *Japanese classification of gastric carcinoma* (1995), (1st edn), with permission from the Japanese Research Society for Gastric Cancer.

of lymph node metastasis in each patient, it has been shown that the incidence of metastasis to an individual node station is dependent on the location and depth of invasion of the primary tumour (Tables 15.1–15.4). In gastric cancer, all nodes should be retrieved from the *en bloc* resection specimen and examined to detect metastasies, because even small, apparently normal nodes sometimes contain them (26.4% of the metastatic nodes are less than 5 mm in their largest dimension: unpublished data of 3141 metastatic nodes from the National Cancer Center Hospital, Tokyo). Table 15.5 shows the reported number of regional lymph nodes

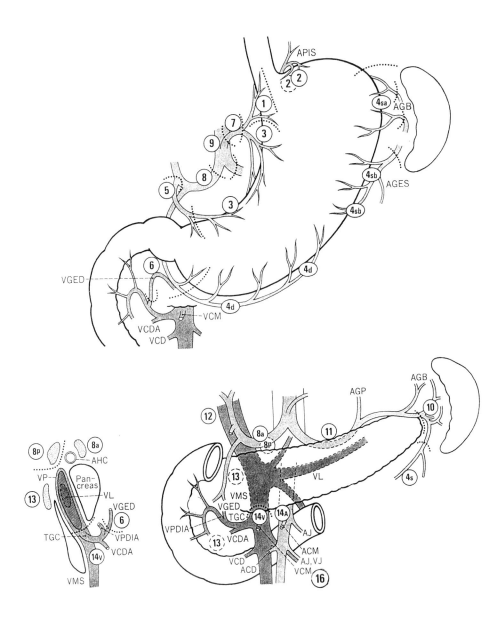

Table 15.1.   Incidence (%) of lymph node metastasis according to the depth of invasion, in tumours located in the antrum (A)

Station	Depth						Overall
	mm	sm	pm	ss	se	si	
1	0	2	1	1	10	8	4
2	0	0	0	11	7	10	5
3	1	8	18	47	51	37	23
4	0.4	9	16	31	44	39	19
5	0	2	4	13	13	10	6
6	2	11	37	46	49	58	26
7	0	3	6	21	32	32	13
8	0.5	2	13	15	31	36	14
9	0	2	5	9	18	12	7
10	0	0	0	0	0	17	3
11	0	1	2	3	8	12	4
12	0	0	5	4	13	8	6
13	0	0	4	0	9	2	6
14	0	0	9	17	14	22	11
16	0	0	0	0	18	20	9

The tumours were treated with curative intent between 1972 and 1986 at the National Cancer Center Hospital, Tokyo.

Abbreviations: mm, mucosal layer, sm, submucosal layer, pm, muscularis propriae; ss, subserosal layer, se, serosal layer, si, surrounding organs invaded.

Table 15.2.   Incidence (%) of lymph node metastasis according to the depth of invasion, in tumours located in the middle third of the stomach (M)

Station	Depth						Overall
	mm	sm	pm	ss	se	si	
1	0.2	0.8	5	18	25	25	8
2	0	0	0	0	7	25	5
3	1	11	28	40	64	61	25
4	0.6	6	20	16	45	63	17
5	0	0	0	2	6	11	2
6	0	2	5	11	27	40	9
7	0.9	4	11	24	35	38	13
8	0.3	2	5	1	18	24	6
9	0	0.8	5	15	15	17	6
10	0	0	7	0	16	30	10
11	0	1	5	2	10	8	4
12	0	0	0	2	5	9	2
13	0	0	0	0	0	11	0.7
14	0	0	0	13	10	50	8
16	0	0	0	14	11	42	9

These tumours were treated between 1972 and 1986 at the National Cancer Center Hospital Tokyo.

Abbreviations are defined in Table 15.1.

Table 15.3. Incidence (%) of lymph node metastasis according to the depth of invasion, in tumours located in the proximal third of the stomach (C)

Station	Depth						Overall
	mm	sm	pm	ss	se	si	
1	0	0	14	35	42	54	27
2	0	0	12	9	21	44	16
3	0	6	32	38	50	50	33
4	0	0	2	9	15	28	10
5	0	0	0	0	3	9	2
6	0	0	3	3	7	13	5
7	2	12	7	24	30	40	21
8	0	2	5	3	9	24	8
9	0	4	5	11	19	21	12
10	0	0	8	8	12	40	14
11	0	4	6	8	15	31	13
12	0	0	0	0	5	0	2
13	0	0	0	0	0	10	2
14	0	0	0	0	0	25	9
16	0	0	0	11	6	25	10

These tumours were treated between 1972 and 1986 at the National Cancer Center Hospital Tokyo. Abbreviations are defined in Table 15.1.

Table 15.4. Incidence (%) of lymph node metastasis according to the depth of invasion, in tumours invading more than two-thirds of the stomach (AMC)

Station	Depth						Overall
	mm	sm	pm	ss	se	si	
1	0	0	14	31	35	51	38
2	0	0	0	25	18	36	23
3	0	22	43	69	71	75	69
4	0	11	29	83	58	72	61
5	0	0	0	17	13	14	13
6	0	11	14	38	46	50	45
7	0	11	14	42	50	55	48
8	0	0	43	33	31	30	29
9	0	0	29	25	21	16	18
10	0	0	14	50	22	42	29
11	0	0	0	0	19	33	22
12	0	0	0	14	8	11	9
13	0	0	0	0	6	14	8
14	0	0	0	0	5	8	6
16	0	0	0	0	27	31	29

These tumours were treated between 1972 and 1986 at the National Cancer Center Hospital Tokyo. Abbreviations are defined in Table 15.1.

Table 15.5.   Number of regional lymph nodes of the stomach. (No. 1–No. 11 (first and second tiers)

| | Surgical specimen nodes retrieved by: | | | | | | Autopsy specimens, reported by Wagner *et al.* (*n* = 80) | | |
| | Japanese surgeon (*n* = 8) | | | Dutch pathologists (*n* = 114) | | | | | |
Station	Mean	Range	SD	Mean	Range	SD	Mean	Range	SD
1	5.5	3–7	1.4	3.2	0–15	2.7	2.2	0–4	0.9
2	2.9	0–10	3.8	2.1	0–7	2.1	2.0	0–5	1.1
3	12.0	3–36	10.6	4.8	0–16	3.7	4.5	0–14	3.1
4	12.6	6–21	5.4	4.7	0–16	3.9	1.2	0–7	1.6
5	1.0	0–4	1.3	0.8	0–5	1.1	2.2	0–5	1.1
6	6.0	5–7	0.8	3.9	0–17	2.8	2.7	0–8	1.8
7	4.0	0–8	2.4	3.0	0–10	2.5	2.3	0–5	2.0
8	4.0	2–7	1.7	2.5	0–12	2.4	2.3	0–6	2.0
9	5.3	3–9	2.2	3.0	0–13	2.6	4.2	0–15	3.3
10	2.5	0–6	2.8	1.2	0–9	1.7	2.2	0–6	1.3
11	5.7	0–21	7.3	2.0	0–15	2.7	2.0	0–9	2.0
Total	59.8	36–105	24.1	27.3	3–71	14.4	27	17–44	6.0

Significantly more nodes were retrieved from the similar specimen of Dutch patients by the Japanese surgeon than by Dutch pathologists. The average number of the latter is almost same as that reported by Wagner *et al.* (1991) from autopsy material.

from the stomach (Wagner *et al.* 1991; Bunt 1993). In the rules, lymph node stations are classified into three or four tiers, according to the incidence of metastasis, and this correlates principally with the distance from the primary lesion.

1.2.   Gastric cancer: localized or systemic disease?

Radical resection for gastric cancer comprises adequate resection of the stomach together with lymph node dissection. Local extension of the lesion is either by direct infiltration or by lymphatic permeation. In many Western countries, carcinoma with lymph node metastasis is regarded as a systemic disease, an opinion supported by observations in various cancers (Cady 1984). In gastric cancer, however, there are many reports, mainly from Japan, suggesting that lymph node metastasis does not always imply systemic disease and that systematic lymph node dissection may still result in a cure (Maruyama *et al.* 1987; Shiu *et al.* 1987; Soga *et al.* 1979; Sasako *et al.* 1995).

1.3.   Do Japanese and Western tumours differ?

To counter the favourable results from Japan it has been suggested that gastric cancer in Japan is a localized disease and the tumours seen in the West are fundamentally different (Fielding 1989). There is, however, no evidence for this view; indeed, a report comparing Japanese and Western gastric cancers has not shown a difference (Bonenkamp *et al.* 1993). However, patients do present earlier in Japan. The proportion of early gastric cancers is over 50% in many Japanese institutions, much higher than in the West where early gastric cancer accounts for only 5–15% in most series (Bogomeletz 1984; Briganze *et al.* 1986; Green *et al.* 1988). However, when compared stage for stage, Japanese and Western tumours behave exactly the same if they are treated by extended surgery (Bollschweiler *et al.* 1993). A recent molecular biological study has shown that there was no difference in expression of onco- and tumour-suppressor genes between Japanese and British gastric cancer (McCulloch *et al.* 1995).

1.4.   A logical operation for gastric cancer: D2 gastrectomy

Based on the above facts it is logical to remove not only the cancer and surrounding normal stomach, but also the lymph nodes to which the tumour drains, including those along the hepatic, splenic, and coeliac arteries. This is known as the D2 radical gastrectomy with extended lymph node dissection, and has been practised as standard surgery in Japan for the past 30 years. If the theories of lymphatic drainage and local disease are correct this operation should give an improved five-year survival and cure.

1.5.   Results of the D2 gastrectomy

To evaluate the survival results of surgical treatment, a total of 6730 patients with primary gastric carcinoma treated between 1962 and 1991 at the National Cancer Center Hospital, Tokyo (NCCH), were analysed. Operative procedures were a distal gastrectomy in 4508 patients, a total gastrectomy in 1474, a proximal gastrectomy in 402, an atypical partial gastrectomy in 38, a gastrojejunostomy (bypass) in 74, exploratory laparotomy in 139, and other procedures in 95. Survival results, according to the depth of invasion and lymph node metastasis, and to histological type and depth of invasion, were analysed by reviewing the patients treated with curative intent between 1977 and 1991.

Five-year survival rates in all patients were 55.4%, whereas those with incurable cancer were 2.2% in total and 2.4% when resected. Among incurable cases, one- and two-years survival rates were 21.2%, 7.0% for patients with liver metastasis and 24.5%, 7.4% for those with peritoneal dissemination at the time of surgery.

Stage for stage survival results are shown in Table 15.6. Five-year survival rates are improving even stage for stage, when the period is divided into three decades. A notable increase of stage Ia patients and decrease of stages IIIb and IV is observed. In most stages, a steady increase of five-year survival rates is clearly demonstrated. More detailed analysis according to pT and pN is shown in Table 15.7, reviewing only those patients treated with curative intent. Many patients with n2 disease are surviving a long period after surgery, if the tumour does not invade the serosa, which suggests that lymph node metastasis does not always imply systemic disease in gastric cancer.

Table 15.6.   Five-year survival rates of patients (%) with gastric carcinoma, treated at the gastric surgery division inclusively, according to TNM stage and periods

TMN stage	1962–71	1972–81	1982–91	Overall
Ia	89.0 (420)	92.0 (638)	92.4 (1103)	91.5 (2161)
Ib	80.0 (205)	84.3 (210)	89.8 (266)	84.6 (681)
II	61.7 (280)	72.4 (239)	76.2 (245)	69.3 (764)
IIIa	39.6 (268)	56.4 (234)	58.9 (208)	50.4 (710)
IIIb	27.6 (279)	29.3 (229)	36.5 (189)	30.6 (697)
IV	2.2 (590)	7.7 (428)	7.5 (449)	5.4 (1467)
Total	44.3 (2049)	54.9 (2140)	65.9 (2541)	55.4 (6730)

The figures in the parentheses are the number of patients at each stage.

Table 15.7.   Five-year survival rates of patients (%) with gastric carcinoma curatively resected according to the combination of the lymph node stage and depth of invasion, by the Japanese classification (1977–1991)

Stage and depth	n0	n1	n2	n3–4	Overall
T1 m sm	92.6 (1445)	89.9 (118)	86.4 (47)	50.0 (2)	92.2 (1612)
T2 pm ss	88.7 (266)	80.9 (162)	59.8 (115)	11.4 (23)	77.5 (566)
T3	63.8 (146)	60.1 (184)	35.6 (244)	10.3 (60)	47.1 (634)
T4	46.0 (24)	44.4 (30)	22.7 (65)	19.8 (33)	29.9 (152)

Figures in parentheses are the number of patients at each stage.

Prognostic relevance of histological type has been reported. In our series (Table 15.8), like many other Japanese series (Iriyama *et al.* 1993), poorly differentiated groups have significantly better survival than well-differentiated groups in cases of early gastric cancer, although the incidence of lymph node metastasis is much higher in the former group (14.0% vs. 8.2%). In contrast, if the tumour invades the serosa,

Table 15.8.   Five-year survival rates according to the depth of invasion and histological type, same period, exclusively curatively resected cases

Stage	Well-differentiated	Poorly differentiated
	90.6	94.8
T1	(1019)	(593)
	75.8	79.4
T2	(291)	(275)
	50.2	45.0
T3	(251)	(382)
	28.2	31.0
T4	(71)	(81)
	79.0	73.1
Total	(1632)	(1331)

'Well-differentiated' includes papillary adenocarcinoma, well-differentiated tubular adenocarcinoma, and moderately differentiated tubular adenocarcinoma. 'Poorly differentiated' includes poorly differentiated adenocarcinoma, signet-ring cell carcinoma, and mucinous adenocarcinoma.
   Figures in parentheses are the numbers of patients at each stage.

poorly differentiated groups have a worse prognosis than well-differentiated groups because of the higher tendency of peritoneal metastasis. When lymph node metastasis is successfully treated by extended nodal dissection, prognosis is more dependent on the risk of peritoneal dissemination.

1.6.   Is stage migration a confounding factor?

To compare end-results of surgery, evaluation should be carried out stage by stage. Due to the efforts of both the JRSGC and UICC, the staging system in Japan and the TNM classification of the UICC (1987) are similar and comparable. Only a few American papers still use the AJCC staging system (AJCC 1992). However, even using the same staging system 'stage migration' can be a problem. This happens when more accurate information for staging is available (Feinstein *et al.* 1985). Additional information leads some patients to move from an earlier to a more advanced stage, which usually improves the results of both groups, with more patients in the more advanced stage, but without any effect on the results of the individual case and the entire group.

   This can happen in both pre- and postoperative staging. Recent applications of computed tomography (CT) scanning, magnetic resonance imaging (MRI), and intraoperative ultrasonography (US) produce more accurate information about liver and distant nodal metastases. However, extended lymph node dissection gives much more information regarding micrometastases in the lymph nodes draining the stomach. The exact method of examining the excised nodes is also very important. When only a few enlarged nodes are retrieved for examination, many positive nodes will be missed, because metastatic nodes from gastric cancer often look normal in size and substance. Also, if more than one section of each node is examined the rate of detection of metastases increases. The method of determining depth of invasion is also important; examination of a semi-continuous section of the lesion can detect the deepest level of invasion. When only one slice of the lesion is examined, the T-factor may be shifted to an earlier stage.

Any possible confounding effect of stage migration can be overcome. The incidence of metastasis and the prognosis of the patients who had lymph node metastasis are shown in Table 15.9. Survival rate is calculated irrespective of metastasis to other nodal stations, including the paraaortic nodes, which are regarded as distant metastases in the TNM classification. Thus, by evaluating the survival effect without any concept of stage, thus circumventing the stage migration effect, suggests the net efficacy of lymph node dissection including the second tier of nodes for advanced gastric cancer (Table 15.10). The data in this table confirm the efficacy of D2 dissection.

1.7. Is D2 gastrectomy feasible surgery for the Western patient?

The above data give strong evidence for the efficacy of extended lymph node dissection in gastric cancer. Final confirmation will be made following the results of

Table 15.9.   Incidence of lymph node metastasis and five-year survival rates of those having nodal metastasis in each station, according to the tumour location (from Sasako *et al.* 1995)

Station	A (distal third)		M (middle third)		C (proximal third)		AMC (entire stomach)	
	Incidence	5YSR	Incidence	5YSR	Incidence	5YSR	Incidence	5YSR
1	6.2	25.0	15.0	52.6	38.0	31.7	32.7	11.3
2	7.1	0.0	3.4	25.0	22.0	23.2	18.2	8.0
3	40.9	42.2	44.8	58.7	45.1	37.9	66.0	17.8
4	34.2	42.3	26.8	48.4	14.5	20.5	53.1	19.0
5	10.5	37.5	2.4	33.3	3.0	0.0	14.2	18.8
6	46.3	46.0	14.6	26.8	6.8	6.3	37.7	18.7
7	23.4	34.9	22.6	46.5	26.9	19.7	44.4	18.5
8	24.5	30.6	11.0	41.5	10.2	20.0	30.6	19.2
9	12.8	30.4	11.0	47.5	16.0	20.5	18.5	20.7
10	3.8	0.0	11.9	33.3	17.4	21.6	21.6	7.4
11	6.7	15.4	6.3	21.4	16.1	11.4	20.6	3.7
12	9.0	29.6	1.6	33.3	2.5	0.0	4.4	0.0
13	8.3	0.0	0.0	0.0	2.5	0.0	5.6	0.0
14	14.6	14.3	8.7	0.0	10.0	0.0	4.5	0.0
16	13.1	18.2	7.4	0.0	12.1	0.0	26.5	11.1

Incidence was calculated by dividing the number of patients with metastasis in each station by the number of patients who underwent dissection of that station. Survival rates of positive patients in each station were calculated irrespective of nodal metastasis to other stations.
5YRSR, 5-year survival rate.

Table 15.10.   Index of estimated benefit from lymph node dissection in each station, according to the tumour location (from Sasako *et al.* 1995)

Station	Upper third	Middle third	Lower third	Entire stomach
1	12.0	7.9	1.6	3.7
2	5.1	0.9	0.0	1.5
3	17.1	26.3	17.3	11.7
4	3.0	13.0	14.5	10.1
5	0.0	0.8	3.9	2.7
6	0.4	3.9	21.3	7.0
7	5.3	10.5	8.2	8.2
8	2.0	4.6	7.5	5.9
9	3.3	5.2	3.9	3.8
10	3.8	4.0	0.0	1.6
11	1.8	1.3	1.0	0.8
12	0.0	0.5	2.7	0.0
13	0.0	0.0	0.0	0.0
14	0.0	0.0	2.1	0.0
16	0.0	0.0	2.4	2.9

☐, first tier; ▨, second tier; ▨, third tier; ■, fourth tier.

First, second, third and fourth tiers are n1–n4 by the Japanese classification, respectively. Each index roughly corresponds the percentage of patients who will benefit from dissection of each station. Aggregation of the numbers in the second tier implies the benefit of D2 dissection over D1.

the MRC (Cuschierri 1986) and Dutch gastric cancer study group trials (Sasako *et al.* 1992). These are the first sizeable randomized controlled trials (RCT), comparing the so-called D2 gastrectomy and conventional limited D1 gastrectomy. Due to the relatively low incidence of the disease in Western Europe both are multicentre trials for which quality control of the surgery is difficult. From the author's (M.S.) personal experience, as the quality controller and tutor in the extended lymph node dissection in the Dutch trial, I would suggest that this type of trial comparing intricate, complex surgical techniques, should be carried out among no more than 15 major hospitals. Despite an enormous effort in quality control, the overall mortality in the Dutch trial is much worse than in the Japanese series, although there was no significant difference in morbidity. However, morbidity and mortality following D2 dissection was significantly worse than that after D1 dissection in the Dutch trial (Bonenkamp *et al.* 1995). There is also an interesting report by McCulloch (1994) regarding differences in operative mortality in a British institute, suggesting that gastrectomy for carcinoma of the stomach should no longer be practised by UK general surgeons.

Patients in Japan are, on average younger, thinner, and have a lower incidence of cardiorespiratory disease than patients in the West, and in the major Japanese centres the D2 gastrectomy has an operative mortality of less than 1%. There is some concern that in the West, although extended lymph node dissection might be oncologically effective, the increased morbidity and mortality may nullify this beneficial effect. We await the outcome of the above trials with great interest in order to determine the efficacy of extended surgery. Several recent papers from Western specialist centres have reported an acceptable mortality of this type of surgery in Western populations (Shiu *et al.* 1989; Sue-Ling *et al.* 1993; Pacelli *et al.* 1993), and confirm that gastric cancer should be only treated by experienced surgeons in Western countries.

1.8.   Preoperative prediction of lymph node metastases and choice of dissection

At the NCCH, Maruyama has compiled a computer-based database based on the pathological data from 3040 patients. With a knowledge of tumour size, position, and depth of invasion (judged preoperatively by endoscopy and double contrast barium meal, or endosonography) it is possible to predict accurately the likelihood of lymph node metastasis in each of the 16 lymph node stations. This enables the correct level of lymph node dissection to be determined. Applicability of this programme to Western patients is already shown by Bollschweiler *et al.* (1992). This may be particularly important in the West where, due to the possibly increased morbidity using the D2 dissection, it may be better to treat those gastric cancers with a computer-predicted low incidence of lymph node metastases with the D1 dissection, which may offer the best compromise between oncological constraints and the realities of surgery in the Western patient.

1.9.   The place of the D3 and D4 'super-extended' lymphadenectomy

With the exception of dissection of the lymph nodes in the hepatoduodenal ligament and on the superior mesenteric vein for antral tumours, more extended lymph node dissection seems to add little benefit (Table 15.10). Tables 15.9 and 15.10 show that dissection of these areas can provide benefits for antral tumours only. Dissection of the lymph nodes on the posterior aspect of the pancreatic head has not been shown to confer benefits for any type of tumour, although classified as the third tier in the general rules of the JRSGC. Therefore, the so-called D3 (R3) dissection should be used only for antral tumours, with dissection of the retro-pancreatic nodes being an option.

Paraaortic lymph node dissection seems beneficial for certain types of tumours but it is still not known whether the increased mobidity and mortality can be justified by survival benefit. This is an issue that can only be resolved by a random-ized controlled trial.

1.10.   The place of combined resection of other organs

Extension of resection to include adjacent organs is less attractive due to the pos-sible increase in major complications. The left upper abdominal evisceration (LUAE) was advocated by Kajitani *et al.* (1981) and modified by Furukawa *et al.* (1988). This operation enables a true *en bloc* resection, but peritoneal dissemina-tion still cannot be controlled well by it (Ohyama *et al.* 1994). Furukawa *et al.* (1988) reported better long-term survival data of LUAE in stage III Borrmann type

4 cancer than ordinary D2 dissection (total gastrectomy with PS). In several institutes, pancreaticoduodenectomy has been attempted in tumours having massive invasion of the duodenum and/or the pancreatic head, or those having macroscopic metastasis to the lymph nodes attaching to the pancreatic head. In their series, Nishi *et al.* (1993) reported an operative mortality of 6.7% and five-year survival rate of 9% in 94 patients who underwent this operation. However, Yonemura *et al.* (1991) reported excellent results using this procedure when combined with right hemicolectomy. Survival gain was most impressive in the patients with a tumour invading the pancreatic head; a five-year survival rate of 55% in 13 patients was achieved in their series.

Organs that might be invaded by direct tumour extension are the transverse colon, the transverse mesocolon, the pancreatic head, body or tail, the gallbladder, the liver, the diaphragm, the left adrenal gland, the spleen, the duodenum, and the oesophagus. Combined resection of the pancreas and the oesophagus increase morbidity and may increase mortality (Paolini *et al.* 1986; Finley and Inculet 1989). Resection of other organs, which do not necessarily increase postoperative morbidity, should be attempted if there is no evidence of distant metastasis, including cytologically detected cancer cells in the peritoneal cavity. Surgery for tumours invading the lower oesophagus is discussed in Section 4.1.

2.   THE D2 GASTRECTOMY: TECHNICAL ASPECTS

2.1.   Partial or total gastrectomy?

There has been a long debate concerning indications for total gastrectomy (TG) *de principe* (Gennari *et al.* 1986; Lindhal *et al.* 1988; Butler *et al.* 1989; Bozzetti 1992). Oncological gain by carrying out a total gastrectomy is: (a) 2–3 cm more proximal margin on the lesser curve and 10–15 cm on the greater curve; (b) complete dissection of the left cardial (No. 2), short gastric vessels (No. 4sa), splenic hilus (No. 10), and splenic artery nodes (No. 11). According to the results shown in Table 15.10, dissection of these nodal stations seems to be of little value for antral cancer, which was also shown by a Hong Kong trial (Robertson *et al.* 1994). Another randomized trial comparing total and subtotal gastrectomy for antral tumours failed to show an advantage for total gastrectomy (Gouzi 1988). If the proximal edge of the tumour is further than 3 cm from the cardia in early cancer, or well-circumscribed advanced tumours, or 6 cm in advanced tumours of infiltrative type, subtotal dissection is adequate (Bozzetti *et al.* 1992). If the tumour is located close to the greater curvature and beyond Demel's point, total gastrectomy is necessary because the lymph drainage from such a tumour feeds into the splenic hilus and flows along the splenic artery. In the case of linitis plastica, total gastrectomy is also recommended, even if it is apparently located to the lower gastric body.

The main problem of routine use of subtotal resection for gastric cancer of the lower half of the stomach is the poor quality of preoperative assessment of the proximal extension of the tumour. There are two types of proximal extension: mucosal and submucosal or deeper extension. Stepwise biopsy of the body is only useful in detecting mucosal invasion and endoscopic judgement of submucosal or deeper extension requires a lot of experience. Endoscopic ultrasonography is very useful in assessing this type of extension, while double contrast barium meal is better than endoscopy at diagnosing rigidity, swelling, and oedema of the wall. Considering the different biological behaviour of intestinal- and diffuse-type cancer, several surgeons recommend a surgical margin of at least 8 cm in diffuse-type, as opposed to 4 cm for intestinal-type (Gall and Hermanek 1985).

2.2. The D2 distal gastrectomy technique

First, Kocher's manoeuvre is performed allowing examination of the paraaortic nodes and, in addition, this procedure is necessary for the reduction of anastomotic tension if Billroth I reconstruction is planned. Then, complete or partial excision of the greater omentum together with the lesser sack (either complete or limited to the right side) lead to the mesenteric root where Henles' surgical trunk is recognized by following the accessory right colic vein, and the right gastroepiploic vein is ligated and divided at its origin. Changing the level of dissection, we come to the anterior surface of the pancreas by dissecting its capsule, which is continuous with the anterior sheet of the mesocolon. In this procedure, the gastroduodenal artery is easily found and by following it caudad, the origin of the right gastroepiploic artery is found by vision but not by palpation. After its ligation and division, the gastroduodenal artery can now be traced to its origin from the common hepatic artery. Visualization of this junction is the last step of this phase of the dissection. Attention is now turned to the lesser omentum. It is incised along the attachment to the left lobe of the liver, from right to left, and the right edge of the oesophageal hiatus is exposed. Then coming back on to the hepatoduodenal ligament, its serosa is incised from the left edge across two-thirds of its width, then downwards to the superior border of the duodenum. Several branches to the first portion of the duodenum from the gastroduodenal artery are then ligated and dissected on the organ. The hepatoduodenal ligament, left to the gastroduodenal artery, is cleared and the origin of the right gastric artery is found, ligated, and divided. The duodenum is divided and the stomach is reflected upwards and to the left. Now, the lymphatics and connective tissue around the coeliac axis and its branches are cleared. With the pancreas pulled caudad, gently but effectively by an assistant, connective tissue is incised along the superior border of the pancreas from the gastroduodenal artery to the middle part of the splenic artery (6–8 cm to the left of the coeliac axis). The left gastric vein may pass through this area, so caution is mandatory. Dissection is carried out from right to left, starting on the proper hepatic artery. Following the common hepatic artery, the termination of the coeliac axis is discerned. Continuing meticulous dissection of the connective tissue above the pancreas to the left, the splenic artery is identified and then the posterior gastric artery, the first major branch from the splenic artery to the stomach, is discerned. In most distal gastrectomies, dissection along the splenic artery is stopped at this artery, which might be preserved in antral tumours but is often ligated and divided for tumours of the lower body. Stripping off all the retroperitoneal tissue on the crura and the coeliac ganglions upwards and towards the coeliac artery, the origin of the left gastric artery is easily exposed, then ligated and divided. Dissection of the tissue behind the stomach on the crura is continued up to the oesophageal hiatus. The tissue on the lesser curvature close to the oesophagogastric junction is cleared, including the right cardial and a part of the lesser curve nodes. Beginning by incising the covering peritoneum over the lesser curvature fatty tissue, complete dissection is achieved by meticulous ligation and division of all upper branches of the left gastric artery to the stomach. Finally, the root of the left gastroepiploic artery is searched for, by following the inferior border of the tail of pancreas towards the spleen. Although there are various anomalies of the branching off from the splenic artery, it is usually the last branch, near the inferior pole of the spleen.

Following clearance of the stomach wall on the greater curvature down to Demel's point, the stomach is transected by a wide stapler. Billroth I gastroduodenostomy is often used for reconstruction, but Roux-en-Y or Billroth II reconstructions are much safer (leakage rate is 2–4% and nearly 0%, in Billroth I and II, respectively).

2.3. The total gastrectomy technique

In the case of total gastrectomy, procedures following the ligation of the left gastric artery are different. The body of the pancreas is mobilized on the layer continuing to Gerota's fascia, cranidad, and towards the spleen, until the reflexion of the retroperitoneum which is then incised. Thus, complete mobilization of the pancreatic body and tail and the spleen can be performed safely. Then, the splenic artery, already stripped off at its origin, is ligated and divided. The splenic vein is discerned by dividing the fascia covering it behind the organ, and is ligated and divided at the level of coeliac axis. Following it, the parenchyma of the pancreas is divided either by a stapler or a knife. An alternative procedure is the pancreas-preserving technique, where the splenic artery is divided and ligated close to the origin or distal to the point where the dorsal pancreatic artery branches off. In any case, all branches to the spleen and greater omentum are dissected *en bloc*, together with the spleen, which enables a complete dissection of the splenic artery nodes and splenic hilus nodes. This technique can be recommended when the tumour has no direct invasion to the pancreas and there are no visible lymph node metastases attached to the organ. Complete tissue clearance surrounding the abdominal oesophagus (including truncal vagotmy) terminates the dissection, when the oesophagus is transected at 1–2 cm above the cardia.

2.4. Combined resection of surrounding organs in D2 dissection

Should the greater omentum and the lesser sack be excised completely? The combined resection of the lesser and greater omenta together with the lesser sack has been regarded as an essential part of radical gastrectomy (Shiu *et al.* 1980; Schlag

1986). However, the considerable increase in early gastric cancer has led many Japanese surgeons to avoid unnecessary resection of these structures. Indeed, preserving sections of the omentum and the anterior sheet of the mesocolon has not resulted in an increase in the recurrence rate. The clinical value of complete excision of the lesser sack is unclear, even for T3 tumours, because recent knowledge from cytological examination of peritoneal lavage has shown that free cancer cells are already present in the pouch of Douglas even in tumours located on the posterior wall of the stomach. However, for T3 (eventually T4) advanced cancer, in which lymphatic infiltration or direct invasion of the omenta, the anterior sheet of the mesocolon or pancreatic capsule seems to happen frequently, complete omentectomy and excision of the lesser sack is still standard procedure. For tumours diagnosed as T1 tumour or T2, limited to the proper muscle layer, the greater omentum within 3 cm of the epiploic vessels should be resected to enable complete dissection of the lymphatic vessels and lymph nodes along these vessels. At the right end of the lesser sack, anterior and posterior sheets of the mesocolon should be separated and the right section of the anterior sheet should be resected, together with the stomach, to get a proper layer of nodal dissection of the infrapyloric nodes.

When should the spleen be removed? For tumours for which distal (subtotal) gastrectomy is performed, a splenectomy is usually contraindicated. In subtotal or distal gastrectomy, the blood supply to the remnant stomach can come from the left gastric, the posterior gastric, the short gastric arteries, or the cardiooesophagel branch of the left inferior phrenic artery. To maintain sufficient blood supply, either the left gastric or the short gastric arteries should be preserved. The frequency of nodal involvement is much higher and efficacy of node dissection of the left gastric artery nodes is much greater than those of splenic hilus nodes for these tumours. Therefore, the left gastric artery area should be completely dissected and the spleen preserved. For tumours that require a total gastrectomy, splenectomy is usually performed. For early gastric cancers on the lesser curve of the proximal one-third of the stomach, the spleen can be preserved without any increased risk of local recurrence. If an accidental rupture of the spleen during distal D2 gastrectomy necessitates splenectomy for haemostasis, resection of the stomach should be extended to total gastrectomy because of very high risk of necrosis of the remnant stomach. In addition, there are some arguments supporting an immunological advantage for preservation of the spleen (Suehiro *et al.* 1984; Sugimachi *et al.* 1980) but this question is still controversial (Kanayama *et al.* 1985; Takahashi and Fujimoto 1980; Brady *et al.* 1991). The incidence of postsplenectomy infection appears to be very low, 0.04 per 100 person years, in the case of adult patients (Cullingford *et al.* 1991). For each person, therefore, 1.2% for 30 years, which seems acceptable considering the carcinological benefit.

Who should have a distal pancreatectomy? For tumours of the upper third or middle half beyond Demel's point, lymph nodes along the splenic artery are as important as the splenic hilus nodes. A distal pancreatectomy together with splenectomy (PS) has been regarded as standard procedure to dissect these lymph nodes. However, due to a very high incidence of pancreatic juice leakage (40%), and consequent subphrenic abscess formation after this operation, the pancreas-preserving technique (PPT) (dissection of the splenic artery together with lymph nodes without resection of the pancreatic parenchyma) has become popular. This can be an alternative procedure when there is no direct invasion of the pancreas, or macroscopically metastatic nodes along the splenic artery (Maruyama *et al.* 1995). This technique reduces the incidence of pancreatic fistula to as low as 20% in Japanese patients. There is no prospective trial comparing these two types of surgery in terms of morbidity, mortality, and long-term survival. The morbidity of the PPT should be studied in Western patients, because the technique causes more pancreatic fistulae in obese patients whose border of the pancreas is often unclear because it is surrounded by dense adipose tissue.

2.5. Morbidity and mortality after D2 dissection

Morbidity and mortality following D2 dissection depends on the type of resection (i.e. total or distal gastrectomy), and the type of lymph node dissection for the splenic artery nodes. Table 15.11 shows the incidence of surgical complications (Sasako 1990). Incidence of anastomotic leakage and intraabdominal infection are shown in Table 15.12, according to the type of resection and the extent of lymph node dissection. Anastomotic leakage happens most frequently at oesophago-jejenostomy, then gastroduodenostomy, followed by jejunoduodenostomy in the reconstruction by a jejunal interposition. It rarely happens at gastrojejunostomy and jejunojejunostomy. Regarding pancreatic fistulae, these occur most frequently after the PS, followed by the PTT, and rarely following distal gastrectomy. Among non-specific surgical complications, pulmonary infection is one of the major problems following extended surgery of the upper abdominal space. To prevent this, a catheter for continuous epidural anaesthesia with morphine is routinely inserted at many institutions in Japan. For 3–7 days, a small amount (6–12 mg/day) of

Table 15.11. Incidence (%) of surgical complications following gastrectomy (from Sasako 1990)

Complication	TG/PG	DG	Overall
Leakage	17.6	2.7	7.0
Pancreatic fistulae	19.3	0.6	6.0
Intraabdominal abscess	5.5	1.3	1.4
Ileus	1.7	1.3	1.4
Bleeding	2.9	0.7	1.3
Anastomotic stenosis	0.6	1.3	1.1
Mediastinitis	2.3	0.0	0.7
Pyothorax	2.0	0.0	0.6
Wound dehiscence	0.6	0.1	0.3
Pancreatitis	0.6	0.2	0.4
No of complications	47.7	83.4	73.0

Patients treated at the National Cancer Center Hospital Tokyo (1982–87)
TG, total gastrectomy; PG, proximal gastrectomy; DG, distal gastrectomy.

Table 15.12. Incidence (%) of major complications and mortality according to the type of resection and extent of lymph node dissection (Japanese population)

No. of patients		Leakage	Abdom. infection	With complic.	Mortality within 30 days
Overall	1082	4.6	13.0	32.6	0.3
D1	168	6.0	13.1	29.2	0.0
D2	807	3.8	11.6	31.0	0.4
D0/3	107				
TG	310	9.0	30.3	56.1	0.6
D1	44	13.6	25.0	40.9	0.0
D2	212	8.5	31.6	57.5	0.9
D0/3	54				
DG	772	2.8	6.1	23.2	0.1
D1	124	3.2	8.9	25.0	0.0
D2	595	2.2	4.5	21.5	0.2
D0/3	53				

Patients treated at the National Cancer Center Hospital, Tokyo (1987–91).

morphine chloride is continuously infused by balloon infuser. This achieves complete pain control, which enables the patient to take deep breaths and become mobile soon after operation. Table 15.13 shows the morbidity and mortality following D2 dissection in a Western population in the Dutch gastric cancer trial. The incidence of complications is not that much different from that of Japanese hospitals, whereas the mortality rate is much higher than that in Japan. This suggests two possible reasons: Western patients appear less able to survive these complications than the Japanese and management of these is better in Japan because of far greater experience.

Table 15.13. Incidence (%) of major complications and mortality according to the type of resection and extent of lymph node dissection (from Bonenkamp *et al.* 1995). (Dutch population)

No. of patients		Leakage	Abdom. infection	With complic.	Mortality within 30 days
Overall	711	6.5	11.0	33.1	6.6
D1	380	4.2	7.4	24.7	3.9
D2	331	9.1	14.8	42.9	9.7
TG	241	10.0	18.3	43.6	10.4
D1	115	8.7	11.3	33.0	5.2
D2	126	11.1	24.6	53.2	15.1
DG	470	4.7	7.2	27.8	4.9
D1	265	2.3	5.7	20.8	3.4
D2	205	7.8	9.3	36.9	6.8

Results from the Dutch gastric cancer trial of patients treated with curative intent.

2.6. Treatment of postoperative complications following D2 surgery

The use of a prophylactic drainage tube after gastrointestinal surgery is still controversial. In the case of oesophagojejunostomy or gastroduodenostomy, however, using a drainage tube appears to be necessary because of the rather high incidence of leakage and the difficulty of treatment if leakage occurs. We routinely insert a tube drain near the anastomosis. As most leakage from the gastroduodenostomy occurs on the greater curvature, a drainage tube placed through the foramen Winslow is not effective for delayed leakage seen after one week. If there is a high risk of leakage, a drainage tube should be inserted to the greater curvature of the gastroduodenostomy directly through the rectus muscle. For pancreatic fistulae, a drain should be inserted directly to the pancreatic stump. If the PTT is used, pancreatic leakage may occur from the entire tail of the pancreas. Therefore, one drain to the left subphrenic space and/or a drain along the superior border of the pancreas and behind it, is recommended.

The correct strategy for treatment of an abscess secondary to anastomotic leakage is decided depending on the general condition of the patient including presence of fever, leucocyte count, size, shape, and location of the abscess. When there is a drainage tube in place, any minor modification of its position is easily carried out under X-ray fluoroscopy. When this is difficult, a guide wire or a fine-calibre endoscope can be used to lead the drainage tube to the main cavity of the abscess. When there is a large amount of discharge from the abscess, continous irrigation is recommended in order to control infection, especially if the discharge contains bile and pancreatic juice. If there is no drainage tube in place and general symptoms suggest systemic sepsis, a laparotomy should be carried out before the 14th postoperative day, because intraabdominal adhesions can then become an eventually fatal problem during further surgery. Aggressive drainage and continuous irrigation (with 100–200 ml/h saline), with the wound open at least as wide as the abscess cavity, is usually successful in controlling the infection and closing the fistula. If the abscess is small and not expanding, and the general condition of the patient remains good, conservative treatment with decompression by nasogastric tube and complete parenteral nutrition can lead to successful resolution.

For prevention and treatment of a pancreatic fistula and accompanying subphrenic abscess after distal pancreatectomy, a drainage tube should be placed close to the stump. After a PTT, a drainage tube should be inserted into the left subphrenic space. If the amylase concentration of the discharge from the drainage tube is particularly high, even on the 5th postoperative day, continuous suction or intermittent suction is recommended with prophylactic aim. If any abscess or infection develops, continuous suction should be performed until the 12th postoperative day when a fistulography should be carried out to determine the shape and size of abscess or tract. If the drainage is not adequate, the drainage tube should be replaced under fluoroscopic control, with a guide wire or endoscopy, if necessary. Continuous irrigation should then be started, just as in the case of anastomotic leakage.

3. PATIENT FOLLOW-UP

3.1. Pattern of recurrence

The recurrence pattern following curative surgery is shown in Fig. 15.4 (Katai *et al.*
1994). Commonly, recurrence away from the abdominal cavity occurs at the end-
stage of the disease. The most frequent recurrences are peritoneal dissemination,
local recurrence including lymph node and liver metastasis. The pattern depends on
serosal involvement and histological type. Diffuse-type cancer has a strong tendency to develop peritoneal dissemination when the tumour invades to the serosa.
Intestinal-type tumours develop more liver metastasis, the incidence of which is still
lower than that of peritoneal metastasis even for this type of histology. Survival
curves of patients' dying from different recurrence patterns are shown in Fig. 15.5.
Mean survival time is shortest for local recurrence groups, including lymph node
metastasis, then liver metastasis groups, followed by peritoneal metastasis groups,
and, finally, longest for distant metastasis.

3.2. How to follow up patients

Early detection of recurrence is of little practical importance because most recurrences cannot be treated with curative intent. However, some liver and lymph node
metastasis, or local recurrences are worth being resected especially when the
primary tumour had no serosal invasion. As there is no established adjuvant
chemotherapy following curative surgery, patients are usually followed-up without
any adjuvant treatment, except in clinical trials. For T1 or T2 tumours, follow-up
is focused on the liver metastasis. When surgical margins are not long enough, frequent checking by endoscopy and biopsy is important, because most of the local

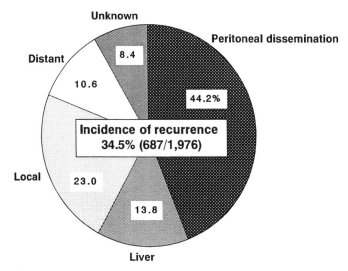

Fig. 15.4.   Predominant mode of recurrence in advanced gastric cancer. Local recurrence includes
lymph node metastases in the gastric bed. (From Katai *et al.* 1994.)

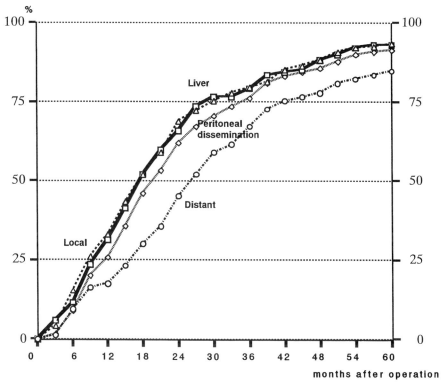

Fig. 15.5. Time intervals between surgery and death according to the mode of recurrence. (From Katai *et al.* 1994.)

recurrence at the surgical margins of T1 or T2 tumours can be resected again with curative intent. For T3 or T4 tumours, in which peritoneal dissemination is the most common pattern of recurrence, its early detection in the large bowel by barium enema study enables early chemotherapy and also provides useful information for patients in order to plan the rest of their lives. Peritoneal dissemination occurring on the retroperitoneum or lymphatic spread on the retroperitoneum sometimes causes stricture of the ureter and hydronephrosis. Insertion of a double-J catheter prevents early development of renal dysfunction by bilateral ureteral occlusion. This is very important especially when patients are expected to receive additional chemotherapy for palliative treatment.

4. SPECIAL PROBLEMS

4.1. Carcinoma of the cardia

Despite the continual decrease in the incidence of gastric cancer, an increased incidence of cardia cancer has been reported by several authors (Blot *et al.* 1991; Rios-Castellanos *et al.* 1992; Pera *et al.* 1993; Hansson *et al.* 1993). Although there should be a 'golden standard' operation in these cases, surgical treatment is still controversial for this type of tumour. There are two major operations of choice: a left thoracoabdominal oblique approach or an abdominal approach with wide opening of the lower mediastinum. The former provides the best operative field, enabling a wide resection of the oesophgeal hiatus and lower mediastinum and a safe oesophagojejunostomy under direct vision. From our results in a series of 58 patients, including incurables, mediastinal node metastasis was observed only in those patients with tumours invading more than 1 cm and being deeper than the proper muscle layer of the oesophagus. The incidence of metastasis was 30% in these cases. Based on these results, a left thoracoabdominal oblique incision was used as our standard surgical procedure from 1987 to 1992 at the NCCH. Only 11 patients with mediastinal node involvement were treated with curative intent and all of them died within five years. Partly because of the small likelihood of cure in patients with mediastinal node metastasis and partly because of the improved safety of high oesophagojejunostomy without thoracotomy, using stapling guns, left thoracotomy is no longer necessary for the treatment of cardia cancer. However, the effectiveness of both techniques is now being investigated in a randomized controlled trial in Japan, studying morbidity, mortality, and survival effects.

4.2. Surgery for gastric stump cancer

Cancer of the gastric stump is becoming an important problem, even though the incidence of distal gastrectomy for benign ulcers decreased markedly following widespread treatment with antiH2 drugs. Based on the high risk estimated in a cohort study, much attention has been given to detecting this type of cancer in its early stage. As a result, an increasing number of early or curable cancers of the gastric remnant have been reported (Sasako *et al.* 1991; Pointner *et al.* 1988; von Holstein *et al.* 1991; Sowa *et al.* 1993). Radical surgery for stump cancer is principally a total resection of the gastric stump with PS or PTT. Due to the increased incidence of metastasis on the greater curvature, splenic hilus, and splenic artery nodes, thorough lymph node dissection of these areas is more important than in primary cancers of the gastric body (Sasako *et al.* 1991). In cases where reconstruction following gastrectomy was carried out by Billroth II-type surgery, dissection of the stump from the mesocolon should not be attempted unless the tumour is a T1 cancer. Total gastrectomy with PS, combined with transverse colectomy, should be carried out in order to prevent incision into the cancerous invasion to the mesocolon, which cannot be discriminated from adhesion. Lymph nodes in the mesentery of the proximal jejunum anastomosed to the remnant stomach are often metastatic when the anastomosis is invaded by cancer. Therefore, the anastomosed mesentery should be widely resected by dividing the jejunal arteries at their origins. When the reconstruction has been made by Billroth I-type surgery, the proximal portion of the duodenum is often invaded by cancer. To complete a curative resection for T3 or T4 tumours, the duodenum should be resected as distally as possible, principally together with the pancreas body and tail distal to the portal vein.

4.3. Surgery for distant metastasis

In paraarotic lymph node metastasis, in cases where some of paraaortic nodes are swollen preoperatively, these patients should be first treated by neo-adjuvant chemotherapy. Macroscopic metastasis to this area indicates a very minor likelihood of cure. On the other hand, patients with lymph node metastases to the paraaortic area resected by a prophylactic wide dissection of these nodes showed five-year survival rates of 10–20%. A randomized controlled trial, comparing D2, versus D2 with paraaortic nodal dissection, is being carried out, in Japan, in order to evaluate the efficacy of the systematic dissection of paraaortic nodes.

In contrast to colon cancer, most liver metastases from gastric cancer are usually multiple and not resectable. The data from the NCCH (Ochiai *et al.* 1994) showed that the rate resectability was approximately 10%. Among 284 patients with liver metastasis at the time of primary surgery, liver resection was attempted for 20 patients only. Including metachronous liver metastasis, 30 patients underwent liver resection: 21 were treated with curative intent and 4 of them survived more than five years. From analyses of prognostic indicators in these patients, liver metastasis should be resected when the primary tumour has no serosal invasion, in the case of synchronous metastases. Where there are metachronous metastases, hepatic resection should be attempted if the primary tumour had no serosal involvement and that no (or only one) vessel involvement (lymphatic or venous) is observed. Synchronous liver resection for metastatic tumours could be tried, even when the primary tumour has serosal invasion, depending on the risk of hepatic resection, because any type of chemotherapy, which is the alternative treatment for this condition, can be carried out as an adjuvant treatment following hepatic resection.

REFERENCES

AJCC (American Joint Committee on Cancer) (1992). Manual of staging of cancer, (4th edn). Lippincott, Philadelphia.

Blot, W.J., Devesa, S.S., Kneller, R.W., and Fraumeni, J.F. Jr. (1991). Rising incidence of adenocarcinoma of the esophagus and gastric cardia. *JAMA*, **265**, 1287–9.

Bogomeletz, W.V. (1984). Early gastric cancer. *Am. J. Surg. Pathol.*, **8**, 381–91.

Bollschweiler, E., Boettcher, K., Hoelscher, A.H., Sasako, M., Kinoshita, T., Maruyama, K., *et al.* (1992). Preoperative assessment of lymph node metastases in patients with gastric cancer: evaluation of the Maruyama computor program. *Br. J. Surg.*, **79**, 156–60.

Bollschweiler, E., Boettcher, K., Hoelscher, A.H., Sasako, M., Kinoshita, T., Maruyama, K., *et al.* (1993). Is the prognosis for Japanese and German patients with gastric cancer really different? *Cancer*, **71**, 2918–25.

Bonenkamp, J.J., van de Velde, C.J.H., Kampschöer, G.H.M., Hermans, J., Hermanek, P., Bemelmans, M., *et al.* (1993). Comparison of factors influencing the prognosis of Japanese, German, and Dutch gastric cancer patients. *World J. Surg.*, **17**, 410–15.

Bonenkamp, J.J., Songun, I., Hermans, J., Sasako, M., Welvaart, K., Plukker, J.T.M., *et al.* (1995). Randomized comparison of D1 and D2 dissection for gastric cancer in 1078 Dutch patients: morbidity does make a difference. *Lancet*, **345**, 745–8.

Bozzetti F. (1992). Total versus subtotal gastrectomy in cancer of the distal stomach: facts and fantasy. *Eur. J. Surg. Oncol.*, **18**, 572–9.

Bozzetti, F., Bonfanti, E., Regalia, E., Andreola, S., Doci, G., La Malfa, G., *et al.* (1992). How long is a 6 cm margin of resection in the stomach? *Eur. J. Surg. Oncol.*, **18**, 481–3.

Brady, M.S., Rogatko, A., Dent, L., and Shiu, M.H. (1991). Effect of splenectomy on morbidity and survival following curative gastrectomy for carcinoma. *Arch. Surg.*, **126**, 359–64.

Bringaze, W.L., Chappuis, C.W., Cohn, I., and Correa, P. (1986). Early gastric cancer, 21-year experience. *Ann. Surg.*, **204**, 103–7.

Bunt, A.M.G. (1993). Lymph node retrieval in a randomized trial on Western (R1) versus Japanese (R2) type surgery in gastric cancer. In *Gastric cancer staging*, pp. 47–58. Pasmans, The Hague.

Butler, J.A., Dublow, T.J., Trezona, T., Klassen, M., and Nejdl, R.J. (1989). Total gastrectomy in the treatment of advanced gastric cancer. *Am. J. Surg.*, **158**, 602–6.

Cady, B. (1984). Lymph node metastases. Indicators, but not governers of survival. *Arch. Surg.*, **119**, 1067–72.

Cullingford, G.D., Watkins, D.N., Watts, A.D.J., and Mallon, D.F. (1991). Severe late post-splenectomy infection. *Br. J. Surg.*, **78**, 716–21.

Cuschieri, A. Gastrectomy for gastric cancer: definitions and objectives. *Br. J. Surg.*, **73**, 513–4.

Feinstein, A.R., Sosin, D.M., and Wells, C.K. (1985). The Will Rogers phenomenon, Stage migration and new diagnostic techniques are a source of misleading statistics for survival in cancer. *N. Engl. J. Med.*, **312**, 1604–8.

Fielding, J. (1989). Gastric cancer: different diseases. *Br. J. Surg.*, **76**, 1227.

Finley, R.J. and Inculet, R.I. (1989). The results of esophagogastrectomy without thoracotomy for adenocarcinoma of the esophagogastric junction. *Ann. Surg.*, **210**, 535–43.

Furukawa, H., Hiratsuka, M., and Iwanaga, T. (1988). A rational technique for surgical operation on Borrmann type 4 gastric carcinoma: left upper abdominal evisceration plus Appleby's method. *Br. J. Surg.*, **75**, 116–9.

Gall, F.P. and Hermanek, P. (1985). New aspects in the treatment of gastric carcinoma—a comparative study of 1636 patients operated on between 1969 and 1982. *Eur. J. Surg. Oncol.*, **11**, 219–25.

Gennari, L., Bozzetti, F., Bonfanti, G., Morabito, A., Bufalino R., Doci R., *et al.* (1986). Subtotal versus total gastrectomy for cancer of the lower two-thirds of the stomach: a new approach to an old problem. *Br. J. Surg.*, **73**, 534–8.

Gouzi, J.L., Huguier, M., Fagniez, P.L., Launois, B., Flamant, Y., Lacaine, F., *et al.* (1988). Total *versus* subtotal gastrectomy for adenocarcinoma of the gastric antrum. A French prospective controlled study. *Ann. Surg.*, **209**, 162–6.

Green, P.H.R., O'Toole, K.M., Slonia, D., Wang, T., and Weg, A. (1988). Increasing incidence and excellent survival of patients with early gastric cancer: experience in a United States Medical Center. *Am. J. Med.*, **85**, 658–61.

Hansson, L.E., Sparén, P., and Nyrén, O. (1993). Increasing incidence of carcinoma of the gastric cardia in Sweden from 1970 to 1985. *Br. J. Surg.*, **80**, 374–7.

Iriyama, K., Miki, C., Ilunga, K., Osawa. T., Tsuchibashi, T., and Suzuki, H. (1993). Prognostic significance of histological type in gastric carcinoma with invasion confined to the stomach wall. *Br. J. Surg.*, **80**, 890–2.

JRSGC (Japanese Research Society for Gastric Cancer) (1993). *Japanese classification of gastric carcinoma*. English edition, (ed. Mitsuma, N., Omori, Y., and Miwa, K.). Kaneharo Tokyo.

Kajitani, T., Takagi, K., and Ohashi, I. (1981). Radical surgery for gastric cancer (left side lymph node dissection). *Geka Rinsho*, **23**, 412–7. (In Japanese)

Kanayama, H., Hamazoe, R., Osaki, Y., Shimizu, N., Maeta, M., and Koga, S. (1985). Immunosuppressive factor from the spleen in gastric cancer patients. *Cancer*, **56**, 1963–6.

Katai, H., Maruyama, K., Sasako, M., Sano, T., Okajima, K., Kinoshita, T., *et al.* (1994). Mode of recurrence after gastric cancer surgery. *Dig. Surg.*, **11**, 99–103.

Lindhal, A.K., Harbitz, T.B., and Liavag I. (1988). The surgical treatment of gastric cancer: a retrospective study with special reference to total gastrectomy. *Eur. J. Surg. Oncol.*, **14**, 55–62.

Maruyama, K., Okabayashi, K., and Kinoshita, T. (1987). Progress in gastric cancer surgery in Japan and its limits of radicality. *World J. Surg.*, **11**, 418–25.

Maruyama, K., Sasako, M., Kinoshita, T., Sano, T., Katai, H., and Okajima, K. (1995). Pancreas-preserving total gastrectomy for proximal gastric cancer. *World J. Surg.*, **19**, 532–6.

McCulloch, P. (1994). Should general surgeons treat gastric carcinoma? An audit of practice and results, 1980–1985. *Br. J. Surg.* **81**, 417–20.

McCulloch, P., Ochiai, A., O'Dowd, G.M., Nash, J.R.G., Sasako, M., and Hirohashi, S. (1995). Comparison of the molecular genetics of c-*erb*-B2 and p53 expression in stomach cancer in Britain and Japan. *Cancer*, **75**, 920–5.

Nishi, M., Ohta, K., and Nakajima, T. (1993). Combined resection. In *Gastric cancer*, (ed. M. Nishi *et al.*), pp. 306–18. Springer, Tokyo.

Ochiai, T., Sasako, M., Mizuno, S., Kinoshita, T., Takayama, T., Kosuge, T., *et al.* (1994). Hepatic resection for metastatic tumours from gastric cancer: analysis of prognostic factors. *Br. J. Surg.*, **81**, 1175–8.

Ohyama, S., Nakajima, T., Ota, K., Ishihara, S., Wakabayashi, K., and Nishi, M. (1994). Left upper abdominal evisceration for advanced gastric cancer. *Jpn. J. Cancer Chemother.*, **21**, 1781–6. (In Japanese)

Pacelli, F., Doglietto, G.B., Bellantones, R., Alfieri, S., Sgadari, A., and Crucitti, F. (1993). Extensive versus limited lymph node dissection for gastric cancer: a comparative study of 320 patients. *Br. J. Surg.*, **80**, 1153–6.

Paolini, A., Tosato, F., Cassese, M., De Marchi, C., Grande, M., Paoletti, P., *et al.* (1986). Total gastrectomy in the treatment of adenocarcinoma of the cardia; review of the results in 73 resected patients. *Am. J. Surg.*, **151**, 238–43.

Pera, M., Cameron, A.J., Trastek, V.F., Carpenter, H.A., and Zinsmeister, A.R. (1993). Increasing incidence of adenocarcinoma of the esophagus and esophagogastric junction. *Gastroenterology*, **104**, 510–13.

Poitner, R., Schwab, G., Köningstrainer, A., Bodner, E., and Schmid, K.W. (1988). Early cancer of the gastric remnant. *Gut*, **29**, 298–301.

Rios-Castellanos, E., Sitas, F., and Jewell, D.P. (1992). Changing pattern of gastric cancer in Oxfordshire. *Gut*, **33**, 1312–17.

Robertson, C.S., Chung, S.C.S., Woods, S.D.S., Griffin, S.M., Raimes, S.A., Lau, J.T.F., *et al.* (1994). A prospective randomized trial comparing R1 subtotal gastrectomy with R3 total gastrectomy for antral cancer. *Ann. Surg.*, **220**, 176–82.

Sasako, M. (1990). Gastric cancer. In *Complications and its management after cancer surgery of digestive organs*, (ed. K. Hojo), pp. 39–53. Kanehara, Tokyo. (In Japanese)

Sasako, M., Maruyama, K., Kinoshita, T., and Okabayashi, K. (1991). Surgical treatment of carcinoma of the gastric stump. *Br. J. Surg.*, **78**, 822–4.

Sasako, M., Maruyama, K., Kinoshita, T., Bonenkamp, J.J., van de Velde, C.J.H., Hermans, J., *et al.* (1992). Quality control of surgical technique in a multicenter, prospective, randomized, controlled study on the surgical treatment of gastric cancer. *Jpn. J. Clin. Oncol.*, **22**, 41–8.

Sasako, M., McCulloch, P., Kinoshita, T., and Maruyama, K. (1995). Therapeutic value of lymph node dissection for gastric cancer: a new method of evaluation circumventing the stage migration effect. *Br. J. Surg.*, **82**, 346–51.

Schlag, P. (1986). Consideration for surgical treatment of gastric cancinoma. *Eur. J. Surg. Oncol.*, **12**, 235–9.

Shiu, M.H., Papacristou, D.N., Kosloff, C., and Eliopoulos, G. (1980). Selection of operative procedure for adenocarcinoma of the midstomach. *Ann. Surg.*, **192**, 730–7.

Shiu, M.H., Moore, E., Sanders, M., Huvos, A., Freedman, B., Goodbold, J., *et al.* (1987). Influence of the extent of resection on survival after curative treatment of gastric carcinoma. *Arch. Surg.*, **122**, 1347–51.

Shiu, M.H., Perrotti, M., and Brennan, M.F. (1989). Adenocarcinoma of the stomach: a multivariate analysis of clinical, pathologic and treatment factors. *Hepatogastoroenterology*, **36**, 7–12.

Soga, J., Kobayashi, K., Saito, J., Fukimaki, M., and Muto, T. (1979). The role of lymphadenectomy in curative surgery for gastric cancer. *World J. Surg.*, **3**, 701–8.

Sowa, M., Kato, Y., Onoda, N., Kubo, T., Maekawa, H., Yoshikawa, K., *et al.* (1993). Early cancer of the gastric remnant with special reference to the importance of follow-up of gastrectomized patients. *Euro. J. Surg. Oncol.*, **19**, 43–9.

Sue-Ling, H.M., Johnston, D., Martin, I.G., Dixon M.F., Lansdown, M.R.J., McMahon, M.J., *et al.* (1993). Gastric cancer: a curable disease in Britain. *Br. Med. J.*, **307**, 591–6.

Suehiro, S., Nagasue, N., Ogawa, Y., Sasaki, Y., Hirose, S., and Yukaya, H. (1984). The negative effect of splenectomy on the prognosis of gastric cancer. *Am. J. Surg.*, **148**, 645–8.

Sugimachi, K., Kodama, Y., Kumashiro, R., Kanematsu, T., Noda S., and Inokuchi K. (1980). Critical evaluation of prophylactic sprenectomy in total gastrectomy for stomach cancer. *Gann*, **71**, 704–9.

Takahashi M. and Fujimoto S. (1980). Clinical studies on the correlation between immunologic status and total gastrectomy combined with splenectomy. *Jpn. J. Surg.*, **10**, 100–4.

UICC (1987). *TNM classification of malignant tumours*, (4th edn). Springer, Berlin.

von Holstein, C.S., Eriksson, S., and Hammar, E. (1991). Role of re-resection in early gastric stump carcinoma. *Br. J. Surg.*, **78**, 1238–41.

Wagner, P.K., Ramaswamy, A., Rüschoff, J., Schimitz-Moormann, P., and Rothmund, M.(1991). Lymph node counts in the upper abdomen: anatomical basis for lymphadenectomy in gastric cancer. *Br. J. Surg.*, **78**, 825–7.

Yonemura, Y., Ooyama, S., Matumoto, H., Kamata, T., Kimura, H., Takegawa, S., *et al.* (1991). Pancreaticoduodenectomy in combination with right hemicolectomy for surgical treatment of advanced gastric carcinoma located in the lower half of the stomach. *Int. Surg.*, **76**, 226–9.

16

Palliative surgery

Asgaut Viste

1. INTRODUCTION

Advanced gastric cancer not being amenable for curative resection is found in varying frequencies around the world. In Western countries a potential curative resection is performed in 40–60% of patients, compared to 75–80% in Japan. The benefit of palliative surgery for stomach carcinoma is controversial. Two questions are commonly raised: (1) should a resection be performed whenever possible; and (2) what is the survival advantage of a palliative resection?

2. THE OBJECTIVES OF PALLIATIVE SURGERY

The aims of palliative surgery are relief of symptoms, improvement of quality of life, and prolongation of comfortable survival without producing new symptoms or incurring excessive mortality or morbidity. The following factors should always be kept in mind: it is impossible to palliate a patient who has no symptoms; and that after effective palliation the patient will till have to face the period of terminal illness leading up to death. The cost–benefit of an operation should be evaluated carefully taking into account pre-existing or imminent symptoms compared to operative morbidity and mortality and postoperative symptoms. Generally, major surgery is followed by at least two to three months of physical debility, and the patient should therefore have a life-expectancy of at least six months to have any benefit from surgery. Consequently, it is our policy not to offer a patient with distant metastases and no symptoms any surgical treatment.

Symptoms which can be palliated include pain, vomiting, dysphagia, and bleeding. Pain might be caused by an ulcer, obstruction or infiltration into neighbouring structures, and if caused by obstruction, surgery may be indicated. Vomiting is a distressing symptom and is a clear indication for palliation when caused by a distal stenosis. Dysphagia and bleeding can often be treated by endoscopic measures, such as laser treatment or sclerotherapy. Resection is, however, sometimes required to control fatal bleeding from a cancerous ulcer, which is more commonly seen in case of Borrmann types 2 and 3 advanced cancer with massive necrosis of the tumour.

In older patient series morbidity and mortality rates following palliative surgery were unacceptably high (Dupont et al. 1978; Inberg et al. 1975). The patient should, however, not accept a morbidity or mortality rate much over—if any—that of curative surgery. In a national multicentre study we have shown that complications and mortality rates do not differ significantly between patients undergoing a potentially curative resection versus those treated palliatively (Viste *et al.* 1988). This holds even if extensive operations like total gastrectomies are performed (Saario *et al.* 1986).

3. PALLIATIVE SURGICAL PROCEDURES

For gastric cancer these can be divided into two main groups: resections and bypass procedures. Proximal tumours constitute a major problem, where the main symptom most often will be dysphagia due to obstruction. For these tumours laser treatment will be an alternative, and as surgical resection will imply a total gastrectomy, which should only be considered in relatively young patients with a rather long life-expectancy.

As for prolongation of life, several studies have shown that tumour resection is the treatment of choice when palliative procedures are indicated (Bozzetti *et al.* 1980; Ekbom *et al.* 1980; Meijer *et al.* 1983; Haugstvedt *et al.* 1989). However, the available data supporting this conclusion are obtained in retrospective series, and even if multivariate analyses are being performed, it might always be suspected that patients having a bypass have the most extensive disease or are more debilitated than those having a resection.

The most difficult question that is not yet answered, is whether palliative resection, in fact, improves quality of life. There are many patients with gastric carcinomas who do not suffer from obstructive symptoms; their main complaints are weight loss, anorexia, lassitude, and general malaise. So far, it is not known if these symptoms are improved by palliative resection. Following surgery, these patients have a 10 to 14-day in hospital stay and it still takes at least 2 months before they recover from surgery. A large proportion of them will die from advanced disease during the following 3–4 months.

When palliative surgery is undertaken for distal tumours, resection should be performed whenever possible (Korenaga *et al.* 1988; Haugstvedt *et al.* 1989). The palliative effect of this procedure is more effective than that of bypass, and the morbidity or mortality should not be greater. However, the question of whether tumour load, or tumour bulk reduction affects survival is still open. Koga *et al.* (1980) found an improved survival in patients with liver metastases when the stomach tumour was resected, and in another report from Japan, Korenaga *et al.* (1988) documented a better outcome in patients having a one organ involvement compared to patients with three organ involvement. However, there are no randomized studies comparing the outcome for patients having such tumours removed versus not removed.

When the tumour is not resectable, a gastrojejunostomy is an available option. In some series, this operation carries an unacceptable mortality of 17–37% (Inberg *et al.* 1975; ReMine 1979). This formidable mortality rate may indicate the poor nutritional and immune status of these advanced cancer patients, but as the above-mentioned studies are not randomized, results may simply be due to selection bias, with more advanced cases treated with bypass procedures.

As for the technical details concerning the operative procedure the gastrojejunostomy should be performed in the simplest way possible; ante colic on the front wall of the stomach. The anastomosis should be rather long in order not to be blocked by tumour extension, and it can easily be performed with a linear stapler or with a running one-layer suture. There is no need for a Braun's enteroanastomosis.

The effect of gastrojejunostomies is sometimes disappointing. The reason for this might be that they are placed too high on the stomach to drain properly, or the poor drainage is associated with tumour involvement of autonomic nerves. This is also the reason why we never perform a prophylactic palliative gastrojejunostomy.

When the palliative operation is a planned procedure, and not encountered as a surprise during attempted radical surgery, a laparoscopic gastrojejunostomy performed with an end-GIA stapler device should be considered. The potential benefit of a minimally invasive procedure could be of special importance for patients with an advanced cancer disease.

REFERENCES

Bozzetti, F., Bonfanti, G., Audisio, R.A., Doci, R., Dossena, G., *et al.*, Prognosis of patients after palliative surgical procedures for carcinoma of the stomach. *Surgery, Gynecology and Obstetrics*, **164**, 151–4.

Dupont, J.B., Lee, J.R., Burton, G.R., and Cohn, I. (1978). Adenocarcinoma of the stomach: Review of 1497 cases. *Cancer*, **41**, 941–7.

Ekbom, G.A. and Gleysteen, J.J. (1980). Gastric malignancy. Resection for palliation. *Surgery*, **88**, 476–81.

Haugstvedt, T., Viste, A., Eide, G.E., and Soreide, O. (1989). The survival benefit of resection in patients with advanced stomach cancer: The Norwegian multicenter experience. *World Journal of Surgery*, **13**, 617–22.

Inberg M.V., Heinonen, R., Rautokokko, V., and Viikari, S.J. (1975). Surgical treatment of gastric carcinoma. A regional study of 2590 patients over a 27-year period. *Archives of Surgery*, **10**, 703–7.

Koga, S., Kawaguchi, H., Kishimota, H., Tanaka, K., Miyano, Y., *et al.* (1980). Therapeutic significance of noncurative gastrectomy for gastric cancer with liver metastases. *American Journal of Surgery*, **140**, 356–9.

Korenaga, D., Okamura, T., Baba, H., Saito, A., and Sugimachi, K. (1988). Results of resection of gastric cancer extending to adjacent organs. *British Journal of Surgery*, **75**, 12–15.

Meijer, S., De Bakker, A.J.G.B., and Hoitsma, H.F.W. (1983). Palliative resection in gastric cancer. *Journal of Surgical Oncology*, **23**, 77–80.

ReMine W.H. (1979). Palliative operations for incurable gastric cancer. *World Journal of Surgery*, **3**, 721–9.

Saario, I., Schroder, T., Tolppanen, E.M., and Lempinen, M. (1986). Total gastrectomy and esophagogastrectomy. *American Journal of Surgery*, **151**, 244–6.

Viste, A., Haugstvedt, T., Eide, G.E., and Soreide, O. (1988). Postoperative complications and mortality after surgery for gastric cancer. *Annals of Surgery*, **207**, 7–13.

17

Endoscopic treatment

Shigeaki Yoshida

1. INTRODUCTION

The roles of therapeutic endoscopy for gastric cancer are generally classified into four categories: (1) cancer removal; (2) recanalization of neoplastic obstruction; (3) hemostasis of cancer bleeding; and (4) other endoscopic palliation. Table 17.1 shows the leading methodologies applied in each category. High-frequency electric current (HFEC), laser irradiation, microwave coagulation, or local injection of anticancer agents can be indicated for the removal of cancer. For recanalization of a cancerous obstruction, laser irradiation, microwave coagulation, endoscopic bougienage, or prosthesis can be used. Against cancer bleeding, local injection of pure alcohol, heat probe, microwave coagulation, HFEC, or low-power laser irradiation is available. Endoscopic drainage of digestive juice can be given as an example of another palliative treatment.

Cancer removal is the most important endoscopic treatment, particularly in early gastric cancer (EGC) having neither lymph node nor distant metastases. It can

Table 17.1. Roles and methodologies of endoscopic treatment in patients with gastric cancer

---

Removal of cancerous lesion
- high-frequency electric current: endoscopic resection (ER), polypectomy
- laser: vaporization, laserthermia, photodynamic therapy (PDT)
- microwave coagulation
- injection of anticancer agent

Recanalization of neoplastic obstruction
- laser vaporization (Nd:YAG, KTP, CO_2, diode, etc.)
- microwave coagulation
- prosthesis for cardiac stenosis

Hemostasis of cancer bleeding
- heat probe
- pure alcohol injection
- microwave coagulation
- low-power laser
- high-frequency electric current (coagulation wave)

Other endoscopic palliation
- percutaneous endoscopic gastrotomy for cardiac cancer patients

---

provide a cure for cancer without the need for laparotomy. Others uses of endoscopy are non-curative and can be divided into two categories: (1) relative curative removal; (2) and non-curative palliation. The former includes the removal of EGCs with submucosal invasion, or small cancers in an advanced stage which are unlikely to metastasize. The latter indicates tumor reduction for recanalization of neoplastic obstruction due to the advanced stage of the gastric cancer.

2. EARLY GASTRIC CANCER: CURATIVE ENDOSCOPIC RESECTION

2.1. Background

Endoscopic diagnosis of EGC without metastasis

Table 17.2A shows the incidence of metastasis by endoscopic appearance and size, in the 1430 cases of well-documented solitary EGC, treated at the National Cancer Center Hospital, Tokyo during 1962–86. The endoscopic appearance was classified into polypoid, ulcerative, gastritis-like, and advanced cancer-like types, according to the definitions given in Chapter 4. From Table 17.2, it appears that no metastasis is seen from a plateau-like elevation (type IIa) of polypoid EGCs less than 20 mm, and in gastritis-like EGCs less than 10 mm. With respect to Lawrence's histological classification, metastasis is not present in intestinal-type of gastritis-like EGCs of less than 20 mm, as shown in Table 17.2B. Therefore, the preoperative diagnosis of

Table 17.2. Incidence of metastasis in early gastric cancer: its relation to endoscopic appearance, size, and histological type

	≦1.0 cm	1.1–2.0 cm	2.1 ≦ cm	Total
A. Endoscopic appearance				
Polypoid	0 (0/11)	8 (5/64)	18 (24/133)	20 (14/70)
I	0 (0/2)	6 (1/16)	25 (13/52)	20 (14/70)
IIa	0 (0/6)	0 (0/25)	11 (4/36)	5 (4/85)
IIa + IIc	0 (0/3)	17 (4/23)	16 (7/45)	15 (11/71)
Gastritis-like	0 (0/53)	2 (1/57)	4 (4/110)	2 (5/210)
Ulcerative	4 (2/50)	6 (9/153)	12 (75/630)	10 (86/833)
Advanced cancer-like	–	38 (3/8)	21 (30/143)	22 (33/151)
B. Endoscopic appearance and histological type				
Gastritis-like				
Intestinal-type	0 (0/42)	0 (0/34)	4 (3/67)	2 (3/143)
Diffuse-type	0 (0/11)	4 (1/23)	2 (1/43)	3 (2/77)
Ulcerative				
Intestinal-type	0 (0/32)	4 (3/81)	11 (28/254)	8 (31/367)
Diffuse-type	11 (2/18)	8 (6/72)	13 (47/376)	12 (55/466)

From the National Cancer Center Hospital (1962–86).

lymph node metastasis in ECG can be estimated from the endoscopic appearance, size, and histological type (biopsy results) of the lesion.

Methodologies in endoscopic removal of EGC

Endoscopic cancer removal is initially attained by colorectal polypectomy using high-frequency electric current (HFEC) (Deyhle *et al.* 1973). In 1974, it was used in the treatment of pedunculated or hemipedunculated EGCs in Japan. Laser endoscopy was the next focus, and many EGC cases of poor risk for surgery have been treated since 1980 (Oguro and Tajiri 1986). In 1984, Tada and co-workers devised a cancer treatment methodology of endoscopic mucosal resection (EMR) using HFEC, as an application of endoscopic snare polypectomy ('strip biopsy') (Tada *et al.* 1987: Takemoto *et al.* 1989). As it is technically simple and ensures histological assessment of the resected specimen at laparotomy, it is now widely used in Japan for the treatment of EGC. In addition Hirao *et al.* (1988) devised another technique called ERHSE (endoscopic resection with local injection of hypertonic saline epinephrine solution), in which mucosal resection by an endoscopic knife using HFEC is enhanced by hemostasis with the injection of HSE (hypertonic saline epinephrine). However, although its therapeutic efficacy is much more reliable than that of strip biopsy, it requires considerable skill.

2.2.   Endoscopic Mucosal Resection (EMR) with strip biopsy

Indications

A prospective study was carried out at the NCCH from November 1987 to 1993 to assess the feasibility and the efficacy of EMR using strip biopsy for 50 consecutive operable ECG cases. Table 17.3 shows the eligibility criteria of this study. The size of the lesion was restricted to a maximum diameter of 15 mm by X-radiation or endoscopic measurement together with an assessment of lateral cancerous invasion. The histological type was limited to intestinal-type EGC and the endoscopic appearance to gastritis-like ECGs, or those with a plateau-like elevation (type IIa). The location of the lesion is essential for EMR manipulation and it was defined as being where the resection can be performed completely, and those lesions located on the cardiac junction or pyloric ring were excluded. The treatment was approved following a preoperative meeting and informed patient consent.

Table 17.3.   Eligibility criteria in the NCCH prospective study of endoscopic resection in early gastric cancer

---
1. Less than 15 mm in maximum diameter
2. With superficial types IIa or IIc
3. With no ulcerative findings including fold convergency
4. Located in an easily manipulated area
5. Not located on the cardiac orifice or pyloric ring
6. Informed consent

Technique

Figure 17.1 shows, schematically, the strip biopsy technique. A two-channel endoscope is required for manipulating the catching forceps and cutting snare independently. About 2–5 ml of saline is first injected into the submucosal layer of the cancerous area in order to make the lesion both elevated and prevent damage due to overtransmission of heat into the deeper area. Second, the lesion is grasped tightly and pulled gently with catching forceps which have already passed through the loop of the cutting snare inserted from other endoscope channel. Then, the cutting snare loop is opened and fastens on to the surrounding mucosa of the lesion which has been pulled by the catching forceps. Gastric mucosa, including EGC, is resected with HFEC in the same way as with polypectomy. After the resection, the snare is pulled out, and the specimen, grasped by the catching forceps is retrieved by pulling the endoscope.

Handling the resected specimen

The correct diagnosis of cancer extension is very important for assessing therapeutic efficacy and the resected specimen should be handled carefully. In the author's technique, the specimen is stretched on a polystyrene sheet soon after retrieval, and soaked in 15% formalin solution for 48–72 hours. Following fixation, the specimen is stained with Karachi-Hematoxylin and the cancer margin is traced under stereomicoscopic observation. Finally, the specimen is cut at intervals of 2 mm in order to include the shortest distance between the cut end of the specimen and the cancer margin, as shown in Figs 17.2a–c.

Assessment of therapeutic efficacy and subsequent treatment

Therapeutic efficacy is assessed histologically. When cancerous invasion is limited within mucosa without any vascular permeation, and not extended to the horizontal cut end of the specimen (cut end-negative), the treatment result is assessed as

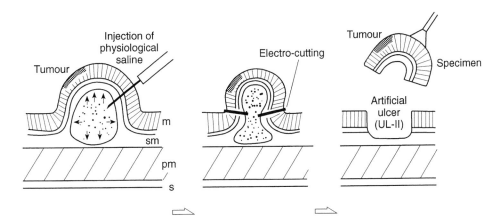

Fig. 17.1. Schematic illustration of strip biopsy.

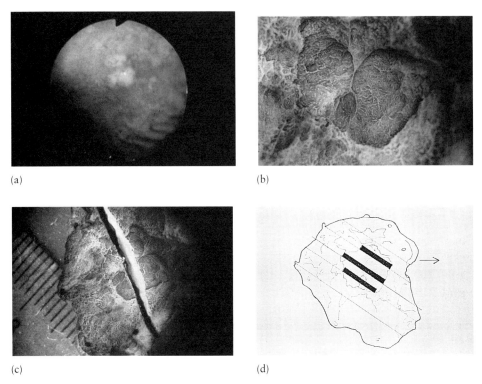

(a)　　　　　　　　　　　　　　　　　(b)

(c)　　　　　　　　　　　　　　　　　(d)

Fig. 17.2.　(a) Endoscopic appearance of an early gastric cancer treated with endoscopic resection. A whitish small elevated lesion is located in the posterior wall of the upper gastric body near the greater curvature. The diagnosis of a well-differentiated type of tubular adenocarcinoma was made by biopsy from this tiny elevation. (b) Stereomicroscopic appearance of the resected specimen. (c) The specimen was cut along the line including the maximum diameter of the lesion. (d) A diagram illustrating cancer extension. Mucosal cancer was detected from the three cut lines including tiny granules seen with stereomicroscopic observation.

'complete'. Although cut end-positive or cut end-negative criteria differ slightly among investigators, they can be generally classified into three groups: (1) 'negative; ew (−)', where more than 5 non-cancerous tubules are detectable in the cross-section at nearest to the end of the specimen; (2) 'relative negative; ew (±)', where less than 4 non-cancerous tubules are seen; and (3) 'positive; ew (+)', where cancerous invasion has reached to the margin of the specimen. Clinically, (1) and (2) are regarded as 'cut end-negative'.

In the case of incomplete resection, patients undergo surgery. Local excision is indicated in those with mucosal cancer without vascular permeation, and gastrectomy with D2 lymph node dissection in those with submucosal cancer, or of mucosal cancer with vascular permeation. In the case of complete resection, patients are followed-up every three months for the first year, every six months for the second year, and every twelve months thereafter. When a recurrence is identified during follow-up examination, patients undergo surgery with D2 lymph node dissection.

Treatment results

No complications were observed in the 50 cases of the prospective NCCH study. Figure 17.3 shows the treatment results. Of the 50 cases, 36 (72%) were either of ew (−) or (+−), and the rest 14 ew (+) because of slip of the snare or unclear margin of the lesion, etc. As the former included 4 cases of submucosal cancer, the complete resection rate was calculated as 64% (32/50), which is nearly the same with those reported by the other investigators (Takahashi *et al.* 1993). The 14 cases of ew (+) included one case of submucosal cancer, and in the remaining 13 cases, local excision was carried out except for 2 cases who rejected surgery (one received laser treatment and the other follow-up study). The 5 cases of submucosal cancer received subsequent surgery, and no lymph node metastasis was detected from either of these. Of the 16 surgical cases 6 (38%) showed remaining cancer cells on the resected specimen histologically. No recurrent cases had occurred by 1995.

From these results, the authors concluded that EMR using strip biopsy is clinically feasible for the treatment of operable EGC under patient-informed consent. Indeed, to date, more than 200 cases of EGC including non-NCCH study patients have been treated with EMR using strip biopsy at the NCCH, showing that about 25–30% of EGC is treated endoscopically.

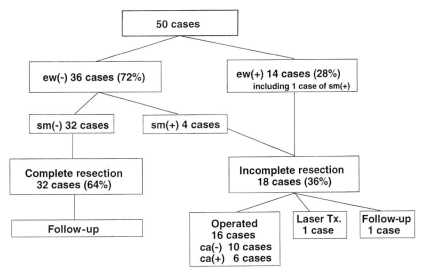

Fig. 17.3. Results of treatment in the NCCH prospective study of 50 consecutive cases of endoscopic resection in early gastric cancer.

2.3. Endoscopic cesection with local injection of hypertonic saline epinephrine solution (ERHSE)

Technique

ERHSE is carried out by using the following procedures:

(1) dye-spraying endoscopy for accurately determining the invasive area;
(2) enclosing the lesion with marking points using coagulation waves;
(3) injection of more than 10 ml of HSE for hemostasis and adequately exfoliating mucosa from submucosa;
(4) mucosal incision along the marking point with an endoscopic knife using 150 watts of HFEC cutting wave;
(5) removing the marginal mucosa incised endoscopically from the submucosa;
(6) resecting the specimen with a snare using blend of cutting and coagulation electric waves; and
(7) retrieval of the resected specimen.

Treatment results

In ERHSE, the resecting area can be created at will and a much larger specimen (i.e. over 4 cm in size) can be obtained, unlike EMR with strip biopsy where the specimen size is limited for a once only resection because of the limited size of the snare loop. Uchizawa *et al.* (1991), who have considerable experience, obtained very high complete resection rates (90%: 144/160) and very low complication rates, in which perforation was observed in only 3 out of 160 cases (surgery was not necessary except for 1 case), and bleeding was completely controlled with HSE. In spite of this, the technique is not widely used in Japan because of the necessity of highly skilled manipulation, and the length of surgery in instances of perforation and bleeding.

3. LASER ENDOSCOPY: A TREATMENT FOR GASTRIC CANCER

Although EMR is a useful technique, its efficacy is limited to superficial lesions. Laser endoscopy is indicated for deeper invasive cancers and for both curative treatment and non-curative palliation of gastric cancer.

3.1. Types of laser

These lasers are classified into two groups, according to the anticancer mechanism: the treatment using the physical effect of heat, as in Nd: YAG lasers; and treatment using the photodynamic effects of laser irradiation with hematoporphylin derivatives (HpD) (photodynamic therapy: PDT).

The Nd:YAG laser

Coagulation and vaporization   A high-power Nd:YAG laser is commonly used for vaporization or coagulation of cancerous tissue. It is delivered through a non-contact endoprobe at 40–60 watts and a duration of 0.5 seconds, and through a contact endoprobe at 15–30 watts and duration of 1–2 seconds. The frequency of the laser irradiation varies, depending on the volume of the tumor.

Laserthermia   The Nd:YAG laser can also be a tool for hyperthermia, as an application of contact technique (Brown 1983). The low power (2–3 watts) of the Nd:YAG laser is used with a high diffusion endoprobe penetrating into the cancerous lesion. The anticancer mechanism obtained differs considerably from that of high-power radiation (see also Daikuzono *et al.* 1988).

The photodynamic reaction

Following the discovery of a photodynamic reaction by Dougherty and co-workers in 1978, a selective anticancer therapy using this particular reaction (PDT) was accomplished with use of an argon dye laser (ADL) as an activator. In PDT, HpD, a photosensitive agent, having high affinity for cancer cells, is given intravenously at 2.5–3.0 mg/kg over 60–72 hours before ADL radiation, thus ensuring a high concentration in cancer cells.

The anticancer effect of PDT obtained from the stimulation of HpD by ADL radiation is generally weak because of the lower penetration of the laser beam. Recently, an excimer dye laser (EDL) with 40 kilowatts as peak power was applied to PDT, and more encouraging results, particularly on deeper invasive ECGs, are reported (Mimura *et al.* 1992).

Because HpD is a photosensitizer, patients receiving PDT should be isolated from daylight and confined in a darkened room for about 2–3 weeks following injection. This is an unavoidable disadvantage of this treatment.

3.2.   Results of laser endoscopy

In laser endoscopy, resected specimens are not obtained and therapeutic efficacy (i.e. possible residual cancer cells or lymph node metastasis) is estimated from indirect evaluation criteria only (e.g. no cancer cells in the biopsy specimen, or no recurrence for a long period after the treatment).

Table 17.4 shows treatment results from a 1986 nation-wide survey of laser endoscopy for the cases with an endoscopic diagnosis of EGC. Of the total 824 cases, 736 (89%) were treated with the Nd:YAG laser. Of the 568 cases followed-up for more than one year after the last treatment, no recurrence of gastric cancer was observed in 452 (effective rate = 80%), and in the remaining 116, cancer recurred during that period (Oguro and Tajiri 1986). Similar results were also obtained from a NCCH study (Tajiri and Oguro 1991), and it appeared that out of the 50 evaluated lesions, 46 of less than 2 cm were effectively treated, and 3 of the remaining 4 revealed remnant cancer cells during the follow-up period. These results may indicate that small EGCs without metastasis can be cured with endoscopic treatment other than EMR, but in the larger or deeper invasive EGCs, there are some difficulties in obtaining cures in all cases by laser treatment.

In Japan, because of its uncertain therapeutic efficacy, laser therapy has been generally indicated for patients with deeper invasive EGC who have a poor risk for

Table 17.4. Treatment results of laser endoscopy for cases with endoscopic diagnosis of early gastric cancer (1986)

Type of laser	Therapeutic effects*			Total
	Complete	Incomplete	Unclear	
Nd:YAG	401	108	227	736
PDT	30	3	22	55
Other	21	5	7	33
Total	452	116	256	824

* *Complete*: cancer negative for more than one year after the treatment. *Incomplete*: cancer positive after the last treatment. *Unclear*: less than one-year follow-up.

surgery. As the results in Table 17.4 indicate, a considerable number of patients treated died of other diseases several years after laser treatment, and it is still unclear whether the actual incidence of recurrence is due to distant or lymph node metastasis.

3.3   Laser endoscopy as palliation

The utility of laser palliation in advanced cancer is mainly focused on the recanalization of neoplastic obstructions, in particular, cardiac stenosis. In this case, PDT is not usually indicated and almost all cases are treated with an Nd:YAG laser. In a Japanese series, therapeutic success of recanalization was achieved in 61% of the 334 patients with esophageal or cardiac cancer and the effectiveness of endoscopic laser hemostasis was reported as 84% of the 134 cases with cancer causing gastrointestinal bleeding (Oguro and Tajiri 1986). Results of an international investigation of 1359 patients receiving laser palliation against inoperable cancer stenosis of the upper gastrointestinal tract showed that the average success rate of the initial treatment was appreciably better than 80% (Daikusono and Joffee 1985). The majority of those responding to the treatment had received a combination of laser and bougienage, depending on the degree of the stenosis.

At the NCCH, endoscopic palliation using the Nd:YAG laser has been administered on 15 cases of advanced gastric cancer in order to alleviate stenosis. Of the 15 patients, 9 were treated by non-contact methods and 6 by contact endoprobe. Of the 9 cases having non-contact method, in only 5 cases was this treatment effective. The remaining 6 patients who had imminent complete obstruction in the esophagocardiac region were treated with contact endoprobe, and normal eating patterns were achieved in all 6 cases by one month following treatment. In this procedure, a rounded endoprobe was used to vaporize the lesions, and no excessive tissue damage or other ill effects were observed (Tajiri and Oguro 1978).

As shown above, the advantage of contact irradiation over the non-contact method was apparent in therapeutic efficacy. Recently, however, a new non-contact irradiation method has been developed, using the endoscope with a transparent cap attached to the distal end. This provides a high therapeutic efficacy as the transparent cap maintains a constant distance between the tip of quarz fiber and the lesion.

Although using laser endoscopy in inoperable cancer stenoses of the upper gastrointestinal tract allows the rapid elimination of dysphasia, frequent recurrence of stenosis due to regrowth of cancer is unavoidable. Further procedures are required, such as subsequent brachytherapy or prosthesis. Combined therapeutic modalities are necessary in order to control the recurrent stenosis.

3.4. Complications of laser endoscopy

According to a Japanese nation-wide survey, the laser endoscopy complication rate in gastrointestinal cancers was reported as 2.9%, overall. The most frequent complication was that of bleeding, as reported in 2.5% (45 cases), and perforation was reported in 0.3% (5 cases). At the NCCH, only 3 cases had bleeding complications during laser endoscopy. Utilizing a pure ethanol injection works well in all cases and, so far, perforation has not been experienced.

4. FUTURE DIRECTIONS

As reported by Yamao *et al.* (1996), intramucosal EGCs, particularly those without lymphatic vessel invasion, histological ulceration, and larger tumor size (> 3 cm) have an extremely low incidence of regional lymph node metastasis (0.36%: 1/277), indicating that they can be cured by simple removal of cancerous tissue. Because of this, EMR is becoming widely used. Recently devised EMR techniques, such as using a knife or a suction method, where the mucosa is sucked into the endoscopic cap, has been applied in order to resect much larger specimens. In addition, laparoscopic surgery is now being used in gastric cancer treatment (Ohgami *et al.* 1994). Recent statistics on EGC show that intramucosal cancers of the intestinal type have few metastases regardless of the size of lesion, indicating that they can be cured by simple removal of cancerous tissue.

On the other hand, laser endoscopic techniques have also improved and high-power lasers, such as the EDL or Er:YAG lasers are expected to provide a high efficacy of treatment results in deeper invasive gastric cancer. In the near future, therefore, the majority of gastric cancers, particularly those at the early stage, may be managed endoscopically thus avoiding any surgical damage.

REFERENCES

Brown, S.G. (1983). Tumor therapy with the Nd:YAG laser. In *Neodyium-YAG laser in medicine and surgery*, (ed. S.N. Joffee, M. Muckerheide, and L. Goldman), pp. 52–8, Elsevier, New York.

Daikuzono, N. and Joffee, S.N. (1985). Artifical sapphire probe for contact photocoagulation and tissue vaporization with the Nd:YAG laser. *Med. Instrum.*, **19**, 173–8.

Daikuzono N., Tajiri H., Suzuki S., *et al.* (1988). Laserthermia: A new computer-controlled contact Nd:YAG system for interstitial local hyperthermia. *Lasers Surg. Med.* **8**, 254–8.

Deyhle, P., Largiader, F., Jenny, S., *et al.* (1973). A method for endoscopic electroresection of sessile colonic polyps. *Endoscopy*, **5**, 38–40.

Dougherty, T.J., Kaufman, J.E., Doldfarb, A., Weishaupt, K.R., Boyle, D.G., and Mittelman, A. (1978). Photoradiation therapy for the treatment of malignant tumors. *Cancer Res.* **38**, 2628–35.

Hirao, M., Takakuwa, R., Kawashima, H., *et al.* (1988). ERHSE (endscopic resection with local injection of hypertonic saline epinephrine solution) for the treatment of early gastric cancer. *Stom. Intes.*, **23**, 399–409. (In Japanese with English summary)

Mimura, S., Ichii, M., and Okuda, S. (1992). Photodynamic therapy for early gastric cancer using excimer dye laser. In *Photodynamic therapy and biomedical lasers*, (ed. P. Spinelli, D. Fante, and R. Marchesini), pp. 272–6. Elsevier, Amsterdam.

Ohgami, M., Kumai, K., Otani, Y., *et al.* (1994). Laparoscopic wedge resection of the stomach for early gastric cancer using lesion-lifting method. *Dig. Surg* **11**, 64–7.

Oguro Y. and Tajiri H. (1986). The present status of YAG laser medicine in Japan— endoscopic laser treatment for GI cancer. In *Nd-YAG laser in medicine and surgery*, (ed. Y. Oguro, K. Atsumi, and S.N. Joffe), pp. 3–9. Professional Postgraduate Services, Tokyo

Tada, M., Karita, M., Yanai, M., *et al.* (1987). Treatment of early gastric cancer using strip biopsy, a new technique for jumbo biopsy. In *Recent topics of digestive endoscopy*, (ed. T. Takemoto and K. Kawai), pp. 137–42. Japan Excerpta Medica, Tokyo

Tajiri, H. and Oguro, Y. (1978). Contact Nd:YAG laser treatment of gastrointestinal cancer. In *Advances in Nd:YAG laser surgery*, (Ed. S.N. Joffee and Y. Oguro), pp. 74–8 Springer, New York.

Tajiri, H. and Oguro, Y. (1991). Laser endosocpic treatment for upper gastrointestinal cancers. *J. Laparoendoscop. Surg.*, **1**, 71–8.

Takahashi, H., Fujita, R., Sugiyama, K. *et al.* (1991). Endoscopic therapy of early gastric cancer—Comparison of endoscopic mucosal coagulation and resection. *Dig. Endosc.*, **3**, 215–21.

Takemoto, T., Tada, M., Yanai, H., Karita, M. and Okita, K. (1989). Significance of strip biopsy, with particular reference to endoscopic "Mucosectomy". *Dig. Endosc.*, **1**, 4–9.

Uchizawa, M., Hirao, M., Masuda, K., *et al.* (1991). Evaluation of ERHSE (endoscopic resection with local injection of hypertonic saline epinephrine solution) for the treatment of early gastric carcinoma. *Stom. Intes.*, **26**, 275–82. (In Japanese with English summary)

Yamao, T., Shirao, K., Ono, H., *et al.* (1996). Risk factors for lymph node metastasis from intramucosal gastric carcinoma. *Cancer*, **77**, 602–6.

Part VII: Non-surgical treatment

18

Chemotherapy

P. Preusser, W. Achterrath, H. Wilke, D. Cunningham, and P. Euis

1. INTRODUCTION

Despite a declining incidence, gastric cancer remains one of the leading causes of cancer death (Findlay and Cunningham 1993). Surgery is the treatment of choice in the early stages of gastric cancer. However, since up to 80% of patients at the time of diagnosis present gastric cancer which is too far advanced for curative resection, it seems that the disease disseminates early (Findlay and Cunningham 1993; Preusser *et al.* 1988). Therefore, since the 1980s, chemotherapy has been more frequently used in patients with unresectable, locally advanced, or metastatic disease. (Middleton and Cunningham 1995; Wils *et al.* 1994).

Since 1993, two randomized studies have been carried out in order to define the therapeutic value of modern chemotherapeutic regimens versus best supportive care (Pyrhönen *et al.* 1995; Middleton and Cunningham 1995). In both studies, chemotherapy was associated with a statistically significant improvement in median time to disease progression and median survival time. Median survival times of 3 months and 10–12 months were reported for best supportive care and chemotherapy, respectively. Additionally, chemotherapy improved the quality of life compared to treatment with best supportive care only.

The therapeutic outcome obtained with single- and multi-agent chemotherapy are reported in this chapter.

2. SINGLE-AGENT CHEMOTHERAPY

In the analysis of the antineoplastic activity of single drugs one has to consider that response rates published in earlier reviews are often based on summarized results or drug-orientated phase II studies which included mostly heterogenous patient populations and only few patients per tumor type. Furthermore, in the older drug and disease-orientated phase II studies, inclusion criteria and response evaluations were less accurate than today. Re-evaluations of several older agents in more recent studies showed that their antitumor activity was overestimated (Louvet *et al.* 1991; Miller *et al.* 1981; Preusser *et al.* 1988).

The discrepancy in response rates of older and newer studies may occur due to less accurate diagnostic techniques (ultrasonography, computed tomography, etc.) and less strict response criteria and patient selection (Preusser *et al.* 1988; Scher

et al. 1987; Cocconi 1994). The newer studies mostly comprise patients with measurable disease; response and response duration have been evaluated according to
World Health Organization (WHO) criteria (Scher *et al.* 1987; Cocconi 1994).

In the last decade, numerous antineoplastic agents have been investigated as first
line chemotherapy in well-designed disease-orientated phase II trials with ≥14
patients per study. These studies are carried out in accordance with more sophisti-
cated statistical considerations and frequently 14 to 19 patients are initially
enrolled (Edler 1993; Lee *et al.* 1979; Simon 1989).

If no response occurs in the first cohort of patients, the conclusion is drawn that
the response rate is less than 20% with 95–99% confidence and that further investigations with this given agent in this specific tumor type are of less interest. If one
response or more are observed in the first cohort, additional patients have to be
enrolled to estimate the antitumor activity of an agent more precisely (Edler 1993;
Lee *et al.* 1979; Simon 1989). Approximately 25 or 45 patients are necessary to
estimate the response rate within ±20% or ±15% with approximately 95%
confidence (Cullinan *et al.* 1985). The single agents that, as first line chemotherapy
in advanced or metastatic gastric cancer, produce overall response rates of ≥15%
are shown in Table 18.1.

Table 18.1.   First line single agent activity in advanced gastric cancer
(≥14 patients per study)

Drug	No. of patients	Overall remission rate: no. of patients (%)	Study
5-Fluorouracil (5FU)	108	25 (23%) (15–31%)[a]	Kim *et al.* 1995 Preusser *et al.* 1988
S1[b]	28	15 (54%) (35–73%)[a]	Wilke *et al.* 1992
Docetaxel	33	8 (24%) (9–39%)[a]	Sulkes *et al.* 1994
Cisplatin	14	5 (36%) (10–62%)[a]	Preusser *et al.* 1988
Irinotecan	15	5 (33%) (0–57%)[a]	Kambe *et al.* 1993
Etoposide	35	7 (20%) (6–34%)[a]	Ajani *et al.* 1993 Preusser *et al.* 1988
Adriamycin	124	21 (17%) (22–23%)[a]	Preusser *et al.* 1988
Epiadriamycin	58	12 (21%) (10–32%)[a]	Findlay and Cunningham 1991
Mitomycin C	211	63 (30%) (24–36%)[a]	Preusser *et al.* 1988
BCNU	55	10 (18%) (8–28%)[a]	Preusser *et al.* 1988
Triazinate	26	6 (15%) (1–29%)[a]	Findlay and Cunningham 1991

[a] 95% confidence limits; [b] oral combined preparation of Tegafur.

More recent studies suggest that S1, cisplatin, irinotecan, docetaxel, 5FU, etoposide, and anthracyclines may be more active than the other agents shown in Table 18.1. This hypothesis is limited because the standard deviations in the response rates of the most of these agents are too high for making a final conclusion. Relatively low overall response rates in the range of 6–14% and 5–16% have been reported for Epi-ADM (Coombes *et al.* 1994; Loehrer *et al.* 1994; and 5FU (Coombes *et al.* 1994; Colucci *et al.* 1995; Loehrer *et al.* 1994), respectively, in newer randomized trials. Therefore, it appears necessary seems to be important to reconsider their role in the treatment of gastric cancer. Furthermore, controversial results have been reported regarding the enhancement of the antitumor activity of 5FU by biochemical modulation with folinic acid and/or interferon (Louvet *et al.* 1991; Berenberg *et al.* 1995; Wilke *et al.* 1992; Hudes *et al.* 1995; Schipper and Wagner 1996).

The quest for new agents with activity against metastatic gastric cancer has been relatively frustrating. In newer phase II studies, response rates in the range of 0–10% have been achieved with idarubicin, aclacinomycin, mitoxantrone, bisantrene, amsacrine, vindesine, raxozane (Preusser *et al.* 1988), carboplatin (Preusser *et al.* 1990; Beer *et al.* 1987; Einzig *et al.* 1985), Trimetrexate, (Hantel *et al.* 1994*a*), piroxantrone (Hantel *et al.* 1994*b*), fluradabine phosphate (Kilton *et al.* 1994), Brequinar (Moore *et al.* 1993), Paclitaxel (Einzig *et al.* 1995), and Gemcitabine (Guchelaar *et al.* 1996).

Second line chemotherapy for gastric cancer is therapeutic problem because overall response rates of 20% have been reported for only a few agents. These are: cisplatin (Hantel *et al.* 1994), irinotecan (Kambe *et al.* 1993), and docetaxel (Taguchi 1994) (Table 18.2). Fol 5FU, adriamycin, and triazinate showed moderate activity. However, Tomudex, methotrexate, mitoxantrone, etoposide, carboplatin, and razoxane seem to be less active or inactive (Table 18.2).

3. COMBINATION CHEMOTHERAPY

Several efforts have been made to develop multi-agent combinations with higher antitumor activity than the more frequently used single agents. Numerous regimens using two to four drugs have been investigated in non-randomized and randomized trials. The comparison of the antitumor activity obtained with both the same regimens and different combinations in non-randomized trials is limited because of the following reasons:

(1) identical combinations have been administered in different dose schedules;
(2) heterogenous patient population with different prognostic factors for response and survival;
(3) different precise diagnostic techniques; and
(4) different criteria for response and response duration.

The comparison of results obtained with the same combinations in non-randomized phase II trials and randomized phase III studies demonstrated lower response rates mainly in the randomized trials. Even for the same combinations, widely different response rates have been reported in several randomized studies.

Table 18.2.   Single agent activity as second line chemotherapy in gastric cancer

Drug	No. of patients	Overall remission rate: no. of patients (%)	Study
Cisplatin	115	23 (20%) (12–28%)[a]	Preusser *et al.* 1988
Irinotecan	45	9 (20%) (8–32%)[a]	Kambe *et al.* 1933
Docetaxel	15	3 (20%) (0–40%)[a]	Taguchi *et al.* 1994
Fol/5FU	17	3 (17%) (0–35%)[a]	Vanhoefer *et al.* 1994
Adriamycin	78	13 (17%) (8–26%)[a]	Preusser *et al.* 1988
Triazinate	26	4 (15%) (1–29%)[a]	Preusser *et al.* 1988
Methotrexate	28	3 (11%) (0–22%)[a]	Preusser *et al.* 1988
Carboplatin	30	2 (7%) (0–9%)[a]	Preusser *et al.* 1988
Tomudex	33	0	Cunningham *et al.* 1996
Razoxane	19	0	Preusser *et al.* 1988
Mitoxantrone	16	0	Preusser *et al.* 1988
Etoposide	11	0	Preusser *et al.* 1988

[*] 95% confidence limits.

4. NON-RANDOMIZED TRIALS

4.1. Two drug combinations

The first generation of two-drug combinations mainly used 5FU in combination with alkylating agents, such as nitrosoureas, Mitomycin C, or Adriamycin (Preusser *et al.* 1988) (Table 18.3). Overall response rates in the range 22–31% range have been reported for 5FU with the alkylating agents, Adriamycin and mitomycin C (Preusser *et al.* 1988), whereas a less than 10% overall response has been achieved with the combination of 5FU and Adriamycin. The median survival times achieved with all of these regimens ranged from 3 to 8 months (Preusser *et al.* 1988).

During the 1980s, promising antitumor activity was reported in several phase II studies for cisplatin as first and second line chemotherapy in metastatic gastric cancer (Preusser *et al.* 1988). These results led to the development of the second generation of two drug regimens containing 5FU in combination with cisplatin or carboplatin (Preusser *et al.* 1988; Berenberg *et al.* 1995).

The combination of 5FU/cisplatin is more frequently used as first line chemotherapy in advanced gastric cancer because of its relatively high antitumor activity. The summarized data of six phase II studies showed that this regimen produced a 41% overall response with a median survival time of 4–9 months for all patients

Table 18.3. Results of two drug regimens in advanced gastric cancer (≥14 patients per study)

Regimen	No. of patients	No. of studies	CR no.: (%)	CR + PR: no. (%)	mR (mths)	mS (mths)	Study
ADM/5FU	124	3	0	7 (6%) (2–10%)[*]	n.s.	5	Preusser *et al.* 1988
ADM/Mitomycin C	76	2	5 (7%)	17 (22%) (12–32%)[*]	5	4–5	Preusser *et al.* 1988
5FU/Mitomycin C	103	2	n.s.	25 (24%) (16–32%)[*]	3–4	4	Preusser *et al.* 1988
5FU/Methyl-CCNU	180	2	n.s.	36 (20%) (14–26%)[*]	3	3	Preusser *et al.* 1988
5FU/BCNU	62	1	n.s.	19 (31%) (19–43%)[*]	10	8	Preusser *et al.* 1988
5FU/Carboplatin	20	1	0	9 (45%) (23–67%)[*]	n.s.	9	Shirai *et al.* 1993
5FU/Cisplatin	291	6	12 (4%)	120 (41%) (35–47%)[*]	n.s.	4–9	KRGCGC 1992 Lacave *et al.* 1991 Preusser and Wilke 1993 Rougier *et al.* 1994 Shirai *et al.* 1995
Fol/5FU/Cisplatin	75	2	8 (11%)	42 (56%) (45–67%)[*]	n.s.	8/11–14[*]	Wilke *et al.* 1995 Ychou *et al.* 1994
Fol/5FU/MTX	28	1	1 (4%)	12 (43%) (23–63%)[*]	7	9	Romero *et al.* 1996
Fol/Doxifluiridin/MTX	21	1	1 (5%)	8 (38%) (17–59%)[*]	n.s.	n.s.	Aschele *et al.* 1996
Fol/5FU/Etoposide	84	2	8 (10%)	38 (45%) (34–56%)[*]	4–8	8–12	de Braud *et al.* 1993 Preusser and Wilke 1993 Louvet *et al.* 1991

[*] 95% confidence limits.

CR, complete remission; PR, partial remission; mR, median remission; mS, medium survival.

(KRGCGC 1992; Lacave *et al.* 1991; Preusser and Wilke 1993; Rougier *et al.* 1994; Shirai *et al.* 1995). Comparable antitumor activity has been reported for the combination of 5FU and carboplatin in a phase II study (Preusser *et al.* 1988). The antineoplastic activity of 5FU/carboplatin is possibly overestimated because of the small number of patients and because carboplatin demonstrates only marginal activity in gastric cancer (Preusser *et al.* 1990; Beer *et al.* 1987; Einzig *et al.* 1985). Therefore, the lower limit of 95% confidence interval may be the true response rate for this combination (Shirai *et al.* 1993).

Another innovation in chemotherapy for gastric cancer was the exploitation of some biochemical modulators of 5FU involving folinic acid and/or methotrexate (Cocconi 1994). The third generation of two drug regimens mainly used Fol/5FU in combination with cisplatin or etoposide (de Braud *et al.* 1993; Preusser and Wilke 1993; Louvet *et al.* 1991; Wilke *et al.* 1995; Ychou *et al.* 1994). 56% overall response, including a 11% complete remission and a median survival time of 11–14 months, has been achieved with Fol/5FU/cisplatin (Wilke *et al.* 1995a; Ychou *et al.* 1994). The combination of Fol/5FU/etoposide produced, compared to above combinations, a slightly lower overall response rate, but the complete response rate and median survival time were within the same range (de Braud *et al.* 1993; Preusser and Wilke 1993; Louvet *et al.* 1991; Wilke *et al.* 1995b; Ychou *et al.* 1994).

A comparison of the first-generation regimens to the two second and third-generation combinations showed that the addition of cisplatin or etoposide to 5FU or Fol/5FU improved the antitumor activity in all studies of 5FU-based regimens regarding overall response rates, complete response rates, and sometimes median survival times (de Braud *et al.* 1993; KRGCGC 1992; Lacave *et al.* 1991; Preusser *et al.* 1988; Preusser and Wilke 1993; Louvet *et al.* 1991; Rougier *et al.* 1994; Wilke *et al.* 1995b; Ychou *et al.* 1994; Shirai *et al.* 1995).

4.2. Multidrug combinations

Only those studies with ≥ 45 patients were evaluated because this number allows an estimation of standard deviations of response rates within a range of ± 15%, and lower, with approximately 95% confidence (Table 18.4).

The combination of 5FU/ADM/Mitomycin C (FAM) was most widely used as a first-generation regimen in the 1980s. Results of FAM in various dose schedules are reported from more than 750 patients with a cumulative overall response rate of 28% including 2% complete remission. The median remission duration was 5–10 months and the median survival time of the whole group was 6–10 months.

The addition of BCNU to FAM and the replacement of Mitomycin C by methyl-CCNU did not enhance the antitumor activity compared to the original regimen (Preusser *et al.* 1988; Preusser and Wilke 1993). In contrast, the substitution of Mitomycin C by BCNU or cisplatin revealed increases of overall response rates without improving median remission duration and median survival time (Figoli *et al.* 1991; Preusser *et al.* 1988; Preusser and Wilke 1993). Due to the low anti-tumor activity and the delayed toxicity associated with FAM, several so-called second generation multidrug combinations have been developed.

Table 18.4. Results of more frequently used three or four drug combinations (≥45 patients per combination) in advanced gastric cancer

Regimen	No. of patients	No. of studies	CR no.: (%)	CR + PR: no. (%)	mR (mths)	mS (mths)	Study
FAM	755	18	12 (2%) (1–3%)*	209 (28%) (25–31%)*	5–10	6–10*	Figoli et al. 1991; Preusser et al. 1988; Preusser and Wilke 1993
FAMe	83	3	10 (12%) (5–19%)*	20 (24%) (15–33%)*	5	6–8	Preusser et al. 1988; Preusser and Wilke 1993
FAM + BCNU	75	3	3 (4%) (0–8%)*	23 (31%) (20–42%)*	4–6+	8	Preusser et al. 1988
FAB	85	2	5 (6%) (1–11%)*	42 (49%) (38–60%)*	9	7	Preusser et al. 1988; Preusser and Wilke 1993
FAP	187	8	9 (5%) (2–8%)*	68 (36%) (29–43%)*	5–7	6–13	Preusser et al. 1988; Preusser and Wilke 1993
FAMTX	217	4	24 (11%) (7–15%)*	118 (54%) (47–61%)*	5–9	3–10	Murad et al. 1993; Preusser et al. 1988; Preusser and Wilke 1993; Louvet et al. 1991
FEMTXP	48	1	5 (10%) (1–19%)*	23 (48%) (34–62%)*	8+	10	Conroy et al. 1993; Louvet et al. 1991
EAP	582	15	49 (8%) (6–10%)*	243 (42%) (38–46%)*	5–7	3–16	Preusser et al. 1988; Preusser and Wilke 1993; Ridolfi et al. 1993; Louvet et al. 1991; Roth et al. 1996; Bajetta et al. 1994; Clark et al. 1995
5FU/Pt/Epi-ADM	399	4	49 (12%) (9–15%)*	206 (52%) (47–57%)*	7–10	8–9+	Delfino et al. 1991; Di Lauro et al. 1995; Findlay et al. 1994; Cervantes et al. 1993; Zaniboni et al. 1995
Fol/5FU/Pt/Epi-ADM	84	2	13 (15%) (7–23%)*	57 (68%) (58–78%)*	7	9–14	Cascinu et al. 1995; Cascinu et al. 1994
Fol/5FU/Pt/ADM	46	2	3 (7%) (0–15%)*	24 (52%) (37–67%)*	7	14	Vaughn et al. 1995; Errichani et al. 1995
Fol/5FU/Pt/Etoposide	117	3	13 (11%) (5–17%)*	63 (54%) (46–62%)*	5	9–11	Cheng et al. 1996; Gonzalez-Baron et al. 1995; Wilke et al. 1994

* 95% confidence limits. (See Table 18.3 for explanation of abbreviations.)

The second-generation three drug regimens, such as FAMTX or FEMTX, EAP, and 5FU/Pt/Epi-ADM, are widely used and the summarized results acquired with each of these regimens are based on the analysis of more than 250 patients treated in clinical studies (see Table 18.4). Response rates in the range of 40–50%, including approximately 10% complete remissions with a median remission duration of 5–10 months and a median survival time for the whole group of 8–16 months, were reported for the second-generation regimens in most studies.

The third generation of three drug combinations consisted of Fol/5FU and cisplatin as a basis and extended these basic regimens with by the addition of anthracyclines or etoposide (Cascinu *et al.* 1995; Vaughn *et al.* 1995; Errihani *et al.* 1995; Cheng *et al.* 1996; González-Barón *et al.* 1995; Wilke *et al.* 1994; Bajetta *et al.* 1994). All these regimens produced a more than 50% overall response rate with a median survival time within the range of 9–14 months. This therapeutic outcome is similar to that obtained by the basic combination in terms of overall response rates, complete response rates, median remission duration, and median survival time (Cascinu *et al.* 1994, 1995; Vaughn *et al.* 1995; Errihani *et al.* 1995; Wilke *et al.* 1995*b*; Ychou *et al.* 1994; Cascinu *et al.* 1994; Taguchi 1994).

Both the second and the third generation of three drug regimens produce higher complete and overall response rates than the older standard FAM. The comparison of complete and overall response rates obtained with the second- and third-generation regimens revealed no significant differences in most studies, but the results of a few studies did show some advantage rates (see Tables 18.3 and 18.4). The impact of the second- and third-generation three drug regimens on the median remission duration is less evident. The comparison of median survival time obtained with FAM and the second-generation combinations showed no significant differences (See Tables 18.3 and 18.4). However, there are several studies with third-generation regimens which suggest that this regimen seems to be slightly superior to FAM as well as the second -generation regimens, in terms of median survival time (Cascinu *et al.* 1994, 1995; Vaughn *et al.* 1995; Errihani *et al.* 1995; Wilke *et al.* 1994, 1995; Ychou *et al.* 1994; Cheng *et al.* 1996; González-Barón *et al.* 1995; Cascinu *et al.* 1994).

5. RANDOMIZED TRIALS

Single agents versus single agents or combinations

Table 18.5 shows 10 two- to three-arm randomized trials comparing single agents to single agents and/or combination chemotherapies, and 9 two- or three-arm randomized trials comparing single agents to multi-agent combinations.

The single-agent activity of 5FU and epirubicin was investigated in two more recent two- or three-arm randomized studies (Coombes *et al.* 1994; Loehrer *et al.* 1994). Overall response rates of 5% and 10% and 6% and 14% have been reported for 5FU and Epi-ADM, respectively (Coombes *et al.* 1994; Wilke *et al.* 1992).

The combination of 5FU/Epi-ADM produced only 12% overall responses in one of these studies whereas 41% overall responses have been reported for this combination in another randomized trial (Preusser *et al.* 1988; Loehrer *et al.* 1994).

Table 18.5. Results of randomized trials comparing single agents or single agents with polychemotherapies in advanced gastric cancer

Regimen	No. of patients	CR + PR (%)	mS (mths)	Study
5FU	25	16	5, 5	Coombes *et al.* 1994
Epi-ADM	28	14	5, 5	
5FU	30	20	n.s.	Preusser *et al.* 1988
5FU/Epi-ADM	32	41	n.s.	
5FU	40	5	5	Loehrer *et al.* 1994
Epi-ADM	16	6	7	
5FU/Epi-ADM	33	12	7	
Fol/5FU	31	29	8	Colucci *et al.* 1995
Fol/5FU/Epi-ADM	31	41	10	
ADM	37	22	4	Preusser *et al.* 1988
5FU/Mitomycin C	53	32	4, 5	
5FU/Methyl-CCNU	49	24	4	
ADM	70	13	5	Preusser *et al.* 1988
FAB[a]	75	40	8	
5FU	41	15	7	Preusser *et al.* 1988
FAM/BCNU	41	22	7	
5FU	14	21	10	Preusser *et al.* 1988
FAM	17	24	9	
5FU	51	18	7	Wils 1992
5FU/ADM	49	27	7	
PAM	51	38	7	
5FU	54	26	8	Kim *et al.* 1995
FAM	57	25	7	
5FU/Pt[b]	55	51	9	

[a] FAB statistically superior to ADM in terms of overall response rate and median survival time.
[b] 5FU/cisplatin statistically superior to 5FU and FAM in terms of overall response rate.
(See Table 18.3 for explanation of abbreviations.)

The single-agent activity of both Adriamycin and 5FU, had been investigated in two and four older randomized studies (Kim *et al.* 1995; Preusser *et al.* 1988; Wils 1992). Response rates of 13–22% and of 15–26% have been obtained in these studies with Adriamycin (Preusser *et al.* 1988) and 5FU (Kim *et al.* 1995; Preusser *et al.* 1988; Wils, 1992), respectively.

Single-agent 5FU has been compared with FAM ± BCNU in 3 two- or three-arm randomized studies (Preusser *et al.* 1988; Wils 1992). No statistically significant advantages for the multi-agent combinations has been observed in terms of overall response rates and median survival time (Preusser *et al.* 1988; Wils 1992). The antitumor activity of 5FU in combination with the biochemical modulator folinic acid was compared with Fol/5FU/Epi-ADM in one randomized study. 29% and 41% overall responses have been obtained with Fol/5FU and Fol/5FU/Epi-ADM, respectively (Colucci *et al.* 1995).

Only two of nine randomized studies comparing single agents with multi-agent combinations showed a statistically significant therapeutic advantage of combination chemotherapy over single agents. FAB produced statistically significant higher

Chemotherapy

overall response rates and median survival time than ADM (Preusser *et al.* 1988) and Pt/5FU provided statistically higher overall response rates in comparison to FAM and 5FU (Kim *et al.* 1995).

6. MULTI-AGENT COMBINATIONS

More frequently applied multi-agent combinations have been investigated in 8 two- to four-arm randomized studies (Table 18.6). The first-generation regimens FAM or FEM have been compared to other first-generation regimens such as FAM or PAM in two randomized trials. No statistically significant differences in the palliative outcome had been observed in terms of overall response rate and median survival time (Preusser *et al.* 1988; De Lisi *et al.* 1996).

Three randomized studies compared first-generation regimens FAM or FEM to second-generation combinations (Diaz-Rubio *et al.* 1992; Jcli *et al.* 1993; Preusser *et al.* 1988). The results obtained with FAM or FEM and EEP, EAP, and FAMTX revealed statistically significant advantages for the second-generation regimens in

Table 18.6. Randomized trials of first line polychemotherapy in advanced gastric cancer

Regimen	No. of patients	CR (%)	CR + PR (%)	mS (mths)	Study
FAM[a]	46	4	39	7	Preusser *et al.* 1988
FAMe	39	10	28	6	
Mitomycin C/ADM	46	7	28	5	
5FU/MeCCNU	44	3	13	3	
FAM	46	2	28	6	De Lissi *et al.* 1996
PAM	50	8	30	7	
FEM	42	5	17	7	Tsavaris *et al.* 1995
FEM + FA[b]	43	0	26	8	
FAM	79	0	9	7	Wils *et al.* 1991
FAMTX[a]	81	6	41	10	
FAM	43	2	14	7	Jcli *et al.* 1993
EAP[b]	47	13	40	5	
FEM	55	6	13	4	
EEP[a]	43	5	30	8	Diaz-Rubio *et al.* 1992
EAP	30	0	20	6	Kelsen *et al.* 1992
FAMTX	30	10	33	7	
FAMTX[1]	45	ne	20	7	Wilke *et al.* 1995
ELF	42	ne	21	7	
Pt/5FU	44	ne	27	8	
FAMTX	49	n	15	ne	Massuti *et al.* 1995
Fol/5FU/Epi-ADM/Pt	47	n	12	ne	

[a] Overall response rate and median survival statistically significantly better.
[b] Overall response rate statistically significantly higher.
(See Table 18.3 for explanation of abbreviations.) ne: not evaluated, n: not reported.

terms of response rates in all studies (Diaz-Rubio *et al.* 1992; Jcli *et al.* 1993; Wils *et al.* 1991), and in terms of median survival time in two studies (Diaz-Rubio *et al.* 1992; Wils *et al.* 1991). In these studies, EEP and FAMTX were associated with a statistically significant improvement of median survival time when compared to first-generation regimens (Diaz-Rubio *et al.* 1992; Wils *et al.* 1991).

Two randomized trails compared second-generation combinations (Kelsen *et al.* 1992; Wilke *et al.* 1995b), and one study compared second-generation regimens to third-generation combinations (Massuti *et al.* 1995). The trial comparing FAMTX with ELF and Pt/5FU showed overlapping results for all investigated regimens in terms of overall response rates and median survival time but ELF was less toxic than the other regimens. No statistically significant differences were observed in terms of response rates when FAMTX was compared to the third-generation combination Fol/5FU, Epi-ADM/Pt (Massuti *et al.* 1995).

7. SUMMARY

7.1. Single agents

Overall response rates of ≥20% have been reported in more recent non-randomized phase II studies for SI, irinotecan, docetazel, cisplatin, and etoposide as first line chemotherapy in advanced or metastatic gastric cancer (Ajani *et al.* 1993; Kambe *et al.* 1993; Preusser *et al.* 1988; Wilke *et al.* 1992; Sulkes *et al.* 1994). Response rates of ≥20% have been obtained in older disease-oriented phase II studies with 5FU, Adriamycin and Epirubicin (Findlay and Cunningham 1993; (Kim *et al.* 1995; Preusser *et al.* 1988). However, more recent, randomized studies showed that the response rates for these agents are in the rage of 6–16% (Coombes *et al.* 1994; Loehrer *et al.* 1994; Preusser *et al.* 1988). Therefore, it seems to be important to reconsider their role in the first line chemotherapies of gastric cancer.

Controversial results have been reported concerning the antitumor activity of 5FU in combination with biochemical modulators, such as folinic acid or interferon (Berenberg *et al.* 1995; Wilke *et al.* 1992; Hudes *et al.* 1995).

The second line chemotherapy of gastric cancer is clinical problem because response rates of ≥15% have been reported for five agents only: cisplatin (Preusser *et al.* 1988), irinotecan (Kambe *et al.* 1993); docetaxel (KRGCGC 1992), Fol/5FU, and Adriamycin (Vanhoefer *et al.* 1994).

Because of the single-agent activity demonstrated in newer disease orientated phase II studies, the following agents can be considered suitable for first line combination chemotherapy in gastric cancer: 5FU ± folinic acid, cisplatin, irinotecan, etoposide, docetaxel, and anthracyclines such as ADM or Epirubicin.

8. COMBINATION CHEMOTHERAPY

The most widely used first-generation regimen in the 1980s was FAM. The low antitumor activity and the delayed toxicity associated with FAM led to the development of second-generation regimens. The comparison of the results obtained with the first-generation regimens to the more frequently used second-generation combinations, such as FAMTX, cisplatin/5FU, cisplatin 5FU/Epirubicin, EAP, and ELF, revealed statistically significant advantages of second-generation combinations in terms of complete and overall response rates in non-randomized studies (Delfino *et al.* 1991; KRGCG 1992; Lacave *et al.* 1991; Murad *et al.* 1993; Preusser *et al.* 1988; Preusser and Wilke 1993; Louvet *et al.* 1991; Di Lauro *et al.* 1995; Rougier *et al.* 1994; Shirai *et al.* 1995; Cheng *et al.* 1996; González-Barón *et al.* 1995; Wilke *et al.* 1994; Findlay *et al.* 1994; Cervantes *et al.* 1993; Zaniboni *et al.* 1995; Roth *et al.* 1996; Bajetta *et al.* 1994; Clark *et al.* 1995) and randomized studies (Diaz-Rubio *et al.* 1992; Jcli *et al.* 1993; Kim *et al.* 1995; Wils *et al.* 1994).

The impact of the second-generation regimens on median remission duration and median survival is less pronounced. But in two randomized studies the second-generation regimens were associated with a prolongation of the median survival time when compared with FAM or FEM (Diaz-Rubio *et al.* 1992; Preusser *et al.* 1988). All second-generation regimens induced similar results regarding complete response rates, overall response rates, median remission duration, and median survival time in non-randomized and randomized trials (see Table 18.6).

Because of the relatively low toxicity of ELF in comparison to the other second-generation combinations this regimen is regarded suitable for patients at risk (Wilke *et al.* 1995*b*).

The third generation of multi-agent combinations used Fo1/5FU and cisplatin as a basic combination. Antharacyclines or etoposide are more frequently used as third combination partners. All the third-generation regimens produce a more than 50% overall response with a median survival time of 9–14 months.

The impact of anthracyclines or etoposide on the antitumor activity of Fol/5FU/cisplatin is uncertain. The therapeutic outcome obtained with the basic combination and the other third-generation regimens is similar in terms of overall response rates, complete response rates, median remission duration, and median survival time. The comparison of the therapeutic outcome obtained with the more frequently used second-generation regimens, such as FAMTX, EAP, ELF, Pt/5FU ± Epirubicin with the third-generation combinations, such as Fol/5FU/Pt ± Anthracyclines or etoposide, revealed a small advantage in third-generation regimens in terms of overall response rate and median survival time. However, these benefits must be confirmed in randomized trails, and the European Organization for Research and Treatment of Cancer (EORTC) has initiated a randomized study that compares the second-generation regimen FAMTX to the third-generation regimen Fol/5FU/cisplatin and other regimens.

9. REPORTING RESULTS OF CLINICAL TRIALS

For adequate evaluation of chemotherapy there is a need for stratified and randomized trials with a sufficient number of patients with measurable disease. Results should be reported in terms of remission rates, median remission duration, and median survival time according to the guidelines of WHO or SWOG. Toxicity may be graded by these guidelines or by the NCI rating scale. Furthermore, the percentages of 1 to 3 year survivors should be reported. The 95% confidence limits for response rates, median remission duration, and for the percentages of 1- to 3-year survivors and of the toxicities should also be given. The results should be compared with adequate statistical tests in order to achieve an accurate conclusion with supporting evidence (Kaplan and Meier 1958; Miller *et al.* 1981; Preusser and Wilke 1993).

10. FUTURE DIRECTIONS

Despite the declining incidence of gastric cancer, this tumor entity remains a therapeutic problem because more than two-thirds of patients die of this disease.

The analysis of the results of chemotherapy in metastatic disease demonstrates that the second- and third-generation regimens produce significantly higher complete and overall response rates than first-generation combinations. However, the impact on median remission duration and median survival time is less evident. A comparison of the therapeutic value of the more frequently used second-and third-generation regimens show an advantage for the third-generation regimens in terms of overall response rates and median survival time, but these advantages are small and must be confirmed in randomized trials. The incorporation of irinotecan, docetaxel and newer fluoropyrimidines in third-generation regimens and the development of new agents with high antitumor activity will become a major focus of investigation in the chemotherapy of gastric cancer.

In the uphill struggle towards a substantial improvement of response rates, especially in complete response rates by newer chemotherapy regimens should improve survival in advanced or metastatic gastric cancer. A further improvement in the treatment of gastric cancer may be achieved by a stage-and risk-adapted, multimodal treatment including chemotherapy, radiotherapy, and surgery.

Encouraging results were reported in several phase II studies with the second-generation regimens in the preoperative treatment of non-resectable and resectable locally advanced gastric cancer (Wils *et al.* 1994). In the non-resectable stage of disease a median survival time of 14–19 months for all patients and 18–29 months for patients with RO resections was achieved. The percentage of 2 year-survivors is within the range of 30–40%. These results suggest that preoperative chemotherapy may improve the prognosis of patients with non-resectable and resectable locally advanced stomach cancer.

The therapeutic value and the claims for additional treatments of preoperative chemotherapy, such as intraperitoneal chemotherapy and radiation, have to be investigated in future trials.

REFERENCES

Ajani, J., Dumas, P., Pazdur, R., Mansfield, P., and Ota, D. (1993). Phase II trial of oral etoposide in untreated patients with advanced gastric carcinoma. *Proc. Am. Soc. Clin. Oncol.*, **12** (abstr.), 659.

Aschele, C., Guglielmi, A., Tixi, L., Grossi, F., Caroti, C., Rosso, R., *et al.* (1996). High activity and low toxicity of alternating bolus fluorouracil, modulated by methotrexate, and oral doxifluridine, modulated by 6-S-leucovorin, in advanced gastric cancer. *Proceedings of ASCO*, **15** (abstr.), 545.

Bajetta, E., Di Bartolormeo, M., de Braud, F., Bozzetti, F., Bochicchio, A.M., Comella, P., *et al.* (1994). Etoposide, doxorubicin and cisplatin (EAP) treatment in advanced gastric carcinoma: a multicentre study of the Italian Trials in Medical Oncology (ITMO) group. *Eur. J. Cancer*, **30A**, 596–600.

Beer, M., Cavalli, F., Kaye, S.B., Lev, L.M., Clavel, M., Smyth, J., *et al.* (1987). A phase II study of carboplatin in advanced or metastatic stomach cancer. *Eur. J. Cancer Clin. Oncol.*, **23**, 1565–7.

Berenberg, J.L., Tangen, C.M.S., Macdonald, J.S., Hutchins, L.F., Natale, R.B., Oishi, N., *et al.* (1995). Phase II study of 5-fluorouracil and folinic acid in the treatment of patients with advanced gastric cancer. *Cancer*, **76** (suppl. 5), 715–19.

Cascinu, S., Fedeli, A., Luzi Fedeli, S., and Catalano, G. (1994). Intensive weekly chemotherapy for advanced gastric cancer using 5-fluorouracil, cisplatin, epirubicin, 6S-leucovorin and granulocyte-colony-stimulating factor. In *Cancer treatment: An update*, (ed. P. Banzet, J.F. Holland, D. Khayat, and M. Weil), pp. 405–10. Springer Verlag,

Cascinu, S., Cordella, L., Del Ferro, E., Fronzoni, M., and Catalano, G. (1995). Neuroprotective effect of reduced glutathione on cisplatin-based chemotherapy in advanced gastric cancer: A randomized double-blind placebo-controlled trial. *J. Clin. Oncol.*, **13**, 26–32.

Cervantes, A., Villar-Grimalt, A., Abad, A., Anton-Torres, A., Belón, J., Dorta, J., *et al.* (1993). 5-fluorouracil. Folinic acid, epidoxorubicin and cisplatin (FLEP) combination chemotherapy in advanced measurable gastric cancer. A phase II trial of the Spanish Cooperative Group for Gastrointestinal Tumor Therapy (TTD). *Annals Oncol.*, **4**, 753–7.

Cheng, A.L., Yeh, K.H., Chen, Y.C., Lin, J.T., Chen, B.R., Liu, M.Y., *et al.* (1996). PE-HDFL An effective combination chemotherapy for advanced gastric cancers. *Proceedings of ASCO*, **15** (abstr.), 1582.

Clark, J.L., Küçük, Ö., Neuberg, D.S., Benson III, A.B., Taylor IV, S.G., Pandya, K.J., *et al.* (1995). Phase II trial of etoposide, doxorubicin, and cisplatin combination in advanced measurable gastric cancer. *Am. J. Clin. Oncol.*, **18**, 18–324.

Cocconi, G. (1994). Chemotherapy of advanced gastric carcinoma: To be completely re-written? *Annals Oncol.*, **5**, 8–11.

Colucci, G., Giotta, F., Maiello, E., Cifarelli, R.A., Leo, S., Giuliani, F., *et al.* (1995). Efficacy of the association of folinic acid and 5-fluorouracil alone versus folinic acid and 5-fluorouracil plus 4-epidoxorubicin in the treatment of advanced gastric carcinoma. *Am. J. Clin. Oncol.*, **18**, 519–24.

Conroy, T., Wils, J., Paillot, B., Wagener, D.J.T., Burghouts, J.T.M., Fickers, M.M.F., *et al.* (1993). Association de 5-FU, methotrexate a haute dose, epirubicine et cisplatine (FEMTX-P) dans les cancers gastriques metastatiques, inoperables ou en recidive locale. *Cancer*, **80**, 255–60.

Coombes, R.C., Chilvers, C.E.D., Amadori, D., Medi, F., Fountzilas, G., Rauschecker, H., *et al.* (1994). Randomized trial of epirubicin versus fluorouracil in advanced gastric cancer. *Annals Oncol.*, 5, 33–6.

Cullinan, S.A., Moertel C.G., Fleming, Th.R., Rubin, J.R., Krook, J.E., Everson, L.K., *et al.* (1985). A comparison of three chemotherapeutic regimens in the treatment of advanced pancreatic and gastric carcinoma. *JAMA*, 253, 2061–6.

Cunningham, D., Zalcberg, J., Smith, I., Gore, M., Pazdur, R., Burris, H., III, *et al.* and the Tomudex International Study Group (1996). Tomudex (ZD 1694). A novel thymidylate synthase inhibitor with clinical antitumor activity in a range of solid tumors. International Study Group. *Annals Oncol.*, 7, 179–82.

de Braud, F., Bajetta, E., Di Bartolomeo, M., and Buzoni, R. (1993). Etoposide, leucovorin and fluorouracil (ELF) regimen in the treatment of advanced gastric cancer (ACG). An Italian trial in medical oncology (ITMO) study. *Proc. Am. Soc. Clin. Oncol.*, 12 (Abstr.), 632.

De Lisi, V., Cocconi, G., Angelini, F., Cavicchi, F., Di Constanzo, F., Gilli, G., *et al.* (1996). The combination of cisplatin, doxorubicin, and mitomycin (PAM) compared with the FAM regimen in treating advanced gastric carcinoma. *Cancer*, 77, 245–50.

Delfino, C., Caccia, G., Fein, L., and Chirino, M.(1991). Cisplatin (C), epirubicin (E), and 5-fluorouracil (F) in patients (pts) with advanced gastric cancer (AGC). *Eur. J. Cancer*, 27 (suppl. 2, abstr.), 457.

Di Lauro, L., Capomolla, E., Vici, P., Carpano, S., Gionfra, T., Amodio, A., *et al.* (1995). Cisplatin, epirubicin and fluorouracil (PEF) for advanced measurable gastric carcinoma. *Proceedings of ASCO*, 14 (abstr.), 503.

Diaz-Rubio, E., Jimeno, J., Aranda, E., Massuti, B., Camps, C., Cervantes, A., *et al.* (1992). Etopiside (E) + epirubicin (E) + cisplatin (P) combination chemotherapy (EEP) in advanced gastric cancer negative impact on clinical outcome. *Annals Oncol.*, 3, 861–3.

Edler, L. (1993). Phase-II-Studien in der Onkologie: Wieviele Patienten sind erforderlich? *Tumordiagn.u.Ther.*, 14, 1–9.

Einzig, A., Kelsen, D.P., Cheng, E.,Sordillo, P., Heelan, R., Winn, R., *et al.* (1985). Phase II trial of carboplatin in patients with adenocarcinomas of the upper gastrointestinal tract. *Cancer Treat. Rep.*, 69, 1453–4.

Einzig, A.I., Lipsitz, S., Wiernik, P.H., Benson, A.B., III (1995). Phase II trial of Taxol in patients with adenocarcinoma of the upper gastrointestinal tract (UGIT). *Invest. New Drugs*, 13, 223–7.

Errihani, H., Musset, M., Cvitkovic, E., Soulie, P., Regensberg, R., Jasmin, C., *et al.* (1995). Combination of monthly THP-Adriamycin, cisplatin, FU/FA and Mitomycin C (THP-FFPM) in metastatic gastric carcinoma (MGC). *Proceedings of ASCO*, 14 (abstr.), 495.

Figoli, F., Galligioni, E., Crivellari, D., Frustraci, S., Talamini, R., Sorio, R., *et al.* (1991). Evaluation of two consecutive regimens in advanced gastric cancer. *Cancer Invest.*, 9, 257–62.

Findlay, M. and Cunningham, D. (1993). Chemotherapy of carcinoma of the stomach. *Cancer Treat. Rev.*, 19, 29–44.

Findlay, M., Cunningham, D., Norman, A., Mansi, J., Nicolson, M., Hickish, T., *et al.* (1994). A phase II study in advanced gastroesophageal cancer using epirubicin and cisplatin in combination with continuous infusion 5-fluorouracil (ECF). *Annals Oncol.*, 5, 609–16.

Gastrointestinal Malignancies, January 9–12, 1995, pp. 50.

González-Barón, M., Feliu, J., Espinosa, E., Garcia-Giron, C., Chacon, I., Garrido, P., *et al.* (1995). Treatment of advanced gastric cancer with the combination fluorouracil, leucovorin, etoposide, and cisplatin: A phase II study of the ONCOPAZ cooperative group. *Cancer Chemother. Pharmacol.*, **36**, 255–8.

Guchelaar, H.-J., Richel, D.J., and van Knapen, A. (1996). Clinical, toxicological and pharmacological aspects of Gemcitabine. *Cancer Treat. Rev.*, **22**, 15–31.

Hantel, A., Tangen, C.M., Macdonald, J.S., Richman, S.P., Pugh, R.P., and Pollock, Th. (1994*a*). Phase II trial of Trimetrexate in untreated advanced gastric carcinoma. *Invest. New Drugs*, **12**, 155–7.

Hantel, A., Tangen, C., Gluck, W.L., and Macdonald, J.S. (1994*b*). Phase II trial of piroxantrone in gastric carcinoma. *Invest. New Drugs*, **12**, 159–61.

Hudes, G., Lipsitz, S., Grem, J., Kugler, J., Weiner, L., and Benson, A. III (1995). Phase II study of interferon α-2A (IFN) in combination with 5-fluorouracil (5-FU) plus calcium leucovorin (LV) in metastatic or recurrent gastric carcinoma: An eastern cooperative oncology group study. *Proceedings of ASCO*, **14**, 467.

Jcli, F., Karaoguz, H., Dincol, D, Günel, N., Demirkazik, A., Üner, A., *et al.* (1993). Comparison of EAP and FAM combination chemotherapies in advanced gastric cancer. *Proc. Am. Soc. Clin. Oncol.*, **12** (abstr.), 619.

Kambe, M., Wakui, P., Nakao, I., Futatsuki, K., Sakata, Y., Yoshino, M., *et al.* (1993). A late phase II study of Irinotecan (CPT-11) in patients with advanced gastric cancer. *Proc. Am. Soc. Clin. Oncol.*, **12** (abstr.), 584.

Kaplan, H.S. and Meier. P.(1958). Nonparametric estimation from incomplete observations. *Am. Stat. Assoc. J.*, **53**, 457–80.

Kelsen, D., Atiq, O.T., Saltz, L., Niedzwiecki, D., Ginn, D., Chapman, D., *et al.* (1992). FAMTX versus etoposide, doxorubicin, and cisplatin: A random assignment trial in gastric cancer. *J. Clin. Oncol.*, **4**, 541-N8.

Kilton, L.J., Ashenhurst, J.B., Wade, J.L.III, Schilsky, R.L., Shiomoto, G., Blough, R.R., *et al.* (1994). Phase II study of fludarabine phosphate for gastric carcinoma. An Illinois Cancer Center Trial. *Invest. New Drugs*, **12**, 163–6.

Kim, N., Park, Y., Heo, D., Suh, C., Kim, S., Park, K., *et al.* (1995). A phase III randomized study of 5-fluorouracil and cisplatin versus 5-fluorouracil, doxorubicin, and mitomycin C versus 5-fluorouracil alone in the treatment of advanced gastric cancer. *Cancer*, **12**, 3813–18.

(KRGCGC) (Kyoto Research Group for Chemotherapy of Gastric Cancer) (1992). A randomized, comparative study of combination chemotherapies in advanced gastric cancer. 5-fluorouracil and cisplatin (FP) versus 5-fluorouracil, cisplatin, and epirubicin (FPEPIR). *Anticancer Res.*, **12**, 1983–8.

Lacave, A.J., Elaron, F.J., Anton, L.M., Estrada, E., De Sande, L.M.G., Palacio, I., *et al.* (1991). Combination chemotherapy with cisplatin and 5-fluorouracil 5-day infusion in the therapy of advanced gastric cancer: A phase II trial. *Annals Oncol.*, **2**, 751–4.

Lee, Y.J., Staquet, M., Simon, R., Catane, R., and Muggia, F. (1979). Two-stage plans for patient accrual in phase II cancer clinical trials. *Cancer Treat. Rep.*, **63**, 1721–6.

Loehrer, P.J., Sr., Harry, D., and Chlebowski, R.T.(1994). 5-Fluorouracil vs. epirubicin vs. 5-fluorouracil plus epirubicin in advanced gastric carcinoma. *Invest. New Drugs*, **12**, 57–63.

Louvet, C., de Gramont, a., Demuynck, B., Nordlinger, B., Maisani, J.E., Lagadec, B., *et al.* (1991). Short report, high-dose folinic acid, 5-fluorouracil bolus and continuous infusion in poor-prognosis patients with advanced measurable gastric cancer. *Annals Oncol.*, **2**, 229–30.

Massuti, B., Cervantes, A., Aranda, E., Abad, A., Anton, A., Jara, C., *et al.* (1995). A phase III multicenter randomized study in advanced gastric cancer (GC): fluorouracil + leucovorin + epirubicin + cisplatin (FLEP) versus fluorouracil + adriamycin + methotrexate + leucovorin (FAMTX). *Second International Conference on Biology, Prevention and Treatment of Gastrointestinal Malignancies*, 9–12 January, (abstr.) p. 50.

Middleton, G. and Cunningham, D. (1995). Current options in the management of gastrointestinal cancer. *Annals Oncol.*, **6**, (suppl. 1), 17–26.

Miller, A.B., Hoogstraten, B., Staquet, M., and Winkler, A. (1981). Reporting results of cancer treatment. *Cancer*, **47**, 207–14.

Mitomycin C, and leucovorin (FEM-LV) in advanced gastric carcinoma (AGC). A randomized trial. *Second International Conference on Biology. Prevention and Treatment of Gastrointestinal Malignancies*, 9–12, January, (abstr.), p. 70.

Moore, M., Maroun, J., Robert, F., Natale, R., Neidhart, J., Dallaire, B., *et al.* (1993). Multicenter phase II study of brequinar sodium in patients with advanced gastrointestinal cancer. *Invest. New Drugs*, **11**, 61–5.

Murad, A.M., Santiago, F.F., Petroianu, A., Rocha, P.R.S., Rodrigues, M.A.G., and Rausch, M. (1993). Modified therapy with 5-fluorouracil, doxorubicin, and methotrexate in advanced gastric cancer. *Cancer*, **72**, 37–41.

Preusser, P. and Wilke, H. (1993). New systemic chemotherapy. In *Gastric cancer*, (ed. M. Nishi, H. Ichikawa, T. Nakajima, K. Maruyama, and E. Tahara). Springer Verlag, Berlin.

Preusser, P., Achterrath, W., Wilke, H., Lenaz, L., Fink, U., Heinicke, A., *et al.* (1988). Chemotherapy of gastric cancer. *Cancer Treat. Rev.*, **15**, 257–77.

Preusser, P., Wilke, H., Achterrath, W., Lenaz, L., Stahl, M., Casper, J., *et al.* (1990). Phase II study of carboplatin in untreated inoperable advanced stomach cancer. *Eur. J. Cancer*, **26**, 1108–9.

Pyrönen, S., Kuitunen, T., Nyandoto, P., and Kouri, M. (1995). Randomized comparison of fluorouracil, epidoxorubicin and methotrexate (FEMTX) plus supportive care with supportive care alone in patients with non-resectable gastric cancer. *Br. J. Cancer*, **71**, 587–91.

Ridolfi, R., Giunchi, D.C., Amadori, M., Innocenti, M.P., Maltoni, R., and Amadori, D. (1993). EAP in advanced gastric cancer. *Eur. J. Cancer*, **29A**, 1219–20.

Romero, A., Lacava, J., Sabatini, C., Cuevas, M., Dominguez, M., Rodriguez, R., *et al.* (1996). Biochemical modulation of 5-fluorouracil (5-FU) by methotrexate (MTX) and leucovorin (LV) in patients (pts) with locally advanced (LA) or metastatic (M) gastric carcinoma (GC): A phase II study. *Proceedings of ASCO*, **15** (abstr.), 528.

Roth, A.D., Herrmann, R., Morant, R., Borner, M.M., Honeger, H.P., Bacchi. M., *et al.* (1996). Cisplatin, adriamycin and VP-16 (PAV) in advanced gastric carcinoma (AGC); The SAKK experience. *Proceedings of ASCO*, **15** (abstr.), 518.

Rougier, Ph., Ducreux, M., Mahjoubi, M., Pignon, J.P., Bellefqih, S., Oliveira, J., *et al.* (1994). Efficacy of combined 5-fluorouracil and cisplatinum in advanced gastric carcinomas A phase II trial with prognostic factor analysis. *Eur. J. Cancer*, **30A**, 1263–9.

Scher, H.I., Geller N.L., Muggia, F.M., and Rozencweig, M. (1987). Clinical evaluation of anticancer treatments. Phase II clinical trials. In *Clinical evaluation of antitumor therapy*, (ed. F.M. Muggia and M. Rozencweig), pp. 175–97. Martinus Nijhoff, Boston.

Schipper, D.L. and Wagner, O.J.T. (1996). Chemotherapy of gastric cancer. *Anti-Cancer Drugs*, **7**, 137–49.

Shirai, M., Matsuura, A., Toda, N., Nakamura, T., Kuno. N., Kurimoto, K., *et al.* (1993). Infusional 5-fluorouracil (5-FU) plus weekly carboplatin (CBDCA) chemotherapy for advanced gastric cancer (ACG). *Proc. Am. Soc. Clin. Oncol.*, **12** (abstr.), 618.

Shirai, M., Matsuura, A., Nakamura, T., Toda, N., Shinoda, M., Murakami, M., *et al.*
(1995). Weekly continuous infusion of high-dose 5-FU and low-dose cisplatin for
advanced stomach cancer. *Proceedings of ASCO*, **14** (abstr.), 545.

Sulkes, A., Smyth, J., Sessa, C., Dirix, L.Y., Vermorken, J.B., Kaye, S., *et al.* for the EORTC
Early Clinical Trials Group (1994). Docetaxel (Taxotere™) in advanced gastric cancer
results of a phase II clinical trial. *Br. J. Cancer*, **70**, 380–3.

Taguchi, T. (1994). An early phase II clinical study of RP 56976 (docetaxel) in patients with
cancer of the gastrointestinal tract. *Jpn. J. Cancer Chemother.*, **21** (suppl. 14), 2431–7.

Tsavaries, N., Tentas, K., Mylonkis, N., Bacoyiannis, Ch., Hatzinikolaou, P., Kosmas, C.,
et al. (1995). 5-fluorouracil, epirubicin, mitomycin C (FEM) vs 5-fluorouracil, epirubicin,

Vanhoefer, U., Wilke, H., Weh, H.J., Clemens, M., Harstrick, A., Stahl, M., *et al.* (1994).
Weekly high-dose 5-fluorouracil and folinic acid as salvage treatment in advanced gastric
cancer. *Annals Oncol.*, **5**, 850–1.

Vaughn, D.J., Holroyde, C., Meropol. N.J., Mintzer, D., Armstead, B., Douglass Jr., H.O.,
et al. (1995). A phase II trial of 5-fluorouracil, leucovorin, adriamycin, and cisplatin
(FLAP) in patients with advanced gastric and gastroesophageal junction adenocarcinoma: A Penn Cancer Clinical Trials Group (PCCTG) and Roswell Park Cancer Institute
(RPCI) Trial. *Proceedings of ASCO*, **14** (abstr.), 466.

Wilke, H., Preusser, P., Stahl, M., Meyer, H.J., Fink, U., Achterrath, W., *et al.* (1994). Phase
II study with folinic acid, etoposide, fluorouracil and cisplatin (FLEP) for advanced
gastric cancer. *Onkologie*, **17**, 154–7.

Wilke, H., Korn, M., Köhne-Wömpner, Ch., Fink, U., Vanhoefer, U., Stahl, M., *et al.*
(1995*a*). Weekly high-dose 24-hours infusions of 5-FU (HD-FU) and folinic acid (FA)
plus biweekly cisplatin (C) are highly active in advanced gastric cancer. *Onkologie*, **18**
(suppl. 2), 306.

Wilke, H., Wils, J., Rougier, Ph., Lacave, A., Van Cutsem, E., Vanhoefer, U., *et al.* (1995*b*).
Preliminary analysis of a randomized phase III trial of FAMTX versus ELF versus
cisplatin/FU in advanced gastric cancer (GC). A trial of the EORTC Gastrointestinal
Tract Cancer Cooperative Group and the AIO (Arbeitsgemeinschaft Internistische
Onkologie). *Proceedings of ASCO*, **14** (abstr.), 500.

Wils, J.A. (1992). Chemotherapy for gastrointestinal cancer: New hopes or new disappoint-
ments? *Scand. J. Gastroenterol.*, **194** (suppl.), 87–94.

Wils, J., Meyer, H.-J., and Wilke, H. (1994). Current status and future directions in the
treatment of localized gastric cancer. *Annals Oncol.*, **5** (suppl. 3), 69–72.

Wils, J.A., Klein, H.O., Wagener, D.J. Th., Bieiberg, H., Reis, H., *et al.* for the EORTC
Gastrointestinal Tract Cooperative Group (1991). Sequential high dose methotrexate
and fluorouracil combined with doxorubicin—A step ahead in the treatment of advanced
gastric cancer: A trial of the European Organization for Research and Treatment of
Cancer, Gastrointestinal Tract Cooperative Group. *J. Clin. Oncol.*, **9**, 827–31.

Ychou, M., Fedkovic, Y., Christopoulou, A., Saint-Aubert, B., Rouanet, Ph., Astre, C., *et al.*
(1994). Combination of 5-FU, leucovorin and cisplatin (CDDP): An efficient low-toxic
chemotherapy in advanced gastric adenocarcinoma. In *Cancer treatment: An update*, (ed.
P. Banzet, J.F. Holland, D. Khayat, and M. Weil), pp. 396–8. Springer Verlag, Berlin.

Zaniboni, A., Barni, S., Labíanca, R., Marini, G., Pancera, G., Giaccon, G., *et al.* (1995).
Epirubicin, cisplatin, and continuous infusion 5-fluorouracil is an active and safe
regimen for patients with advanced gastric cancer. *Cancer*, **76** (suppl. 10), 1694–9.

19

Adjuvant and neoadjuvant chemotherapy

P. Ellis and D. Cunningham

1. ADJUVANT CHEMOTHERAPY

Although surgery remains the treatment of choice for localized gastric cancer, five-year survival following curative resection is only approximately 30% (Dupont *et al.* 1978), with relapse a combination of loco- regional and systemic failure. Over the past 30 years, investigators have examined the role of adjuvant chemotherapy in this setting, yet even now its value remains unclear, with no firm evidence for improvement in patient survival.

Early single-agent studies using drugs such as Thiotepa and fluorodeoxyuridine failed to show any survival benefit (Dixon *et al.* 1971; Serlin 1969). Single-agent Mitomycin C has been used extensively as adjuvant therapy particularly in Japan. There have been two randomized trials comparing this agent with surgery alone. One involved the intravenous administration of Mitomycin C 6-weekly within 6 weeks of surgery (Grau *et al.* 1993), while a small Japanese study randomized patients to receive either no additional therapy or intraperitoneal adsorbed Mitomycin C (Hagiwara *et al.* 1992). Both have shown a significant improvement in survival for the treatment group (Table 19.1). Other non-randomized studies from Japan also appear to show an improvement in survival with adjuvant Mitomycin C (Imanaga and Hattori 1977; Nakajima *et al.* 1979). Given the apparent success of single-agent Mitomycin C, one might expect even better results with combination chemotherapy regimes known to be active in advanced disease, however, this has not proven to be so.

There have been four major randomized studies examining the role of 5FU/methyl-CCNU. A study from the Gastrointestinal Tumour Study Group (GITSG) (1982) revealed a significant improvement in median survival (48 months vs. 33 months, $P < 0.03$) for the chemotherapy group, however, three other trials using a similar study design were not able to confirm any survival advantage (Engstrom *et al.* 1985; Higgins *et al.* 1983; Italian Gastrointestinal Tumour Study Group 1988). The British Stomach Cancer Group has undertaken two randomized trials of adjuvant chemotherapy, one randomizing patients to 5FU/Mitomycin C with or without an induction course of 5FU, vincristine, cylophosphamide, and methotrexate, versus surgery alone (Allum *et al.* 1989) and the other comparing surgery alone with adjuvant radiotherapy or FAM (5FU/Adriamycin/Mitomycin C) chemotherapy (Hallisey *et al.* 1994). Neither study was able to demonstrate an improvement in survival. Two other groups, the South West Oncology Group

Table 19.1. Randomized trials of adjuvant chemotherapy in gastric cancer

Study	Treatment arms	Stage	No. of patients	Median survival (mths)	5-yr survival (%)	Significance
Grau et al. 1993	Mitomycin C iv vs. surgery alone	Cur. res.	68 66	–	41* 26*	P <0.025
Hagiwara et al. 1992	Mitomycin C ip vs. surgery alone	T3–T4	24 25	–	69 (3 yrs) 27	P <0.005
GITSG 1982	5FU + Methyl-CCNU vs. surgery alone	Cur. res.	41 47	–	55* (4 yrs) 38*	P = 0.03
Engstrom et al. 1985	5FU + Methyl-CCNU vs. surgery alone	Cur. res.	91 89	36.6 32.7	57 57	n.s.
Higgins et al. 1983	5FU + Methyl-CCNU vs. surgery alone	Cur. res.	66 68	26.5 26.5	38 (3.5 yrs) 39	n.s.
IGITSG 1988	5FU + Methyl-CCNU vs. 5FU + Methyl-CCNU + Levamisole vs. surgery alone	Cur. res.	75 69 69	–	50 50 50	n.s.
Allum et al. 1989	5FU + Mitomycin C vs. 5FU + Mitomycin C + CMVF vs. surgery alone	Cur. res.	141 140 130	–	18* 10 18	n.s.
Hallissey et al. 1994	FAM vs. RT vs. surgery alone	II, III, IVA	138 153 145	18 12 14	18* 9* 13*	n.s.
MacDonald et al. 1992	FAM vs. surgery alone	IB, IC, II, III	83 93	–	Not stated	n.s.
Coombes et al. 1990	FAM vs. surgery alone	Cur. res. except T1 N0	133 148	39 51	46 35	n.s.
Krook et al. 1991	5FU + Adriamycin vs. surgery alone	Cur. res.	61 64	–	32 33	n.s.
Neri et al.	ELF vs. surgery alone	Cur. res.	48 55	20.4 13.6	–	P <0.01

* Estimated from survival curve; n.s., not significant.

(MacDonald *et al*. 1992) and an international co-operative group (Coombes *et al*. 1990) have designed randomized trials using the FAM regimen, including all patients with curative resections except those with $T_1 N_0$ tumours. Neither study was able to demonstrate an overall survival benefit, although the latter study suggested a benefit for T_3 and T_4 tumours on retrospective subgroup analysis. Krook and co-workers, using 5FU and Adriamycin (ADM) as adjuvant treatment, also found no evidence of a survival benefit versus surgery alone (Krook *et al*. 1991). The disappointing results from these combination chemotherapy randomized trials (summarized in Table 19.1) seem to contradict the encouraging results with Mitomycin C.

There have been numerous reports using combined chemotherapy/immunotherapy regimens with immunotherapy agents including cell wall skeleton of bacille Calmette–Guérin (BCG–CWS), nocardia cellwall skeleton (N-CWS), polypetin glycoprotein (PSK), and Levamisole. These have produced conflicting results with many of the studies having been either non-randomized or randomized against a chemotherapy arm rather than having a surgery-alone control arm. Chemotherapy in combination with radiotherapy has also been examined as adjuvant treatment, however, there currently appears to be no survival advantage for radiotherapy alone or in combination with chemotherapy (Hallissey *et al*. 1994; Moertel *et al*. 1984; Bleiberg *et al*. 1989).

Many of the randomized trials of chemotherapy just discussed above, include small patient numbers, sometimes with more than two randomization arms, thus making it difficult to detect small differences in survival. A meta-analysis of adjuvant chemotherapy trials (Hermans *et al*. 1993) has been reported. This reviewed all randomized trials since 1980 with a surgery-alone control arm involving 2096 patients, and found no evidence of a survival benefit for the drug combinations used. The two single-agent Mitomycin C studies (Grau *et al*. 1993; Hagiwara *et al*. 1992) showing a survival benefit for chemotherapy were not included in this analysis.

One very recent prospective randomized study does show more promising results however. Neri *et al*. compared one of the newer chemotherapy regimens 5FU, leucovorin, epidoxorubicin (ELF) with surgery alone in node-positive patients only (Neri *et al*. 1996). They found a significantly improved median survival (20.4 months vs. 13.6 months $P < 0.01$) and delayed time to recurrence for the chemotherapy-treated patients. Further follow-up is required to assess whether there is any clinically relevant effect on long-term survival.

It is difficult to compare directly many of the European and American adjuvant studies with those from Japan. Many of the latter are either non-randomized reports or randomized to a chemotherapy arm (often single-agent Mitomycin C), reflecting the fact that adjuvant chemotherapy is used to be viewed as standard therapy in 1980 in Japan. Despite this, adjuvant treatment appears to offer more successful results than in other parts of the world. Possible reasons for this may include a different natural history of the disease in that country, earlier presentation of disease, and the fact that more aggressive surgery, including extended lymphadenectomy, is often performed in Japan.

Conclusion

Our own view is that there is currently still no definite place for adjuvant chemotherapy in resected gastric cancer, outside the setting of a clinical trial. Clinical research, however, continues in this area particularly as new regimens, such as ELF (Neri *et al.* 19??), FAMTX (5FU/ADM methotrexate) and ECF (Epirubicin/cisplatin/infusional 5FU), appear to show increased activity compared with older regimens previously used in the adjuvant setting. Future studies using these newer regimens, focusing on high-risk groups of patients (e.g. those with serosal penetration and ocal nodal involvement) appear to offer the best chance of demonstrating a definite role for adjuvant chemotherapy in this disease.

2. NEOADJUVANT CHEMOTHERAPY

The relatively disappointing results of adjuvant chemotherapy in gastric cancer, coupled with the development of newer more effective chemotherapy regimens in advanced disease, has led to increasing interest in the use of preoperative chemotherapy in both locally advanced inoperable tumours and in resectable gastric cancer. The aim of this approach is to reduce tumour bulk, thus downstaging the primary tumour and increasing resection rates, and treating micrometastatic disease, thereby, it is hoped, improving survival. However, there are some problems in using this form of treatment in patients with resectable disease. Patients with surgically curable early gastric cancer can be difficult to exclude by current clinical staging methods. These patients would not benefit from preoperative chemotherapy and, potentially, could progress while on this treatment. Newer imaging techniques, such as transluminal endoscopic ultrasound, may help to solve this dilemma.

There have been a number of preoperative chemotherapy studies reported and these are summarized in Table 19.2. Wilke *et al.* (1989) report on 34 patients with unrespectable gastric cancer after failed laparotomy treated with the EAP (etoposide/ADM/cisplatin) regimen: 23 (patients (70%) had a major response, with two further patients having a minor response; 19 of the 25 responders (76%) went forward to surgery, with 15 undergoing complete resection. Of these, 5 patients were found to have pathological complete remission, and the median survival time for all patients was 18 months and for disease-free patients 24 months. Another group have also reported their results with preoperative EAP in potentially resectable gastric cancer (Ajani *et al.* 1993): 48 patients were treated with three cycles of EAP followed by surgery, with a further two cycles of postoperative chemotherapy. The overall response was 31%, with 90% of patients undergoing curative resections. However, there were no pathological complete remissions in this group.

In our own experience with ECF (Findlay *et al.* 1994) 28 of 35 patients (80%) with unresectable disease responded to chemotherapy. Of these, 19 patients went forward for surgery with 10 undergoing complete resection and 4 of these having complete pathological remission: 6 patients were not resectable and 3 had incomplete resections (with positive resection margins.)

Table 19.2. Neoadjuvant chemotherapy for locally advanced gastric cancer

Study	Regimen	Resectability	No. of patients	CR + PR: response (%)	No. of patients having surgery	Complete resection: no. (%)	Complete pathological response
Wilke *et al.* 1989	EAP	Unres.	33	70	20	15 (75)	5
Ajani *et al.* 1993	EAP (pre + post)	Potentially res.	48	31	41	37 (90)	0
Findlay *et al.* 1994	ECF	Unres. or clinically LAD[b]	35	80	19	10 (53)	4
Wils *et al.* 1991	FAMTX	Unres.	19	NS	7	3 (43)	NS
Vershueren *et al.* 1988	MF	Unres.	17	NS	13	7 (54)	NS
Leichman *et al.* 1992	FLC[a]	Potentially res.	38	45	35	29 (83)	3
Roberts *et al.* 1991	Epiribucin, Tegafur (pre + post) *vs.* surgery alone	Potentially res.	92	NS	92	NS	NS (increased disease-free survival with chemotherapy)

[a] Postoperative intraperitoneal floxuridine and cisplatin. [b] Locally advanced disease. (CR + PR), complete remission + partial remission; NS, not stated.

The EORTC randomized study comparing FAM to FAMTX (Wils *et al.* 1991) reported 19 patients with unresectable disease randomized to FAMTX, 7 proceeding to second laparotomy. Of these, 3 had complete resection of their residual disease. Versuchueren *et al.* (1988) used methotrexate and 5FU in 17 patients with un-resectable disease: 7 of 13 patients (53%) going forward to have further surgery were able to be completely resected.

Leichman *et al.* (1992) reported the use of preoperative FLC (infusional 5FU/ leucovorin/cisplatin) in patients with operable gastric cancer not thought to be resectable for cure by clinical staging. In addition, all patients undergoing complete resection received intraperitoneal cisplatin and floxuridine: 33 of 38 (87%) had gastric resection with 29 (76%) having complete resection, and 3 achieving a complete pathological response. Median survival for all patients had not been reached at 17 months.

A Finnish group randomized 92 patients to either surgery alone or pre- and post-operative chemotherapy with Epirubicin and Tegafur (Roberts *et al.* 1991). Although not all details are available in the reported abstract, the groups were comparable with regard to age and stage of disease and at median follow-up of 36 months there was evidence of prolongation of disease-free survival in the chemotherapy arm. There was, however, no difference in overall survival between the two groups at three or five years.

3. CONCLUSION

The results of these initial studies of neoadjuvant chemotherapy in gastric cancer are encouraging. However, it is still too early to determine whether this approach will influence survival in resectable tumours and in locally advanced disease. The increased activity of new chemotherapy regimens and the increased availability of new technology, such as transluminal endoscopic ultrasound, enabling refinement of non-surgical assessment of resectability, will, it is hoped, allow the recruitment of increased patient numbers into randomized trials in an attempt to define the role of this type of therapy in the future. One such randomized trials is currently now in progress in the United Kingdom assessing the use of chemotherapy prior to radical resection in those with locally operable non- metastatic disease, using ECF. A similar trial was carried out in the Netherlands, using FAMTX, but closed much earlier than expected because of very low rate of observed down staging.

REFERENCES

1. Dupont, B., Lee, J.R., Burton, G.R., *et al.* (1978). Adenocarcinoma of the stomach. Review of 1497 cases. *Cancer*, **41**, 941–7.
2. Dixon, W.J., Longmire, W.P. Jr., and Holden, W.D. (1971). Use of triethylenethio-phosphoramide as an adjuvant to the surgical treatment of gastric and colorectal carcinoma, ten year follow up. *Ann. Surg.*, **173**, 26–7.

3. Serlin, O., Wokoff, J.S., Amadeo, J.M., *et al.* (1969). Use of 5-fluorodeoxyuridine (FUDR) as an adjuvant to the surgical management of carcinoma of the stomach. *Cancer*, **24**, 223–9.

4. Grau, J.J., Estape, J., Alcobendas, F., *et al.* (1993). Positive results of adjuvant mitomycin-C in resected gastric cancer. A randomised trial of 134 patients. *Eur. J. Cancer*, **339**, 629–31.

5. Hagiwara, A., Takahashi, T., Kojima, O., *et al.* (1992) Prophylaxis with carbon adsorbed mitomycin against peritoneal recurrence of gastric cancer. *Lancet*, **339**, 629–31.

6. Imanaga, H. and Nakazato, H. (1977). Results of surgery for gastric cancer and effect of adjuvant Mitomycin-C on cancer recurrence. *World J. Surg.*, **1**, 213–24.

7. Nakajima, T., Fukani, A., Ohashi, I., *et al.* (1978). Long term follow up study of gastric cancer patients treated with surgery and adjuvant chemotherapy with Mitomycin-C. *Int. J. Clinic. Pharmacol.*, **16**, 209–16.

8. Gastrointestinal Tumour Study Group (1982). Controlled trial of adjuvant chemotherapy following curative resection for gastric cancer. *Cancer*, **9**, 1868–73.

9. Engstrom, P.F., Lavin, P.T., Douglass, H.O., *et al.* (1985). Postoperative adjuvant 5-fluorouracil plus methyl-CCNU therapy for gastric cancer patients: Eastern Co-operative Oncology Group Study (EST 3275). *Cancer*, **55**, 1868–73.

10. Higgins, G.A., Amadeo, J.H., Smith, D.E., *et al.* (1983). A Veterans Administration Surgical Oncology Group Report. Efficacy of prolonged intermittent therapy with combined 5FU and methyl CCNU following resection for gastric carcinoma. *Cancer*, **52**, 1105–12.

11. Italian Gastrointestinal Tumour Study Group (1988). Adjuvant treatments following curative resection for gastric cancer. *Br. J. Surg.*, **75**, 1100–4.

12. Allum, W.H., Hallissey, M.T., and Kelley, K.A. (1989). Adjuvant chemotherapy in operable gastric cancer. 5 year follow up of first British Stomach Cancer Group Trial. *Lancet*, **1**, 571–6.

13. Hallissey, M.T., Dunn, J.A., Ward, L.C., Allum W.H., for the British Stomach Cancer Group (1994). Trial of adjuvant radiotherapy or chemotherapy in resectable gastric cancer: five year follow up. *Lancet*, **343**, 1309–12.

14. MacDonald, J.S., Gagliano, R., Fleming, T. *et al.* (1992). A phase III trial of FAM (5-fluorouracil, Adriamycin, Mitomycin-C) chemotherapy vs control as adjuvant treatment for resected gastric cancer. A South West Oncology Group trial. *Proc. Am. Soc. Clin. Oncol.*, **11**, 168.

15. Coombes, R.C., Schein, P.S., Chilvers, C.E.D., *et al.* (1990). A randomised trial comparing adjuvant fluorouracil, doxorubicin and mitomycin with no treatment in operable gastric cancer. *J. Clin. Oncol.*, **8**, 1362–9.

16. Krook, J.E., O'Connell, M.J., Wieand, H.S., *et al.* (1991). A prospective randomised evaluation of intensive course 5-fluorouracil plus doxorubicin as surgical adjuvant chemotherapy for resected gastric cancer. *Cancer*, **67**, 2454–8.

17. Moertel, C.G., Childs, D.S., O'Fallon, J.R., *et al.* (1984). Combined 5 fluorouracil and radiation therapy as a surgical adjuvant for poor prognosis gastric carcinoma. *J. Clin. Oncol.*, **2**, 1249–54.

18. Bleiberg, H., Goffin, J.C., Dalesio, O., *et al.* (1989). Adjuvant radiotherapy and chemotherapy in resectable gastric cancer: a randomised trial of gastrointestinal tract cancer co-operative group of the EORTC. *Eur. J. Surg. Oncol.*, **15**, 535–43.

19. Hermans, J., Bonenkamp, J.J., Boon, M.C., *et al.* (1993). Adjuvant therapy after curative resection for gastric cancer: Meta-analysis of randomised trials. *J. Clin. Oncol.*, **11**, 1441–7.

19. Neri, B., de Leonardis, V., Romano, S., *et al.* (1996) Adjuvant chemotherapy after gastric resection in node-positive cancer patients: a multi-centre randomised study. *Brit. J. Cancer*, **73**, 549–52.

20. Wilke, H., Preusser, P., Fink, U., *et al.* (1989). Preoperative chemotherapy in locally advanced and non resectable gastric cancer: a phase II study with etoposide, doxorubicin and cisplatin. *J. Clin. Oncol.*, **7**, 1318–26.

21. Ajani, J.A., Mayer, R.J., Ota, D.M., *et al.* (1993). Pre-operative and post-operative combination chemotherapy for potentially resectable gastric carcinoma. *J. Natl. Cancer Inst.*, **85**, 1839–44.

22. Findlay, M., Cunningham, D., Norman, A., *et al.* (1994). A phase 2 study in advanced gastric cancer using epirubicin and cisplatin in combination with continuous infusion 5-fluorouracil (ECF). *Ann. Oncol.*, **5**, 609–16.

23. Wils, J.A., Klein, H.O., Wagener, D.J., *et al.* (1991). Sequential high dose methotrexate and fluorouracil combined with doxorubicin—a step ahead in the treatment of advanced gastric cancer: a trial of the European organisation for Research and Treatment of Cancer Gastrointestinal Tract Co-operative Group. *J. Clin. Oncol.*, **9**, 827–31.

24. Vershueren, R.J.C., Willemse, P.H.B., Sleijfer, D. Th., *et al.* (1988). Combined chemotherapeutic–surgical approach of locally advanced gastric cancer. *Proc. Am. Soc. Clin. Oncol.*, **7**, 93.

25. Leichman, L., Silberman, H., Leichman, C.G., *et al.* (1992). Preoperative systemic chemotherapy followed by adjuvant postoperative intraperitoneal therapy for gastric cancer: A University of Southern California Pilot Program. *J. Clin. Oncol.*, **10**, 1933–42.

26. Roberts, P.J., Antila, S., Alhava, E., *et al.* (1991). Results of perioperative chemotherapy in patients with radically operated gastric cancer. *Eur. J. Cancer.*, **27**, (suppl. 2), (abstr.), 398.

20

Radiation therapy

J.B. Dubois

Although the incidence of gastric cancer is diminishing, the therapeutic problems posed by this type of tumor remain major. The five-year survival rate for resectable cancers does not exceed 15–20% and has not been modified over the past 20 years despite the development of surgical techniques acting directly on the tumor itself and on the lymphatic drainage areas (Bizer 1983; Gunderson and Sosin 1982). Thus, it would appear legitimate, still faced with a high rate of local and regional recurrence, to combine surgery with another loco-regional therapy such as radiotherapy (Nordman and Kaupinnen 1972; Wisbeck *et al.* 1986).

1. ANATOMICAL AND RADIOBIOLOGICAL DATA

The theoretical tumoricidal dose for gastric cancer is 70 Gy delivered over 7 weeks: 5 fractions of 2 Gy per week. However, healthy gastric tissue cannot tolerate doses greater than 45 Gy for reduced volumes, and of 35–40 Gy when the totality of the stomach is irradiated. Signs of radio intolerance in the small bowel can appear at 25–30 Gy. The totality of the liver also cannot tolerate doses greater than 25–30 Gy. Thus, isolated radiotherapy has no curative possibility for a non-resectable gastric cancer. However, combinations of radiotherapy and surgery are interesting using the doses of 45 Gy delivered during 4.5 weeks in order to cure microscopic subclinical disease in the tumor bed or lymph nodes. It can be expected that this will permit a therapeutic gain by a reduction in local recurrence rates.

2. IRRADIATION METHODS

External beam radiation therapy uses X-ray photons from 10 to 25 MV. The choice of the target volume varies according to whether the patient is inoperable or has undergone complete or incomplete tumor removal. In cases where the patient is inoperable or it is impossible to remove the tumor entirely, the target volume must include the primary tumor and the paratumoral and regional lymph nodes. In cases where there is total excision of the tumor, the target volume is determined according to operative and pathological findings.

During the operation, metal markers can be put in place to guide the choice of the irradiation fields. The portals are usually anteroposterior and posteroanterior symmetrical, with the same axis, sometimes with left and right lateral fields or oblique fields to protect critical organs: kidneys, liver, and the spinal cord.

With external beam radiotherapy doses of 45–50 Gy are delivered at a rhythm of 5×1.8 or 5×2 Gy per week either in a continuous rhythm or, in some cases, with a split-course therapy: 20 Gy in 10 fractions—2 weeks rest-period—20 Gy in 10 fractions.

3. OPTIMIZATION OF THE BIOLOGICAL EFFECTS OF IRRADIATION

As healthy tissue does not tolerate high dosage radiotherapy, it is often difficult to reach the optimal tumoricidal dose. For this reason, several attempts have been made to try and reduce the disadvantages of irradiation to healthy tissues or to increase the effects of irradiation on the tumoral tissues either by avoiding critical organs with intraoperative radiation therapy, or by increasing the radiation effects on tumor cells by combining radiation beams with physical or cytotoxic agents.

4. INTRAOPERATIVE RADIOTHERAPY

Because of anatomical conditions, this therapy is easier in gastric cancer than in any other tumor in the gastrointestinal tract tumor. Intraoperative radiotherapy (IORT), by giving a dose of irradiation directly to the tumoral residue or the tumoral bed, avoids irradiation of healthy tissue and delivers a greater dose to the tumoral zones than traditional external irradiation. Intraoperative radiotherapy is carried out using electrons with variable energy, depending on the thickness of the tissue to be treated. The energy normally varies from 6 to 20 MeV and the doses, calculated on 85% or 90% isodoses, vary from 15 to 20 Gy, according to the histological type and the size of the target volume. The irradiated volumes depend on the surgical procedure carried out and the operative findings (Ogata 1995).

In their experience, Abe *et al.* (1974, 1980) have compared 110 patients treated by surgery alone to 101 treated by surgery and intraoperative radiotherapy of 28–35 Gy. The results show a significant improvement in the number of patients surviving for five years in the group treated by surgery alone: 77% vs. 54.5% for stage II; 44.6% vs. 36.8% for stage III; and 19.5% vs. 0% for stage IV. This study helped to define the selection criteria for the use of IORT in gastric cancer. The contraindications include hepatic and peritoneal extension, tumors with involvement of the anterior surface of the stomach favoring peritoneal seeding, tumor of the gastric body or the oesophago-gastric junction responsible for multidirectional lymphatic drainage, and unresectable tumors.

Our own experience (Dubois 1992) concerns a group of 20 gastric cancer patients who were subjected to complete surgical excision and IORT treatment (20 Gy). Local control was achieved in 12 patients (60%) 6 of these 12 died either of distant metastases or from recurrence outside the IORT field. Persistence of disease in the IORT field was noted in only 2 patients. An overall actuarial three-year survival was observed, as in many other literature series. This study shows, as do others, improvement in local control with IORT, but no improvement in survival time.

The National Institute of Cancer randomized trial (Sindelar and Kinsella 1987)—20 Gy with IORT vs. 50 Gy as a post-operative radiation treatment—has not yet shown a significant increase in survival, but does show a notable improvement in local control and disease-free survival.

There are other ongoing randomized studies, such as the French IORT Group trial (IORT + postoperative radiation therapy after surgery vs. surgery alone), or are in preparation (e.g. EORTC Committee).

5. PHYSICAL RADIOSENSITIZATION

Physical radiosensitization creates intratissular hyperthermia by means of microwaves or radio frequencies allowing a theoretical increase in the radio sensitivity of the tumorous tissues. The hyperthermia can reach temperatures of 40 °C to 42 °C maintained for a minimum period of 45 minutes. Numerous pilot and random studies tend to demonstrate the contribution of hyperthermia to radiotherapy and/or chemotherapy treatments.

6. COMBINATION OF RADIOTHERAPY AND CHEMOTHERAPY

Numerous clinical experiments associating radiotherapy and various chemotherapy drugs, such as 5-fluoro-uracil, (5FU), ametycin (mitomycin C), nitrosoureas, have been carried out with radiochemotherapeutic combinations either sequentially or simultaneously, but the results with inextirpable gastric cancers or incomplete resections have not been very satisfactory. Randomized therapeutic trials have also been published (Moertel *et al.* 1984).

The trial of the Gastro-Intestinal Tumor Study Group (GITSG) (1982) is one of the first randomized studies which compares chemotherapy with 5FU and methyl-CCNU alone or associated with external radiotherapy in two series of 25 Gy separated by a free interval of two weeks, in 90 patients having undergone incomplete surgical excision. The results show a better survival rate in the group treated with combined treatment, but the mean survival rate was never greater than nine months. There was also a marked morbidity rate in the group treated with radiochemotherapy, especially in the first year.

Dent *et al.* (1979) compare chemotherapy with 5FU and Thiotepa to a mono-chemotherapy with 5FU combined with an irradiation of 20 Gy in patients having undergone either complete or incomplete surgical excision. They observed no significant difference in the survival rates of the two groups. This may be due to the small doses of radiotherapy delivered.

Results are more encouraging in cases where surgery was complete. A randomized study by the Mayo Clinic (Gunderson *et al.* 1983), of 62 patients having undergone complete resection but with poor prognosis, compared the association of 5FU and radiotherapy (37.5 Gy in 24 fractions) with no treatment. In this study, a significant difference in survival at five years was noted in favor of the group that was treated (23% vs. 4%). However, these results were not confirmed in a more recent analysis.

The EORTC trial (Slot *et al.* (1989), compared radiotherapy alone (50 Gy/30 fractions/6 weeks) with a combination of the same radiotherapy and 5FU. Three different modalities of administration were used in 115 patients who had undergone a complete tumor excision. There was a mean overall survival of 55 weeks with a slight advantage for the group associating radiotherapy and chemotherapy during 18 months. However, a later study did not confirm this significant result.

Present series are oriented towards a combination of radiotherapy with polychemotherapy (5FU, Adriamycin, mitomycin). The randomized study (no. GI8281) of the GITSG (1982) compares chemotherapy with 5FU, Adriamycin, and methyl-CCNU combined or not combined with radiotherapy. These studies are presently ongoing.

7. THERAPEUTIC INDICATIONS

7.1. Palliative treatment

The result of radiotherapy alone in inoperable patients and in non-resectable gastric tumors are poor. Thus, Holbrook (1974) notes no improvement in survival in a comparative study with an historically untreated group. Moertel *et al.* (1969) observed no five year survival among patients with inoperable gastric cancers having received one external irradiation of 35–40 Gy. Furthermore, Asakawa and Takeda. (1973) observed no survival at two years even for doses of 60 Gy of external radiotherapy alone. In the study by Tsukiyama *et al.* (1988) with 75 advanced inoperable gastric cancers, the mean survival was 26.5 months for complete responses, 7.3 months for partial responses, and 3.2 months for cases with no response to the radiotherapy. Wieland and Hymmen (1970) obtained five year survival rates of 7% with doses of 60 Gy (1.5–2 Gy per fraction), but long-term tolerance remains questionable.

7.2. Curative treatment

Radiotherapy alone is not able to cure gastric cancer. However, the aim of radio-surgical combinations is a curative one. The presence of liver metastases or of other distant metastases excludes the use of radiotherapy. After complete excision of the tumor, doses of 45 Gy are able to sterilize microscopic residual disease whose risk is directly correlated with the degree of parietal (muscular or serious) involvement and regional lymph node extension and with histological grading.

In the case of incomplete excision of lymphatic involvement, the optimization of the effects of external radiotherapy should permit the delivery of the equivalent of 50–55 Gy doses in order to approach the curative tumoricidal dose.

The present development of intraoperative radiotherapy and of radiochemother-apeutic combinations should bring about greater effectiveness of radiotherapy and the recognition of its place, with chemotherapy, in the framework of non-surgical treatments for cancer of the stomach.

REFERENCES

Abe, M., Takahashi, M., Yabumoto, E., Tobe, T., and Mori, K. (1974). Intraoperative radiotherapy of gastric cancer. *Cancer*, **34**, 2034–41.

Abe, M., Takahashi, M., Yabumoto, E., Adachi, H., Yoshii, M., and Mori, K. (1980). Clinical experiences with intraoperative radiotherapy of locally advanced cancers. *Cancer*, **45**, 40–8.

Asakawa, H. and Takeda, T.: (1973). High energy X-ray therapy of gastric carcinoma. *Jap. Soc. Cancer Ther.*, **8**, 362–71.

Bizer, L. (1983). Adenocarcinoma of the stomach. Current results of treatment. *Cancer*, **51**, 743–5.

Dent, D.M., Werner, I.D., and Movis, B. (1979). Prospective randomized trial of combined oncological therapy for gastric carcinoma. *Cancer*, **44**, 385–91.

Dubois, J.B. (1992). Intra-operative radiation therapy in the treatment of gastrointestinal cancer. In *Gastrointestinal Oncology*, (ed. J.D. Ahlgren and J.S. MacDonald), pp. 607–14. Lippincott, Philadelphia.

GITSG (Gastro-Intestinal Tumor Study Group) (1982). A comparison of combination chemotherapy and combined modality therapy for locally advanced gastric carcinoma. *Cancer*, **49**, 1771–7.

Gunderson, L.L. and Sosin, H. (1982). Adenocarcinoma of the stomach: areas of failure in a reoperation series (second or symptomatic look) clinicopathologic correlation and implications for adjuvant therapy. *Int. J. Radiat. Oncol. Biol. Phys.*, **8**, 1–11.

Gunderson, L.L., Hoskins, R., and Cohen A. (1983). Combined modality treatment of gastric cancer. *Int. J. Radiat. Oncol. Biol. Phys.* 7, 585–90.

Holbrook, M.A. (1974). Radiation therapy. in Current concepts in cancer. Gastric cancer: treatment principles. *JAMA*, **228**, 1289–90.

Moertel C.G., Childs D.S., Reitemeier R.J., and Colby M.Y. (1969). Combined Fluorouracil and supervoltage radiation therapy of locally unresectable gastro-intestinal cancer. *Lancet*, **2**, 865–7.

Moertel, C.G., Childs, D.S., O'Fallon, J.R., Holbrook, M.A., Schutt, A.J., and Reitemeier, R.J. (1984). Combined 5-Fluorouracil and radiation therapy as surgical adjuvant for poor prognosis gastric carcinoma. *J. Clin. Oncol*, **21**, 1249–54.

Nordman, E. and Kaupinnen, C. (1972). The value of megavolt therapy in carcinoma of the stomach. *Strahlentherapie*, **144**, 635–40.

Ogata, T. (1995). A 10-year experience of intra-operation radiotherapy for gastric carcinoma and a new surgical method of creating a wider irradiation for cases of total gastrectomy patients. *Int. J. Oncol. Biol. Phys.*, **32**, 341–7.

Sindelar, W.F. and Kinsella, T.J. (1987). Randomized trial of resection and intra-operative radiotherapy in locally advanced gastric cancer. *Proc. Am. Soc. Clin. Oncol.*, **6**, 91 (abstract).

Slot, A., Meerwaldt, J.H., Van Putten, W.L.J., and Treurniet-Donker, A.D. (1989). Adjuvant post-operative radiotherapy for gastric carcinoma with poor prognostic signs. *Radiother. Oncol.*, **16**, 269–74.

Tsukiyama, I., Akine, Y., Kajiura, Y., Ogino, T., Yamashita, K., Egawa, S., *et al.* (1988). Radiation therapy for advanced gastric cancer. *Int. J. Radiat. Oncol. Biol. Phys.*, **15**, 123–7.

Wieland, C. and Hymmen, U. (1970). Megavoltage therapy for malignant gastric tumors. *Strahlentherapie*, **140**, 20–6.

Wisbeck, W.M., Becher, E.M., and Russell, A.H. (1986). Adenocarcinoma of the stomach: autopsy observations with therapeutic implications for the radiation oncologist. *Radiother. Oncol.*, **7**, 13–18.

21

Other treatments

Hisanao Ohkura

1. INTRODUCTION

As there is no dependable treatment that can control metastatic or recurrent gastric cancer of the type which show no indication for surgical or endoscopic resection, some new trials have been reported. Although there has been some success, the results are discrepant and their clinical value remains to be elucidated.

2. IMMUNOTHERAPY

There are two approaches in immunotherapy for gastric cancer. One is specific immunotherapy, or immunotargeting therapy using antibodies specially generated against gastric cancer cells or their products, such as CEA, CA125, and cell membrane antigens. Experimentally, cytotoxic monoclonal antibodies, radioisotope-antibody conjugates, and immunotoxins were given to patients with advanced gastric cancer but no or a little benefit was reported.

The other approach is non-specific immunotherapy, or immunopotentiation by stimulating the immune system of the patient. There have been some clinical trials using immunostimulators and biological response modifiers (BRMs) that enhance cellular immunity, such as BCG, OK432, levamisol, interferons, interleukins, and tumor necrosis factor (TNF). They are administered via the systemic route, orally, endoscopically intratumor, or intraperitoneally (Torisu *et al.* 1983). Some BRMs provided a very good response and enabled a longer survival period in patients having adjuvant immunotherapy, but others did not show any apparent clinical response. BRMs are now studied in combination with surgery or systemic chemotherapy. Large-scale randomized studies in South Korea (Kim *et al.* 1992), and Japan (Nakazato *et al.* 1994) demonstrated longer disease-free periods and longer survival periods following surgery in those receiving immunochemotherapy with OK432 (Picibanil), or with a protein polysaccaride (Krestin), than those receiving chemotherapy alone.

Surgically harvested tissue-infiltrating lymphocytes (TIL), following stimulation with interleukin 2 (IL-2) *in vitro*, are readministered to the patient intraperitoneally for the control of peritonitis carcinomatosa. Lissoni *et al.* (1993) reported that immunotherapy with IL-2 plus pineal hormone, indole melatonin, was effective for advanced gastric cancer and hepatoma.

At present, unfortunately, no state-of-the-art immunotherapy, immunochemo-therapy, or immunoendocrine therapy for gastric cancer exists.

3. HORMONE THERAPY

Tamoxifen, an estrogen receptor competitor, is effective for estrogen-dependent malignancies, such as those of the breast, uterine cervix, and endometrium. As there is a special type of gastric scirrhous-type carcinoma occurring in young females, which has different clinical features and the worst prognosis, its hormone-dependency has been investigated.

There have been several studies on the role of an estrogen receptor in gastric cancer. For example, Tokunaga *et al.* (1989) and Harrison *et al.* (1989) have invest-igated hormone-dependent growth and therapy with antiestrogens. Higher levels of estrogen receptor, as in the breast, was determined in some of the human gastric cancer cell lines. A trial in Japan revealed that oral tamoxifen (40 mg daily) was effective in improving the survival period in young females with scirrhous carci-noma. However, this did not apply to other types of tumor.

No confirmatory result has been reported on the use of somatomedin, secretin, and antigastrins.

Glucocorticoids and chemotherapeutic agents of immunosupressive activity are used for gastric lymphomas in combination. However, no immunosuppressive agents should be given for low-grade B cell gastric lymphomas of mucosa-associated lymphoid tissue (MALT).

In general, glucocorticoids are effective for treating chemotherapy induced nausea and vomiting but not recommended alone for gastric adenocarcinoma. However, they can be given to terminally ill patients as a palliative.

4. OTHER THERAPIES

There have been trials with H2 blockers, 8-C1-cAMP, membrane calcium channel blockers, etc. Some of them have shown very promising results in their action against cultured human gastric cancer cell lines or in animal models. However, none are used routinely in clinics at present. Heparin, urokinase, and some bio-active substances are used in combination with other therapeutic modalities.

Carotenoids are thought to suppress the effect of promoters that affect pre-cancerous cells to cancer and, also exert cytotoxic effects on cancer cells *in vitro* and *in vivo*. Some carotenoids are tried to prevent or treat gastric cancer.

Oral administration of viable *Lactobacillus bifida* sometimes improves dyspepsia of those patients with advanced gastric cancer. This is partly because of the salvaging and normalizing effect of bacterial flora in the stomach and intestine. Some animal models supported that these bacilli enhanced cellular immunity and help to suppress tumor metastasis.

In gastric lymphoma, Wotherspoon *et al.* (1991,1993) have proposed a new entity of disease, low-grade B cell gastric lymphomas of mucosa-associated lymphoid tissue (MALT). This proposal is based on the evidence that gastric lymphoma is usually accompanied by intramucosal infection of a subaerobic bacteria, *Helicobacer pylori* (HP), and that eradication of this bacteria by oral antibiotics regressed this type of tumor (Hussel *et al.* 1993).

REFERENCES

Harrison, J.D., *et al.* (1989). The effect of tamoxifen and estrogen receptor status on survival in gastric carcinoma. *Cancer*, **64**, 1007–10.

Hussel, T., Isaacson, P.G., Crabtree, J.E., *et al.* (1993). The response of cells from low-grade B-cell gastric lymphomas of mucosa-associated lymphoid tissue to *Helicobacter pylori*. *Lancet*, **342**, 571–4.

Kim, J.P., Kwon, J., Sung, T., and Yang, H.K. (1992). Results of surgery on 6589 gastric cancer patients and immunochemosurgery as the best treatment of advanced gastric cancer. *Ann. Surg.*, **216**, 269–79.

Lissoni, P., Barni, S., Tnacini, G., Ardizzoia, A., Rovelli, F., Cazzaniga, M., *et al.* (1993). Immunotherapy with subcutaneous low-dose interleukin-2 and the pineal indole melatonin as a new effective therapy in advanced cancer of the digestive tract. *Br. J. Cancer*, **67**, 1404–7.

Nakazato, H., Koike, A., Saijo, S., Ogawa, N., and Sakamoto, J. (1994). Efficacy of immunochemotherapy as adjuvant treatment after curative resection of gastric cancer. Study group of immunochemotherapy with PSK for gastric cancer. *Lancet*, **343**, 1122–6.

Tokunaga, A., *et al.* (1989). Hormone receptors in gastric cancer. *Eur. J. Cancer Clin. Oncol.*, **19**, 687–9.

Torisu, M., *et al.* (1983). New approach and management of malignant ascites with a streptococcal preparation, Ok-432. Improvement of host immunity and prolongation of survival. *Surgery*, **93**, 357–64.

Wotherspoon, AC., Ortiz-Hidalgo, C., Falzon, M.R., and Issacson, P.G. (1991). *Helicobacter pylori*-associated gastritis and primary B-cell gastric lymphoma. *Lancet*, **338**, 1175–6.

Wotherspoon, A.C., Doglioni, C., Diss, T.C., *et al.* (1993). Regression of primary low-grade B-cell gastric lympyoma of mucosa-associated lymphoid tissue (MALT) type after eradication of *Helicobacter pylori*. *Lancet*, **342**, 575–7.

Part VIII: Palliative care

22

Palliative care and quality of life

Sam Ahmedzai and Chantal Meystre

1. THE RELEVANCE OF PALLIATIVE CARE

To palliate is to relieve the symptoms of a disease, without necessarily modifying the underlying disease process, and without primarily aiming to prolong life. Palliation is therefore very often the only reasonable treatment option in the management of gastric cancer when it presents late, or relapses after initial curative therapy. Many modalities of treatment may be used in palliation, including radiotherapy, drugs, such as analgesics and antiemetics, and techniques of nursing care.

Palliative care is now recognized as a rather broader concept than palliation, being the multidisciplinary management of advanced, progressive disease that is likely to cause death within the foreseeable future, with emphasis on the physical, emotional, social, and spiritual suffering in patients and their family carers (Doyle *et al.* 1993). It is often stated that palliative care should begin when the patient's prognosis is about 12 months, but this definition may vary from country to country. Moreover, prognosis is clearly not easy to predict accurately.

Patients with advanced gastric cancer suffer a variety of symptoms which are amenable to palliation, and the psychosocial aspects of their illness can be helped by consultation with, or referral to a specialist palliative care team. In some countries, a large part of this work is done by hospice services (e.g. in the United Kingdom or the United States); in other countries it is the domain of hospital-based specialist teams; and in yet other countries palliative care may be very poorly developed as a specialty and not available for the majority of patients. The World Health Organization (WHO) cancer control programme attempts to spread the benefits of palliation—especially of rational pain control—and the wider aspects of palliative care, in the appropriate context of different countries' health systems (Stjernswärd 1993).

2. SYMPTOM CONTROL

Patients with advanced gastric cancer suffer a wide range of physical symptoms, including pain, anorexia, nausea and vomiting, dysphagia, early satiety, and weakness. In addition, many patients with advanced malignancy of any primary site tend to develop problems associated with reduced mobility, such as constipation, lethargy, and pressure sores. It is important to be aware that any of these symptoms may, in fact, arise as side-effects of medication or other therapies, and it is helpful to review all the medication of cancer patients frequently to eliminate or reduce unhelpful drugs.

3. PAIN

Pain in gastric cancer is usually related to local infiltration of visceral structures, but it may sometimes be due to distant metastases. The WHO cancer pain relief programme recommends a three-step gradation of analgesia from non-opioid drugs for mild pains, to weak opioids for moderate pain, and strong opioids for severe pain (WHO 1986). The most helpful non-opioid analgesic is paracetamol. Mild and strong opioids vary in availability between countries: typical WHO 'Step 2' mild opioids are codeine dihydrocodeine, tramadol and the most widely used strong opioid for 'Step 3' analgesia is morphine. Unfortunately, many countries have strict limitations on the availability and usage of strong opioids.

Most opioids can be given orally, but absorption of morphine can be unpredictable and first-pass metabolism is responsible for reduced bio-availability. However, these factors are not usually of clinical significance and the large majority of patients can be maintained on regular oral medication until the very late stages of disease. Morphine must be taken 4-hourly if it is in solution, but sustained release preparations may be taken every 12 or 24 hours, with obvious compliance advantages. There is no proven advantage of the parenteral route for morphine or its analogues, unless the patient is unable to swallow medication. In this case, the morphine can be given either 4-hourly by subcutaneous injection, or preferably by continuous infusion via a subcutaneously placed needle, attached to a syringe driver. The advantage of the syringe driver in the terminal stage of disease is that many other drugs can also be given in the same syringe, thus enabling patients to have complete symptom control with only intermittent nursing supervision. Alternative routes for analgesia and other medication in terminal disease include rectal suppositories, and transdermal application via a skin patch (Hancock *et al.* 1993, Ahmedzai and Brooks (in press)).

It is customary to offer patients co-analgesics to assist with the drugs described above. Many patients gain benefit from an added non-steroidal anti-inflammatory drug (NSAID) such as naproxen, ibuprofen, or diclofenac. Care must be taken when using these drugs when there is a history of dyspepsia and it is usually prudent to prescribe them with a gastric mucosal protective agent, such as misoprostol, or a gastric acid-reducing agent, such as an H2-antagonist, if there is a definite history of peptic ulcer. NSAIDs are particularly helpful when pain is associated with bone metastases, as these can be associated with local prostaglandin production.

Pain from upper abdominal viscera may be considerably helped by a neurolytic blockade of the coeliac plexus. For details of this procedure and fuller descriptions of analgesic drugs and co-analgesics, the reader is referred to a modern palliative medicine text (Payne *et al.* 1993). It is nowadays quite feasible and honest to assure the patient that pain should not dominate the terminal part of his/her illness.

4. ANOREXIA

Loss of appetite is a very common feature of many malignant diseases, and may indeed be the presenting complaint. The mechanisms include disordered taste sensation, abnormal metabolic pathways, and psychological factors. Sometimes, the effects of treatments, such as chemotherapy, contribute to anorexia, whereas oropharyngeal candidiasis may be due to either tumor-related or drug-induced immunosuppression. The syndrome of cachexia, which includes severe weight loss and progressive weakness, is a frequent accompaniment. Patients are acutely aware of the social embarrassment of not being able to eat properly, and of a deteriorating body image.

The simplest measures include attention to the presentation of meals, with emphasis on small portions, and avoiding strong tastes or smells. Small amounts of alcohol in the form of sherry or spirits before meals, if the patient is used to it and if alcohol is culturally appropriate, may stimulate appetite. Oral candidiasis should be treated vigorously with antifungal agents such as nystatin, ketoconazole, or fluconazole.

Corticosteroids have been traditionally used as appetite stimulants, but evidence of their benefit is conflicting and any positive effect tends to be short-lived. It is reasonable to given the patient a trial for 5–7 days, and if there has been no definite subjective response, to stop the steroid immediately, in order to prevent long-term adverse effects. Progestogens, such as megestrol acetate and medroxyprogesterone acetate, have been reported to cause significant weight gain when used in patients with breast cancer, and this 'side-effect' has been used to good advantage in other malignant conditions and also in AIDS (Loprinzi *et al.* 1992). At moderate doses, these agents can give good improvement in appetite as well as useful weight gain which may contribute to an improvement in the patient's quality of life. Other agents have been used as appetite stimulants but the evidence for their effectiveness is less convincing.

Nutritional deficiency influences not only the development of gastric cancer but also morbidity during surgical and oncological treatments, and throughout the course of the disease. Early involvement of the dietitian gains useful advice on nutrition, vitamin supplementation, therapeutic, and cultural diets and education of the patient and their carers (Shaw 1992).

5. DYSPHAGIA

Difficulty in swallowing is usually caused by direct occlusion of the oesophagus or gastric inlet by tumor, but can be associated with severe oesophageal candidiasis which may not be seen in the mouth. Physical obstruction by tumor encroaching into the lower oesophagus may be relieved by a prosthesis (stent), intraluminal radiation (brachytherapy), intralesional alcohol or laser therapy if the patient can tolerate endoscopy. However, these treatments are expensive and of limited availability.

Percutaneous endoscopic gastrostomy (PEG) is a reasonable option to consider in some patients, when obstruction is at the level of the cardia or oesophagus. Once a PEG tube has been placed, the patient may freely receive adequate enteral nutrition by intermittent pump, using commercially available liquid feeds. It is possible to provide good palliation of dysphagia and to reverse cachexia like this over many months. Only rarely will parenteral nutrition be appropriate for maintanence feeding in advanced disease.

6. NAUSEA AND VOMITING

Nausea is a frequent problem, and may be due to the adverse effects of drug therapy as well as the disease process. Vomiting can be troublesome especially if it is projectile when there is gastric outflow obstruction. Rational antiemetic therapy, like pain control, requires a knowledge of the cause of vomiting and the site of pathology (Twycross 1995). Drugs that increase gastric peristalsis, such as metoclopramide, may be counter-productive if there is pyloric stenosis. Haloperidol is a good centrally acting antiemetic but can be sedating in higher doses; cyclizine is another helpful agent with similar properties. Serotonin (S-HT3) antagonists (ondasetron, granisetron etc) although expensive are useful where other antiemetics have failed. Both of these can be given orally or by subcutaneous infusion via a syringe driver, in combination with a strong opioid if necessary. If there is evidence of pyloric stenosis or bowel obstruction, the vomiting and associated colicky abdominal pain may be palliated by the use of an anticholinergic agent, such as scopolamine, which can also be given orally or by subcutaneous infusion (Johnson and Patterson 1992).

Octreotide, a long-acting synthetic analogue of the inhibitory hormone somatostatin, is useful for the treatment of intractable symptoms of gastrointestinal obstruction. It may be used alone or in combination with antiemetics and opiods. Mercadante *et al.* (1993), Riley and Fallon (1994), and Khoo *et al.* (1994) report 58% to 85% symptomatic response to octreotide in patients with obstruction and advanced inoperable cancers of various origin including stomach. Doses between 100 μg and 1200 μg daily have been given as either a 12-hourly subcutaneous injection or continuous infusion. When used for palliation of obstructive symptoms octreotide causes few side-effects apart from dry mouth and flatulence.

Octreotide breaks into the cycle of distension, increasing intraluminal secretions, colicky pain, and vomiting by decreasing water, sodium, and chloride secretion at luminal level and increasing water and electrolyte absorption. It may also act directly on gut neurones to inhibit peristalsis and a direct analgesic effect has not been ruled out (Fallon 1994). Octreotide already has an established place for those patients who develop fistulae, dumping syndrome, or chemotherapy induced diarrhoea.

7. EARLY SATIETY

If the stomach is extensively replaced by tumor, or if the liver is enlarged and pressing on it, the patient may complain of early satiety (i.e. feeling full after minimal food or drink). The 'squashed stomach syndrome' is difficult to treat but simple measures like frequent small meals are helpful. A course of high-dose corticosteroids may give short-term relief, but the systemic adverse effects of steroids often supervene.

8. WEAKNESS

Increasing weakness and lassitude are almost inevitable with most advancing solid tumors, and can arise from the anorexia–cachexia syndrome described above; from anaemia; and from adverse effects of therapies such as cytotoxic chemotherapy or even palliative drugs. Anaemia may respond to blood transfusion, especially if there has been rapid blood loss (Gleeson and Spencer 1995). In older patients, the benefits of transfusion are often less marked and cardiac overload may be a hazard. Corticosteroids have traditionally been used as a 'tonic' but there is no good evidence for this effect and the disadvantages usually outweigh any short-term benefit.

It is important to pay attention to the nursing of the patient, and to encourage adjustments in living arrangements so that the need to walk between bed, chair, and bathroom is reduced to a minimum. It is very difficult for most previously active people to accept a major reduction in activity, but planned small changes in lifestyle, made with the help of a physiotherapist or occupational therapist, may be more acceptable.

9. PSYCHOLOGICAL PROBLEMS

Emotional distress and disorders of adjustment or coping are understandably common in cancer patients. Often they can be considered as 'normal' reactions to the disease and to symptoms, such as chronic pain, and only reassurance and verbal support is necessary. In a small proportion of patients, however, psychological problems become true functional disorders such as persistent anxiety state, or depression. These should be treated actively using conventional medication. Benzodiazepines can be used cautiously, and antidepressants like dothiepin have the advantage of being slightly sedating if this is needed. It is rare to need to make a psychiatric referral, but help from a counsellor, who may be a trained social worker, nurse or volunteer, is frequently useful.

10. QUALITY OF LIFE

There is much talk now about 'quality of life'. At one level, it is a very individual perception and varies between patients, and is also affected by culture and family structures. However, it is possible to measure quality of life using standardized and validated instruments (usually self-rated questionnaires), many of which have been designed for use in cancer clinical trials (Ahmedzai 1993; G.I. Ringdal and

K. Ringdal 1993). So far, there have been no large-scale studies of quality of life using this methodology in gastric cancer.

Modern palliative care places emphasis in two areas which can affect the quality of life of the cancer patient. First, it is acknowledged that the patient has a right to information about his/her condition and prognosis, but this should be conveyed sympathetically and in appropriate terms respecting the patient's ability to understand and assimilate. Second, by considering the needs and stresses on relatives, particularly those who provide the constant bedside care in the terminal stage, the quality of life for the whole family can be improved. This has important implications for the well-being of bereaved carers, as their own health as well as future perceptions about cancer may be adversely affected by a difficult period of unsupported caring and grief.

11. TERMINAL CARE

It is often impossible to state exactly when the 'terminal' stage of cancer has been reached. With gastric cancer, it may occupy the last few weeks of life, or it may start from the time of first diagnosis with metastatic disease. It is important to try and anticipate this phase, because the needs of the patient (and the family carers) will change dramatically. In the terminal stage, the emphasis is entirely on providing comfort and symptom relief, and futile efforts to prolong life should be discontinued—but by discussion and explanation, not abruptly and cruelly. Nursing care is of paramount importance, and in most cultures it is possible to share this task between professional staff and the family members, with great psychological (and economic) benefits to both. For many patients and relatives, as well as doctors and nurses, it will never be easy to accept a fatal outcome. However, the experience of modern palliative care is that good preparation for dying, by means of sharing of information and meticulous symptom control, can help to make the death itself more bearable.

REFERENCES

Ahmedzai, S. (1993). Quality of life measurement in palliative care: philosophy, science or pontification? *Progress in Palliative Care*, **1**, 6–10.

Ahmedzai, S., Brooks, D.J. (in press) Transdermal fentanyl versus sustained release oral morphine in cancer pain: preference, efficacy and quality of life. *J. Pain Sympt. Manag.*

Doyle, D., Hanks, G.W.C. and MacDonald N. (1993). Introduction. In *Oxford textbook of palliative medicine* (ed. D. Doyle *et al.*), pp. 3–8. Oxford University Press.

Fallon, M.T. (1994). The physiology of somatostatin and its synthetic analogue, octreotide. *Euro. J. Pall. Care*, **1**, 20–2.

Gleeson, C., Spencer, D. (1995). Blood transfusion and its benefits in palliative care. *Palliative Med.*, **9**, 307–13.

Hancock, B.W., Ahmedzai, S. and Clark, D. (1993). Palliative care of patients with terminal cancer. *Current Opinion in Oncology*, **5**, 655–60.

Johnson, I. and Patterson, S. (1992). Drugs used in combination in the syringe driver—a survey of hospice practice. *Palliative Med.*, **6**, 125–30.

Khoo, D., Hall, E., Motson, R., Riley, J., Denman, K. and Waxman, J. (1994). Palliation of malignant intestinal obstruction using octreotide. *Euro. J. Cancer*, **30A**, 28–30.

Loprinzi, C.L., Goldberg, R.M., and Burnham, N.L. (1992). Cancer-associated anorexia and cachexia. *Drugs*, **43**, 499–506.

Mercadante, S., Spoldi, E., Caraceni, A., Maddaloni, S. and Simonetti, M.T. (1993). Octreotide in relieving gastrointestinal symptoms due to bowel obstruction. *Palliative Med.*, **7**, 295–9.

Payne, R., Gonzales, G., Foley, K.M., Inturrisi, C.E., Hanks, G.W.C., Rawlins, M.D. *et al.* (1993). Management of pain. In *Oxford textbook of palliative medicine*, (ed. D. Doyle *et al.*), pp. 140–274. Oxford University Press.

Riley, J. and Fallon, M.T. (1994). Octreotide in terminal malignant obstruction of the gastrointestinal tract. *Euro. J. Pall. Care*, **1**, 23–5.

Ringdal, G.I. and Ringdal, K. (1993). Testing the EORTC Quality of Life questionnaire on cancer patients with heterogeneous diagnoses. *Quality of Life Research*, **2**, 129–40.

Shaw, C. (1992). Nutritional aspects of advanced cancer. *Palliative Med.*, **6**, 105–10.

Stjernswärd, J. (1993). Palliative medicine—a global perspective. In *Oxford textbook of palliative medicine*, (ed. D. Doyle *et al.*), pp. 3–8. Oxford University Press.

Twycross R. (1995). *Palliative care*. Radcliffe Medical Press, Oxford, pp. 105–117.

WHO (World Health Organization) (1986). *Cancer pain relief*. WHO, Geneva.

Index

BC Cancer Agency
Vancouver Cancer Centre
Library
600 West 10th Ave.
Vancouver, B.C. Canada
V5Z 4E6